**Primary Prevention by Nutrition Intervention in Infancy and Childhood**

Nestlé Nutrition Workshop Series
Pediatric Program, Vol. 57

# Primary Prevention by Nutrition Intervention in Infancy and Childhood

Editors

*Alan Lucas*, London, UK

*Hugh A. Sampson*, New York, N.Y., USA

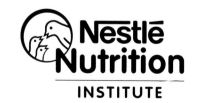

KARGER

**Nestec Ltd., 55 Avenue Nestlé, CH–1800 Vevey (Switzerland)**
**S. Karger AG, P.O. Box, CH–4009 Basel (Switzerland)  www.karger.com**

Printed in Switzerland on acid-free paper by Reinhardt Druck, Basel
ISBN 3–8055–7978–0
ISSN 0742–2806

**Library of Congress Cataloging-in-Publication Data**

Nestlé Nutrition Workshop (57th : 2005 : Half Moon Bay, Calif.)
  Primary prevention by nutrition intervention in infancy and childhood / volume editors, Alan Lucas, Hugh A. Sampson.
    p. ; cm. – (Nestlé Nutrition workshop series. Pediatric program ; v. 57)
  "57th Nestlé Pediatric Nutrition Workshop, which took place in May 2005 at Half Moon Bay, San Francisco"–Foreword.
  Includes bibliographical references and index.
  ISBN 3-8055-7978-0 (hard cover : alk. paper)
  1. Diet therapy for children–Congresses. 2. Diet therapy for infants–Congresses. 3. Medicine, Preventive–Congresses.  I. Lucas, Alan, MD.  II. Sampson, Hugh A.  III. Title.
IV. Series: Nestlé Nutrition workshop series. Paediatric programme ; v. 57.
  [DNLM:  1. Nutrition Therapy–methods–Child–Congresses.  2. Nutrition Therapy–methods –Infant–Congresses.  3. Primary Prevention–methods–Child–Congresses.  4. Primary Prevention–methods–Infant–Congresses. WS 130 N468p 2006]
RJ53.D53N47 2006
618.92′39–dc22

                                                                                      2005027723

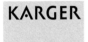 Basel · Freiburg · Paris · London · New York ·
Bangalore · Bangkok · Singapore · Tokyo · Sydney

   The material contained in this volume was submitted as previously unpublished material, except in the instances in which credit has been given to the source from which some of the illustrative material was derived.
   Great care has been taken to maintain the accuracy of the information contained in the volume. However, neither Nestec Ltd. nor S. Karger AG can be held responsible for errors or for any consequences arising from the use of the information contained herein.

# Contents

Contents

Other Potentially Preventable Diseases

LC-PUFAs: Influence on Multiple Health Outcome

Impact of Nutrition on Health Mechanism Aspects

# Foreword

For the 57th Nestlé Pediatric Nutrition Workshop, which took place in May 2005 at Half Moon Bay, San Francisco, the topic 'Primary Prevention by Nutrition Intervention in Infancy and Childhood' was chosen. Early nutrition seems to be involved in the mechanism of control, especially taking into account the role of protein and long-chain polyunsaturated fatty acids (LC-PUFAs). It seems that the new generation of infant formulas already takes those findings into consideration.

We would like to thank the two chairmen, Prof. *Hugh Sampson* and Prof. *Alan Lucas* who are recognized experts in this field, for putting the program together and inviting the opinion leaders in the field of maternal and infant nutrition as speakers.

Our first chairperson, Prof. *Hugh Sampson*, already chaired the 34th Nestlé Nutrition Workshop entitled 'Intestinal Immunology and Food Allergy' in Versailles, France, in June 1993, a topic related to allergy and intestinal immunity. Since then a lot of new data concerning this area have been discovered and the results of the GINI study in Germany have confirmed the hypothesis that mildly hydrolyzed whey-based formulas are effective in the prevention of atopy. Having Professors *von Berg, Björkstén, Zeiger* and *Sampson* around the table was a source of lively exchanges, discussions and ideas resulting in strong and valuable conclusions.

Prof. *Alan Lucas*, our second chairperson, has substantially contributed to our understanding of early nutrition and long-term outcome. With his co-workers *A. Singhal* and *M. Fewtrell*, he is raising new hypotheses in the development of obesity, diabetes, cardiovascular diseases later in life, the so-called 'syndrome X'.

We would also like to thank Mrs. *Linda Hsieh* and her team from Nestlé USA, who provided all logistical support, enabling the participants to enjoy the American hospitality.

*Prof. Ferdinand Haschke, MD, PhD*  
Vice President and Chairman

*Dr. Philippe Steenhout, MD*  
Medical Advisor

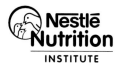

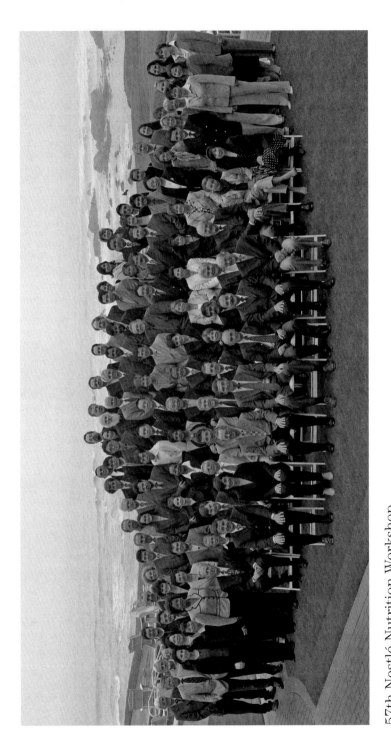

57th Nestlé Nutrition Workshop
Pediatric Program
Half Moon Bay, San Francisco, May 24–28, 2005

# Contributors

## Chairpersons & Speakers

### Prof. Bengt Björkstén

National Institute of Environmental
Medicine
IMM Division of Physiology
Karolinska Institutet
SE–17177 Stockholm
Sweden
Tel. +46 8 52 48 69 56
Fax +46 8 30 06 19
E-Mail bengt.bjorksten@
admin.ki.se

### Dr. Mary Fewtrell

MRC Childhood Nutrition Research
Centre
Institute of Child Health
30 Guilford Street
London WC1N 1EH
UK
Tel. +44 207 905 2389/2251
Fax +44 207 831 9903
E-Mail m.fewtrell@
ich.ucl.ac.uk

### Prof. Lars Å. Hanson

Göteborg University
Department Clinical Immunology
Guldhedsgatan 10
SE–413 46 Göteborg
Sweden
Tel. +46 31 342 4916/+46 31 342
4996
Fax +46 31 342 4621
E-Mail lars.hanson@immuno.gu.se

### Prof. Stephen D. Hursting

Division of Nutritional Sciences
University of Texas at Austin
1 University Station, A2700
Austin, TX 78712
USA
Tel. +1 512 475 7931
E-Mail shursting@mail.utexas.edu

### Dr. Anja Kroke

Research Institute of Child Nutrition
Rheinische Friedrich-Wilhelms-
Universität Bonn
Heinstück 11
DE–44225 Dortmund
Germany
Tel. +49 231 79 22 10 17
Fax +49 231 71 15 81
E-Mail kroke@fke-do.de

### Dr. Martin Kussmann

Nestec Ltd.
c/o Nestlé Research Center
PO Box 44
CH–1000 Lausanne 26
Switzerland
Tel. +41 21 785 9572
Fax +41 21 785 9486
E-Mail Martin.Kussmann@
rdls.nestle.com

Contributors

### Prof. Zvi Laron

Endocrinology & Diabetes Research
Unit
Schneider Children's Medical Center
of Israel
14 Kaplan Street
49202 Petach Tikva, Israel
Tel. +972 3 925 3610
Fax +972 3 535 1295
E-Mail laronz@clalit.org.il

### Prof. Alan Lucas

MRC Childhood Nutrition Research
Centre
Institute of Child Health
30 Guilford Street
London WCN 1EH, UK
Tel. +44 20 905 2389
Fax +44 20 404 7109
E-Mail a.lucas@ich.ucl.ac.uk

### Dr. Claudio Maffeis

Department of Mother and Child
Biology – Genetics
Section of Pediatrics
University of Verona
Piazza L.A. Scuro, 10
IT–37134 Verona, Italy
Fax +39 45 820 0993
E-Mail claudio.maffeis@univr.it

### Dr. Florence Massiera

Laboratoire 'Développement du Tissu
Adipeux'
Centre de Biochimie –
CNRS UMR 6543
Parc Valrose – Faculté des Sciences
FR–06108 Nice Cedex 2, France
Tel. +33 4 92 07 64 39
Fax +33 4 92 07 64 04
E-Mail massiera@unice.fr

### Prof. Hugh A. Sampson

Department of Pediatrics
Jaffe Food Allergy Institute
Mount Sinai School of Medicine
Box 1198
New York, NY 10029-6574
USA
Tel. +1 212 241 5548
Fax: +1 212 426 1902
E-Mail hugh.sampson@mssm.edu

### Dr. Atul Singhal

MRC Childhood Nutrition Research
Centre
Institute of Child Health
30, Guilford Street
London WC1N 1EH
UK
Tel +44 20 7905 2389
Fax +44 20 7831 9903
E-Mail a.singhal@ich.ucl.ac.uk

### Dr. Andrea von Berg

Forschungsinstitut an der
Klinik für Kinder- und
Jugendmedizin
des Marien-Hospital Wesel
Pastor-Janssen-Strasse 8–38
DE–46483 Wesel
Germany
Tel. +49 281 104 1179
Fax +49 281 319 1659
E-Mail vonberg@
marien-hospital-wesel.de

### Dr. Robert S. Zeiger

Kaiser Permanente Medical Center
Department of Allergy-Immunology
7060 Clairemont Mesa Boulevard
San Diego, CA 92111
USA
Tel. +1 858 573 5408
Fax +1 858 573 5251
E-Mail robert.s.zeiger@kp.org

### Prof. Dennis M. Bier

USDA/ARS Children's Nutrition
Center
1100 Bates Street
Houston, TX 77030
USA
Tel. +1 713 798 7022
Fax +1 713 798 7022
E-Mail dbier@bcm.tmc.edu

## Moderators

### *Prof. Steven Abrams*

USDA/ARS Children's
Nutrition Research Center
1100 Bates Street
Houston, TX 77030, USA
Tel. +1 713 798 7124
Fax +1 713 798 7119
E-Mail sabrams@bcm.edu

### *Prof. Craig Jensen*

Baylor College of Medicine
Texas Children's Hospital MC1010.00
6621 Fannin Street
Houston, TX 77030, USA
Tel. +1 832 822 3611
Fax +1 835 825 3633
E-Mail cljensen@
texaschildrenshospital.org

### *Prof. William Klish*

Baylor College of Medicine
Texas Children's Hospital MC1010.00
6621 Fannin Street
Houston, TX 77030, USA
Tel. +1 832 822 3616
Fax +1 835 825 3633
E-Mail wklish@bcm.tmc.edu

### *Prof. Alan Lake*

10807 Falls Rd
Lutherville, Maryland 21093
USA
Tel. +1 410 321 9393
Fax +1 410 825 4945
E-Mail alakeslake@aol.com

### *Prof. José Saavedra*

Nestlé USA, Nutrition Division
800 N. Brand Blvd.
Glendale, CA 91203
USA
Tel. +1 818 549 6774
Fax +1 818 549 5704
E-Mail jose.saavedra@
us.nestle.com

## Invited attendees

Prof. Elza Daniel de Mello/Brazil
Prof. Angela Mattos/Brazil
Dr. Thomas J. Bowen/Canada
Prof. Zave Chad/Canada
Prof. Ernest Seidman/Canada
Dr. Eduardo Atalah/Chile
Dr. Xiaochuan Wang/China
Dr. Dorian Tjesic-Drinkovic/Croatia
Dr. Duska Tjesic-Drinkovic/Croatia
Dr. Jose Luis Abreu/Dominican
  Republic
Prof. Manuel Garcia Sugranes/
  Dominican Republic
Dr. Rafael Aulestia/Ecuador
Prof. Enrique Bolona/Ecuador
Mrs. Aila Paganus/Finland
Prof. Otto Schofer/Germany
Dr. Alexander Andreou/Greece
Prof. Eleftheria Roma/Greece

Dr. Emmanouil Manousakis/Greece
Dr. Eva Micskey/Hungary
Badriul Hegar Syarief/Indonesia
Arinda Yunanto/Indonesia
Prof. Adib Moukarzel/Lebanon
Dr. Olga Zimanaite/Lithuania
Dr. Angel Carlos/Mexico
Dr. Eustorgio Garcia/Mexico
Dr. Raul Garza/Mexico
Dr. Sofia Leyva/Mexico
Dr. Ricardo Reyes Retana/Mexico
Dr. Enrique Rodriguez/Mexico
Prof. Per Finne/Norway
Dr. Alfredo Mora/Panama
Gerado Rivera/Panama
Dr. Rommel Bernardo/Philippines
Dr. Augustus Manalo/Philippines
Prof. Virginia Tanueco/Philippines
Dr. Luis Pereira-da-Silva/Portugal

# Contributors

Dr. Saleh Al-Alaiyan/Saudia Arabia
Dr. Michael Greeff/South Africa
Dr. Manuel Martin Esteban/Spain
Dr. Ine Martinah Mingoen/Suriname
Prof. Mehari Gebre-Medhin/Sweden
Prof. Christian Braegger/Switzerland
Dr. Somporn Chotinaruemol/Thailand
Prof. Zulaika Ali/Trinidad & Tobago
Prof. David Picou/Trinidad & Tobago
Dr. Rajindra Parag/Trinidad & Tobago
Dr. Lynette Welch/Trinidad & Tobago

Dr. Assia Turki-Hammami/Tunisie
Prof. Aziz Sheikh/UK
Dr. Lillian Beard/USA
Dr. Stuart Cohen/USA
Mrs. JoAnn Hattner/USA
Dr. Robert N. Hamburger/USA
Dr. John Kerner/USA
Dr. Ricardo Sorensen/USA
Dr. Ekhard Ziegler/USA
Dr. Bich Chi Pham/Vietnam

## Nestlé participants

Prof. Carlos Nogueira de Almeida/
    Brazil
Mrs. Shaunda Durance-Tod/Canada
Andrea Papamandjaris/Canada
Mrs. Lis Vinther/Denmark
Mr. Elias Papadopoulos/Greece
Veronidia Ventura/Philippines
Prof. Antonio Guerra/Portugal
Mrs. Mabel Labuschagne/South Africa
Dr. Anette Jarvi/Sweden
Dr. Irene Corthesy/Switzerland
Dr. Bianca-Maria Exl-Preysch/
    Switzerland
Dr. Marie-Claire Fichot/Switzerland
Prof. Ferdinand Haschke/Switzerland

Mr. Charly Huber-Haag/Switzerland
Dr. Martin Kussman/Switzerland
Mr. Philippe Steenhout/Switzerland
Prof. Marco Turini/Switzerland
Dr. Peter Van Dael/Switzerland
Mrs. Nicola Bradley/UK
Ms. Cynthia Brown/USA
Ms. Cynthia Busby/USA
Ms. Nina Carroll/USA
Ms. Julie Dunmire/USA
Ms. Kelly Green/USA
Ms. Linda Hsieh/USA
Ms. Kathleen Novak/USA
Ms. Lisa Reavlin/USA
Mr. Ernie Strapazon/USA

Lucas A, Sampson HA (eds): Primary Prevention by Nutrition Intervention in Infancy and Childhood.
Nestlé Nutr Workshop Ser Pediatr Program, vol 57, pp 1–13,
Nestec Ltd., Vevey/S. Karger AG, Basel, © 2006.

# Infant Nutrition and Primary Prevention: Current and Future Perspectives

*A. Lucas*[a], *Hugh A. Sampson*[b]

[a]MRC Childhood Nutrition Research Centre, Institute of Child Health, London, UK; and
[b]Jaffe Food Allergy Institute, Mount Sinai School of Medicine, New York, USA

In the past two decades there has been a major change in focus in the field of nutrition. Previously, the main interest was meeting nutritional needs; now the major emphasis is the impact on health. Indeed, our new understanding of the biological effects of nutrition that influence health has revealed the immense potential for nutrition in primary prevention.

## The Concept of Primary Prevention

Primary prevention is generally considered as the prevention of a disease before it occurs, or reduction of its incidence. However, this concept needs to be expanded here since early nutritional interventions are often targeted towards optimizing neurodevelopmental potential. Therefore, the suggested definition of primary prevention for this Workshop is as follows:
*To prevent or reduce the risk of disease and prevent impairment of cognitive potential*
The means of achieving primary prevention by nutrition is through education, clinical or public health practice or intervention, and through policy, legislation and regulation. However, these strategies are all dependent on the establishment of a solid research base – the focus of this Workshop. Research in primary prevention may and should have a fundamental basis, as considered in several chapters, but ultimately effective prevention strategies depend on formal evidence-based research that establishes the impact of nutrition on health and developmental outcomes.

## Impact of Nutrition on Health

Nutrition has the potential to influence health in a broad variety of ways, which may be usefully categorized as in table 1.

1

**Table 1.** Impact of nutrition on health

| | |
|---|---|
| 1 | Short-term or immediate effects |
| 2 | Long-term effects |
| | 'Programming' during critical periods |
| | Impact of nutrition throughout childhood |
| 3 | Diet as a 'vehicle' for factors that impact on health |

In the following sections I shall give illustrations in each of these categories, taking for convenience data from my own center's work, simply to illustrate some concepts that underlie the large array of examples that will emerge at this Workshop.

## Short-Term or Immediate Effects of Nutrition

Primary prevention may occur *during* a short-term intervention. An important example is the effect of human milk in neonatal intensive care in preventing life-threatening necrotizing enterocolitis (NEC) or neonatal sepsis. For instance, our own study on 926 preterm infants under 1,850 g birth weight [1] showed that in exclusively formula-fed infants confirmed NEC occurred in 7.2%; whereas in those partially or totally human milk-fed NEC occurred in only 2.5 and 1.2%, respectively. Above 30 weeks gestation, when other risk factors for NEC are less common, diet emerged as particularly influential, with 1/20 of the rate of NEC in those fed human milk versus formula. Indeed in a national survey of NEC (unpublished) those above 30 weeks fed predominantly human milk who developed NEC had a mortality of 5%, compared to 26% in those predominantly formula-fed. Further work from a randomized trial [2] and observational data also show a major reduction in neonatal sepsis in those fed human milk.

In general, when appraising the 'prevention potential' for a nutritional intervention, there are three key factors to consider: (a) the quality of evidence available; (b) the size of the effect demonstrated, and (c) the feasibility of the intervention.

In the above example, the evidence that breast milk reduces the risk of NEC or sepsis is based on numerous observational studies, some randomized trial data and biological plausibility; the effect size is large, and in terms of feasibility, counseling of mothers of preterm infants to provide at least some expressed breast milk has been effective. Thus, use of breast milk in neonatal care for primary prevention is widely employed.

## Long-Term Impact of Nutrition

Nutrition as a 'lifestyle' factor throughout childhood has raised considerable interest in relation to a number of disease processes, particularly obesity and associated non-insulin-dependent diabetes in view of the current epidemic – a major focus of this Workshop. Here, however, I shall consider perhaps the fastest growing area of current nutritional research: 'programming', and its relationship to prevention.

Programming was defined by Lucas [3] as the concept that a stimulus or insult, when applied to a critical or sensitive period in development may have a long-term or life-time effect on the structure or function of the organism.

### Background

The concept of 'critical periods' dates back to Spalding's formal description in the 19th century of 'imprinting' in chicks. The first evidence for *nutritional* programming came from the work of McCance [4] in animals in the early 1960s demonstrating in rats the long-term impact of neonatal nutrition on adult size. Since then numerous animal studies including those in primates have shown that in adulthood nutrition may program such outcomes as blood pressure, lipid metabolism, insulin resistance, atherosclerosis, bone health, learning, behavior and even lifespan [3–9].

Given the immense potential for disease prevention raised by this work, corresponding studies in humans have been imperative. In 1982 we initiated the first formal intervention trials, based on the pharmaceutical trial model, to test the programming concept in humans [10], first in preterms then full-term infants. From the later 1980–1990s there was also an explosion of retrospective observational studies relating size in early life (as a putative marker of nutrition) to later disease [11].

### Programming Effects on Cardiovascular Disease

Breastfeeding is now emerging as important in the primary prevention of cardiovascular disease risk [12]. Numerous observational studies in healthy full-term infants have shown that breastfeeding is associated with a later reduction in insulin resistance, blood pressure, LDL cholesterol and obesity – the latter three, the subject of formal meta-analyses. However to confirm causation, studies on preterm infants have been important since it is possible, in those whose mothers elect not to provide breast milk, to conduct formal randomized outcome trials comparing donated banked breast milk with formula. Moreover, because breast milk intake in preterms can be recorded accurately (since it is fed by nasogastric tube), a 'dose-response relationship' between intake and later outcome can be explored – important, if found, in supporting causation.

3

Our own such trials on preterm infants provide experimental evidence that human milk feeding in the neonatal period reduces, later in adolescence, blood pressure, LDL cholesterol, insulin resistance and leptin resistance (metabolic tendency to obesity), and the greater the human milk intake the greater the benefit [13–16]. Thus, extensive evidence in term and preterm infants, now including experimental evidence from formal outcome trials, shows that human milk reduces the key features of the metabolic syndrome – the major risk complex for cardiovascular disease.

In a recent review Singhal and Lucas [12] linked these findings into a broader concept – the postnatal growth acceleration hypothesis. This hypothesis is based on extensive evidence from studies in diverse animal species [17] (from butterflies to primates), human observations [18, 19] and now our own experimental interventions on preterm and full-term infants, that rapid growth acceleration (upward centile crossing) in the early postnatal period increases later cardiovascular disease risk. Thus the advantage for breast milk-fed infants could be related to their slower early growth rate [12].

The potential long-term impact of breast milk feeding or other strategies to prevent early growth acceleration is large. In our trials the impact on later blood pressure of either breast milk in preterm infants or using a standard versus nutrient-enriched formula in small-for-gestational age full-term infants [12] was over 3 mm Hg. Yet, the Framingham study noted that just a 2-mm reduction in population diastolic blood pressure would result in around 100,000 less strokes and coronaries in the US each year. The impact of breast milk on later cholesterol – around a 10% reduction – would, in adults, reduce cardiovascular risk by 25% and mortality 13–14% [12].

*Programming and the Brain*

The programming effect of early nutrition of the brain is equally important in terms of primary prevention. In a randomized trial in preterm infants, use of a standard versus enriched preterm formula (in the early 1980s, when standard formulas were often used) resulted in a major deficit in later IQ, reaching 13 verbal IQ points in males [20]. Those (males and females) fed the standard formula had, at 7–8 years, a 38% incidence of some degree of mental or motor impairment compared to only 15% in the group fed the enriched formula. Our (unpublished) evidence shows that the cognitive effects persist into early adulthood when we have also found differences between randomized groups in the structure of the brain (using MRI scanning with statistical parametric mapping). In term infants, previous studies on the impact of undernutrition on neurodevelopment were observational and confounded by poverty and poor social circumstances. However, the first randomized trials of early nutritional supplementation in developing countries are beginning to demonstrate the long-term cognitive effects of early nutrition [21]. Nevertheless, the effect-size appears greater in those born preterm.

The impact of specific nutrients (e.g. iron, zinc, taurine, long-chain polyunsaturated fatty acids) and of breastfeeding are also receiving much study, and have considerable potential for the prevention of reduced cognitive performance [21].

*Balance of Risks*

It is of interest, however, that whilst a high plane of early nutrition is important for brain development, a lower plane of nutrition and growth appears to favor cardiovascular health, as discussed above. This apparent conflict requires risk-benefit analysis. In preterm infants, the brain is particularly sensitive to the impact of nutrition. For this reason, a high plane of nutrition and growth takes precedence – hence the rationale for breast milk fortifiers and multi-nutrient-enriched preterm formulas in neonatal care. However, in full-term infants, whilst early nutrition appears to have a major impact on later cardiovascular risk, the impact on the brain appears less than in preterms. Whilst further research is needed, these findings in healthy infants suggest slower early growth, as seen with breastfeeding, would be more optimal.

## Diet as a Vehicle for Factors That Impact on Health

The human diet is a complex medium that may act as a vehicle for numerous factors that can influence short and long-term health. These include pathogenic organisms (e.g. HIV in breast milk and *Enterobacter sakazakii* in infant formulas), environmental contaminants (e.g. dioxins, phytoestrogens) and a variety of potentially toxic factors. It is one of the latter, aluminum, I shall cite as an illustrative example here.

Parenteral aluminum has long been known to be neurotoxic. Before its removal from renal dialysis solutions, patients became frankly demented. However, intravenous feeding solutions used in the pediatric population may be significantly contaminated with aluminum, for instance, in calcium gluconate [22]. We tested the hypothesis that in preterm infants, frequently fed intravenously and born at a sensitive stage of brain development and with limited excretory capacity, parenteral aluminum might be especially neurotoxic. A large randomized trial was conducted comparing those fed on regular total parental nutrition (TPN) versus a specially sourced low aluminum TPN including calcium chloride rather than gluconate [22]. At the 18-month follow-up those receiving more than the median number of days of TPN for the cohort (9 days) had a 10-point deficit in the mental development index (MDI) if fed on the standard versus low aluminum solution in the newborn period. Taking the whole cohort, each day of standard TPN solution, as fed in many Western units, was associated with loss of 1 MDI point [22]. This illustrates the importance of achieving high standards of quality control

**Table 2.** Research issues in primary prevention by nutrition in infancy and childhood

---

Critical interactions
Timing of the window
Emergence of the effect
Quality of evidence required
Risk-benefit analyses
Mechanism

---

of feeds for infants in relation to primary prevention. Such control is often best achieved at a legislative or regulatory level.

## Research Issues in Primary Prevention

Whilst the potential for primary prevention via nutrition is high, research in this area is complex. I shall consider here an illustrative selection of key research issues listed in table 2.

## Critical Interactions

Nutrition may interact with genes, subject characteristics, and environmental factors.

*Genetic Factors*
Interaction between early diet and family history for later risk of atopy provides an instructive model. Whilst all observational studies comparing breast and formula feeding are confounded by demographic factors, preterm infants provide an opportunity for randomly comparing human milk (from a milk bank) with formula (see above). In the only such randomized outcome trial for atopy [23], those with a family history of atopy who were randomly assigned to formula versus human milk in the neonatal period had over twice the incidence of eczema, nearly three times the incidence of food and drug reactions and a strong trend of more wheezing at 18 months follow-up. Conversely, in those with a negative family history, there was trend in the opposite direction [23]. Indeed, in a further trial of preterm versus term formula where the former group had higher cow's milk protein intake, in those with a negative family history of atopy, infants receiving the greatest cow's milk protein intake had the lowest incidence of atopy 18 months later [23]. Thus, whether later tolerance or sensitization occurred appeared to be genetically determined.

More work is needed to identify *specific* genes that interact with the diet. In young adults we found that early evidence of the atherosclerotic process (reduced flow-mediated endothelial-dependent arterial dilatation) was dose-related to the plasma n-3 fatty acid level (principally related to fish intake). However, this beneficial effect of fish intake on later vascular health was only seen in glu298asp heterozygotes (30% of the population) of the eNOS gene (influential for vascular health); the glu298glu homozygotes were unaffected [24].

These data illustrate that genetic characterization of family history may be needed in some primary prevention studies to identify the optimal target group for intervention.

*Subject Characteristics*

Not all subgroups within a population are equally affected by diet. In most studies, including our own, on nutrition and later neurodevelopment, males show the major response [20]. This is also seen in the extensive corresponding animal literature [8]. Furthermore, in an unpublished 15- to 18-year follow-up we found that higher verbal IQ after using a nutrient enriched diet (see above) was only seen in appropriate- and not small-for-gestational-age infants.

Thus, again, target subgroups within a population that respond most favorably to the nutritional intervention require identification.

*Environmental Interactions*

One of the most concerning interactions in the programming area is that between infant diet and our subsequent Western environment – probably our Western diet.

In the 1980s Lewis et al. [7] assigned baboons to breast versus formula feeding during infancy and then placed both groups on a 'Western-style' diet, rich in saturated fats, to test whether early nutrition in a Western context could influence later cardiovascular health. In adulthood, the previously breastfed group appeared the disadvantaged one in terms of higher LDL cholesterol, lower HDL, higher cholesterol absorption from the gut and reduced cholesterol excretion. Thus, the previously breastfed baboons appeared to be programmed to 'conserve' cholesterol – perhaps an advantage in the 'wild' on a natural diet. But on a Western diet, this became disadvantageous, emphasized by the postmortem evidence that throughout the arterial tree, the previously breastfed group had around twice the area of early atherosclerosis compared to the previously formula-fed group [7].

Later, Barker [11] noted that whilst breastfeeding was associated with lower rates of ischemic heart disease overall, if prolonged beyond a year in more vulnerable males, it was associated with increased ischemic heart disease. More recently we showed in 400 20- to 30-year-olds that, beyond 3–4 months of breastfeeding (not exclusive), increasing duration was associated with progressive worsening of vascular distensibility 20–30 years later [25]. This is now supported by a further Scandinavian study also showing that vascular health in 10-year-old children was worse in those who were breastfed longer.

These studies [7, 11, 25] collectively raise the hypothesis that breast-feeding, if sufficiently prolonged, is an adverse risk factor for cardiovascular disease when followed by a Western diet. Thus, breastfeeding overall is beneficial for vascular health – but the optimal duration in the West is unknown. Of course, the data impugn our Western diet rather than breast-feeding and prolonged breastfeeding is not in any way challenged in developing countries. There are also other outcome benefits for breastfeeding. Nevertheless, in a Western context, research in this area is now critical.

Taking these interactions collectively, the research implication is that:

*The impact on health of a nutrition intervention may be highly influenced by genes, subject characteristics and by current and future environment.*

## Timing of the Window

Defining the optimal window for nutrition intervention is a key research issue. For cardiovascular programming the period beyond birth (whether term or preterm) appears to be a particularly sensitive one [12]. Conversely, for the brain, gestation appears important so that term infants may be less sensitive (not insensitive) than those born preterm.

With regard to cardiovascular disease, a key research question has been whether prevention is best achieved by prenatal or postnatal intervention. Whilst there is extensive evidence that fetal environment may influence outcome, when birth weight is taken as a measure of fetal growth, its relationship with later cardiovascular risk factors (blood pressure, insulin resistance and LDL cholesterol) is small; whereas the impact of postnatal nutrition based on both experimental and observational studies, is large [12]. Fetal growth manipulation is also difficult to achieve whereas postnatal nutrition can be modified practically. More work is needed, but the postnatal period is emerging as an important one in terms of prevention potential for cardiovascular disease. Thus:

*The efficacy of a prevention strategy may be highly influenced by its timing.*

## Emergence of the Effect

Lewis et al. [9] showed in baboons that overfeeding in infancy resulted only in a temporary increase in body weight which then remained normal throughout 'childhood'. However, those overfed in infancy became progressively obese in adulthood; an excellent example of programming, in which a 'memory' had been retained of the early intervention, yet outcome effects were not expressed until adulthood.

Examples of late-emerging effects are found in humans. In our own trial (cited above) preterm infants randomly assigned to human milk or formula in the neonatal period, showed no difference in blood pressure at 7–8 years, but a major reduction in blood pressure was seen in those fed human milk by 13–16 years [14]. A more disturbing example was found in our randomized trial of a formula with and without long-chain polyunsaturated fatty acids (LCPUFA). In all, 460 full-term subjects were studied including a reference group. Follow-up at 18 months showed no differences in developmental scores between groups [26]; but at 4–6 years, the group given LCPUFA had a significant 6-point reduction in IQ (unpublished). Our other LCPUFA trials show that outcome is dependent on source (see Chapter X), and other sources of LCPUFA have not had this adverse effect. Nevertheless taking these late-emerging programmed effects collectively a clear research message emerges:

*Long-term follow-up is essential in intervention trials of early nutrition to ensure detection of late emerging effects, which may have implications for safety as well as efficacy.*

## Quality of Evidence Required in Studies on Prevention

Many health practices in nutrition are defended only by observational data, which are often confounded (for instance differences in breast- and formula-fed infants). It is difficult therefore to use such data to prove causation and hence underpin health practices.

An example of the difficulty in establishing causation from observational data comes from the observed relationship between birth weight and later insulin resistance, interpreted as fetal programming [15]. However, in our own randomized trial demonstrating experimentally the influence of postnatal diet on later insulin resistance in adolescence, we were able to do an instructive secondary analysis. Birth weight, postnatal growth and, of course, postnatal nutrition were each found to be significantly related to later insulin resistance. However, when all three were placed as independent variables in the same regression model, only postnatal growth remained significantly related to insulin resistance [15]. This suggested that postnatal growth explained the effect of postnatal nutrition, but also the *birth weight* effect. If so, birth weight may be more a proxy for *future* growth (postnatal catch-up, which occurs more at lower birth weight), rather than *fetal* growth, as previously assumed.

As a reflection of the potential dangers of formulating practice recom-mendations on the basis of observational data, retrospective studies had

**Table 3.** Levels of mechanistic research on prevention

Genomics, omics and cell biology
Physiology
Structure
Behavior
Anthropology
Evolution

suggested promotion of postnatal growth would be advantageous for later cardiovascular disease risk [27]; yet experimental studies in both animals and humans have now shown the opposite, as discussed above. In conclusion:

*Wherever possible, experimental studies form a more secure basis for proof of causation and for underpinning practice than observational ones.*

**Risk-Benefit Analyses**

The evidence that more rapid growth favors the brain yet slower growth favors later cardiovascular health indicates the need for risk-benefit analyses in the formulation of health practices, as discussed above. A more general message emerges from this, namely that:

*It may not be safe to devise nutrition policies solely on the basis of the outcome of interest to the investigator. A broader range of outcomes may be needed to define an optimal intervention strategy.*

**Research into Mechanism**

Whilst not the focus of this introductory paper, I shall consider here a few illustrative aspects of mechanistic research. An understanding of mechanism is not a prerequisite for developing effective prevention practices though clearly should be a goal for future development of the field. Such research needs to be a number of levels, as listed in table 3.

Substantial research at a basic biological level is now directed at the descriptive biology and fundamental mechanisms involved in programming and the health impact of early nutrition.

Within the genetic sphere, one area of focus has been the genetic propensity to respond to the nutritional stimulus – that is, nutrient–gene interactions (as discussed above). However, of greater fundamental interest is the converse phenomenon – the impact of nutrition on genetic expression. Lucas [10] proposed that the 'memory' of the original nutritional programming event must be stored in some way to be transmitted through cell generations and expressed later in life. The proposed mechanisms include adaptive changes in gene expression, clonal selection and differential proliferation of cell types within tissues [10]. An understanding of such processes is not only of importance to nutritional programming but to the broader issue of how events in general during early critical periods could have long-term effects.

At a physiological level one key issue is the study of 'coupling mechanisms' that link early nutrition to 'receptors' in sensitive tissues and initiate the physiological changes that will have future health significance. Hormones are likely coupling agents. Factors such as insulin, IgF-1, leptin and gut hormones are known to be influenced or programmed by early nutrition and have plausible effects that could influence health outcomes. Thus, leptin programmed by neonatal nutrition has been shown to influence vascular function [16, 28]. The significantly higher insulin release after a feed in formula-versus breastfed infants in the first week of life is a plausible factor in the later difference in cardiovascular disease risk between these groups [29].

As an example of the importance of exploring mechanism at a *structural* level, our studies showing that neonatal nutrition has long-term impact on a part of the brain co-localized with numeracy skills (unpublished) has led to substantial research showing the impact of early nutrition and specific nutrients, such as taurine, on numeracy [30].

Mechanistic research relating to behavior and social anthropology will be of importance in the understanding of our modern epidemic of obesity. And evolutionary modeling across species has generated fundamental biological hypotheses that underpin human research relevant to health – for instance the postnatal growth acceleration hypothesis [17]. In summary:

*Multilevel mechanistic research is needed to provide a sound underpinning for future prevention strategies.*

## Overview

Thirty years ago it could not have been conceived how immense the potential would become for primary prevention through infant and child nutrition. This chapter only provides illustrative examples of broad areas considered at this Workshop including the programming of obesity, cardiovascular disease, neurodevelopment, bone health, immunity, atopy and cancer.

Research in this area is complex, with many pitfalls, as illustrated in this introduction. Nevertheless, given the major potential to reduce the burden of human disease, substantial worldwide research investment is a high priority.

Perhaps the most important conceptual development from a health perspective is the recognition that nutrition can no longer be seen simply in terms of meeting nutrient needs, but rather, it should be viewed as a therapeutic intervention that influences health and development. Once this conceptual leap is made, it becomes clear, as in other areas of therapeutics, that nutrition practice cannot be based, as it often has been, on theory, politics or uncontrolled observations. Formal evidence-based research is now required to provide a sound basis for primary prevention by early nutrition.

## References

1 Lucas A, Cole TJ: Breast milk and neonatal necrotizing enterocolitis. Lancet 1990;336: 1519–1523.
2 Lucas A, Fewtrell M, Morley R, et al: Randomized outcome trial of human milk fortification and developmental outcome in preterm infants. Am J Clin Nutr 1996;64:142–151.
3 Lucas A: Programming by early nutrition in man. Ciba Found Symp 1991;156:38–55.
4 McCance RA: Food, growth and time. Lancet 1962;ii:671–676.
5 Hahn P: Effect of litter size on plasma cholesterol and insulin and some liver and adipose tissue enzymes in adult rodents. J Nutr 1984;114:1231–1234.
6 Mott GE, Lewis DS, McGill HC: Programming of cholesterol metabolism by breast or formula-feeding. Ciba Found Symp 1991;156:56–76.
7 Lewis DS, Mott GE, McMahan CA, et al: Deferred effects of preweaning diet on atherosclerosis in adolescent baboons. Arteriosclerosis 1988;8:274–280.
8 Smart J: Undernutrition, learning and memory: review of experimental studies. Proc 12th Int Congr Nutr. London, Libbey, 1986, pp 74–78.
9 Lewis DS, Bertrand HA, McMahan CA, et al: Preweaning food intake influences the adiposity of young adult baboons. J Clin Invest 1986;78:899–905.
10 Lucas A: Programming by early nutrition: an experimental approach. J Nutr 1998;128(suppl): 401S–406S.
11 Barker DJ: Fetal origins of coronary heart disease. BMJ 1995;311:171–174.
12 Singhal A, Lucas A: Early origins of cardiovascular disease. Is there a unifying hypothesis? Lancet 2004;363:1642–1645.
13 Singhal A, Cole TJ, Fewtrell MS, et al: Breast-milk feeding and the lipoprotein profile in adolescents born preterm: follow-up of a prospective randomised study. Lancet 2004;363:1571–1578.
14 Singhal A, Cole TJ, Lucas A: Early nutrition in preterm infants and later blood pressure: two cohorts after randomised trials. Lancet 2001;357:413–419.
15 Singhal A, Fewtrell MS, Cole TJ, et al: A Low nutrient intake and early growth for later insulin resistance in adolescents born preterm. Lancet 2003;361:1089–1097.
16 Singhal A, Farooqi IS, O'Rahilly S, et al: Early nutrition and leptin concentrations in later life. Am J Clin Nutr 2002;75:993–999.
17 Metcalfe NB, Monaghan P: Compensation for a bad start: grow now, pay later? Trends Ecol Evol 2001;16:254–260.
18 Stettler N, Zemel BS, Kumanyika S, Stalligns VA: Infant weight gain and childhood overweight status in a multicenter, cohort study. Pediatrics 2002;109:194–199.
19 Soto N, Bazaes RA, Pena V, et al: Insulin sensitivity and secretion are related to catch-up growth in small-for-gestational-age infants at age 1 year: results from a prospective cohort. J Clin Endocrinol Metab 2003;88:3645–3650.
20 Lucas A, Morley R, Cole TJ: Randomised trial of early diet in preterm babies and later intelligence quotient. BMJ 1998;317:1481–1487.
21 Lucas A, Morley R, Isaacs E: Nutrition and mental development. Nutr Rev 2001;59:S24–S33.
22 Bishop NJ, Morley RM, Day JP, Lucas A: Aluminum neurotoxicity in preterm infants receiving intravenous feeding solutions. N Engl J Med 1997;336:1557–1561.
23 Lucas A, Brooke OG, Morley R, et al: Early diet of preterm infants and development of allergic or atopic disease: randomised prospective study. BMJ 1990;300:837–840.
24 Leeson CPM, Hingorani AD, Mullen MJ, et al: Glu298Asp endothelial nitric oxide synthase gene polymorphism interacts with environmental and dietary factors to influence endothelial function. Circ Res 2002;90:1153–1158.

25  Leeson CPM, Kattenhorn M, Deanfield JE, Lucas A: Duration of breast-feeding and arterial distensibility in early adult life: population based study. BMJ 2001;322:643–647.
26  Lucas A, Stafford M, Morley R, et al: Efficacy and safety of long-chain polyunsaturated fatty acid supplementation of infant-formula milk: a randomised trial. Lancet 1999;354:1948–1954.
27  Law CM: Significance of birth weight for the future. Arch Dis Child Fetal Neonatal Ed 2002;86:F7–F8.
28  Singhal A, Farooqi IS, Cole TJ, et al: Influence of leptin on arterial distensibility: a novel link between obesity and cardiovascular disease. Circulation 2002;106:1919–1924.
29  Lucas A, Blackburn AM, Aynsley-Green A, et al: Breast vs. bottle: endocrine responses are different with formula feeding. Lancet 1980;i:1267–1269.
30  Wharton BA, Morley R, Isaacs EB, et al: Low plasma taurine and later neurodevelopment. Arch Dis Child Fetal Neonatal Ed 2004;89:F497–F498.

Lucas A, Sampson HA (eds): Primary Prevention by Nutrition Intervention in Infancy and Childhood.
Nestlé Nutr Workshop Ser Pediatr Program, vol 57, pp 15–30,
Nestec Ltd., Vevey/S. Karger AG, Basel, © 2006.

# Nutritional Interventions in Infancy and Childhood for Prevention of Atherosclerosis and the Metabolic Syndrome

*Atul Singhal*

MRC Childhood Nutrition Research Centre, Institute of Child Health, London, UK

Atherosclerotic cardiovascular disease (CVD) is the leading cause of death and disability, and the most important public health priority in the West [1]. Yet, despite great progress in its clinical management, the prevalence of CVD continues to increase [1]. In the UK alone an estimated 2.7 million people are now living with coronary heart disease – a number that has risen sharply [1]. Consequently, the role of prevention has become a major priority for public health policy and future scientific research [1].

Atherosclerosis is now known to have a long preclinical phase with the development of pathological changes in the arteries of children and young adults well before the clinical manifestations of disease later in adulthood [2]. Nutritional factors have been shown to be particularly influential [2, 3] and affect a lifetime risk of CVD [3]. For instance, both observational and, more recently, experimental studies suggest that nutrition in fetal life ('the fetal origins hypothesis' [4]) and in the early postnatal period [5] influences, or programs, the long-term development of atherosclerosis and its complications. This effect occurs via programming of classical cardiovascular risk factors (e.g. obesity) and also by effects on the vascular biology of early atherosclerosis [6].

Other than via programming, nutrition also has an important direct impact on conventional cardiovascular risk factors in childhood. These risk factors show tracking into adult life [7], affect the earliest stages of atherosclerosis, and have a strong, independent influence on the long-term risk of CVD [8]. Obesity in childhood, for instance, adversely affects adult CVD risk independent of adult weight [8].

Based on the strong evidence for the early origins of atherosclerosis, the American Heart Association has recently published guidelines for the primary prevention of CVD beginning in children and adolescents [9]. The present review focuses on the evidence and rationale for such interventions, emphasizing the role of nutrition in infancy and childhood.

## The Childhood Origins of Atherosclerosis

Autopsy studies of the atherosclerotic changes in the coronary arteries of young men killed in the Korean and Vietnamese wars first stimulated research into the early development of atherosclerosis [10]. Similar studies in children, particularly from the Bogalusa Heart Study, demonstrated a high prevalence of coronary atherosclerosis (up to 90%) by the third decade of life [10]. Strikingly, the presence and extent of atherosclerotic lesions in these reports correlated positively with established risk factors and, in accordance with the Framingham risk score for predicting cardiovascular mortality, their severity was associated with an increase in the number of risk factors [11]. Importantly, these autopsy findings have been confirmed in other populations (e.g. the Pathobiologic Determinants of Atherosclerosis in Youth Study) and extended to atherosclerosis at different vascular sites [12].

Intravascular ultrasound studies have confirmed and extended earlier findings from pathological studies [13]. One such study, performed in heart transplant recipients days after transplantation, found that up to 17% of asymptomatic teenagers had coronary atherosclerosis [13]. Similar observations were made using noninvasive measures of subclinical atherosclerosis, which, unlike coronary arteriography and intravascular coronary ultrasound, can be used in asymptomatic individuals and large population studies. For example, in the Bogalusa Heart Study, carotid intima-media thickness (especially in the carotid bulb) was increased in young adults aged 20–38 years [10]. This marker of atherosclerosis was associated with conventional cardiovascular risk factors and predicted by such risk factors in childhood [10]. Similarly, in 10- to 17-year-olds, arterial distensibility, a marker of arterial wall elasticity and the early atherosclerotic process, was related to lipid profile, blood pressure and parental history of myocardial infarction [10]. In fact, conventional cardiovascular risk factors have been shown to affect vascular health from early in childhood, and Leeson et al. [6] showed an inverse correlation between brachial arterial distensibility and cholesterol concentration from as early as the first decade of life.

Thus, in summary, there is now strong evidence for the presence of subclinical atherosclerosis in children from both pathological studies and ultrasound measures of vascular function. The latter are particularly important because they help elucidate risk factors for atherosclerosis in children, act as markers of the intensity of the burden of CVD, and could identify those at particular risk for future cardiovascular events. Ultimately, these noninvasive techniques could help both in the investigation of mechanisms and the development of rational approaches to prevention.

## The Metabolic Syndrome in the Young

Postmortem studies and noninvasive measures of atherosclerosis both show that the same risk factors contribute to early atherosclerosis in the young as in adults [10]. As in adults, these risk factors correlate with each other and tend to occur in clusters. This clustering, first described in 1988 by Reaven [14] as the 'metabolic syndrome', links obesity, insulin resistance, dyslipidemia and hypertension with an increased risk of atherosclerosis, CVD and type-2 diabetes mellitus. In recent years, a number of new phenotypes have been added including microalbuminuria, endothelial dysfunction, and elevation in C-reactive protein and fibrinogen concentration [15]. However, obesity remains central to the development of the metabolic syndrome and subsequent cardiovascular risk [15].

*Role of Obesity*

As found in adults, obesity plays a major role in the development of the metabolic syndrome in the young. Obesity often precedes the development of other features such as insulin resistance, and each component of the metabolic syndrome worsens with increasing adiposity [16]. Recent evidence suggests that the syndrome is more common than previously suspected, with up to 50% of obese children and adolescents being affected [16].

That obesity (and particularly central obesity) is a major independent risk factor for CVD is well known. For instance individuals with a body mass index (BMI) of $>30\,kg/m^2$ are four times more likely to suffer from CVD than those with a BMI of $<25\,kg/m^2$ [17]. Obesity in children may be particularly detrimental [10]. Childhood obesity predicts the risk of developing a constellation of metabolic, hemodynamic and inflammatory disorders associated with CVD and, importantly, increases cardiovascular risk independent of adult weight [8]. Given that more than 30% of children in the USA are obese (BMI >95th percentile) [18], the current epidemic of childhood obesity has major implications for the prevalence of adult CVD.

The effect of childhood obesity on CVD is more complex than simply its association with conventional risk factors that make up the metabolic syndrome. The observation that insulin resistance cannot explain many newer features of the metabolic syndrome (e.g. features of inflammation) have led to suggestions that insulin resistance and atherosclerosis share common antecedents such as the adverse effects of inflammatory mediators secreted by adipocytes [15]. Adipose tissue could, therefore, have a direct detrimental effect on vascular health and particularly on endothelial cell dysfunction, a critical early event in the atherosclerotic process.

This concept, that adipose tissue is not just a passive energy store but is highly physiologically active, has become increasingly important in understanding the role of obesity in vascular disease. Adipose tissue secretes several biologically active cytokine-like molecules (e.g. C-reactive protein, interleukin-6, and leptin) collectively termed adipokines, which could affect vascular function by their local and distant actions. Leptin in particular, although predominantly involved in the regulation of appetite, has been shown to act via receptors on vascular cells to increase angiogenic activity and oxidative stress, and to promote vascular calcification and smooth muscle cell proliferation [19]. Consistent with this atherogenic action, we showed recently that leptin concentration was associated with lower arterial distensibility, independent of fat mass, inflammatory markers and insulin resistance [19]. These observations suggest that leptin is a key link between obesity and vascular disease. The fact that these findings were in healthy non-obese adolescents further suggests that this link is important early in the atherosclerotic process [19].

## Mechanisms

If we accept that atherosclerosis and the metabolic syndrome have their origins in childhood, then understanding the mechanisms becomes a high priority. Although a detailed discussion of mechanisms is beyond the scope of this chapter, such understanding will be critical in identifying the best interventions.

At its simplest level, the early origins of CVD may represent a genetic predisposition. Clearly, the development of atherosclerosis involves a complex interaction between the vascular endothelium, serum lipids, platelets, and inflammatory and vascular smooth muscle cells; a process in which poorly characterized genes must interact with a changing environment. Obesity, for instance, has been shown to have a 40–70% inheritance in twin studies [18]. Therefore, the same genes that predispose to obesity may be associated with other components of the metabolic syndrome and have a similar effect on atherosclerosis risk in the young as in older individuals.

Along these lines, the thrifty genotype hypothesis was first proposed over 40 years ago to explain the modern emergence of obesity and type-2 diabetes [20]. This hypothesis postulated that genetic selection of individuals, whose energy storage capacity allowed survival during time of famine, predisposed them to obesity and its complications during times of calorie excess (as in the modern world). However, while the development of atherosclerosis must involve complex gene-environmental interactions, family studies suggest only a moderate heritability for endothelial dysfunction (14%), a key early stage in this process [21]. The relative contribution of nature versus nurture for the development of atherosclerosis therefore remains largely unknown.

A second mechanism is the role of nutrition in the development of CVD. Nutrition has a major impact on most cardiovascular risk factors, which collectively account for more than 90% of the population-attributable risk of myocardial infarction (abnormal lipids, smoking, presence of diabetes, hypertension, abdominal obesity, psychological factors, consumption of fruits and vegetables, and alcohol, and regular physical activity) [22]. The same risk factors are important in both sexes, at all ages, and in all regions [22]. Furthermore, nutrition has the same effects on these factors in children as in adults [11] and, importantly, long-term follow-up studies have shown clear evidence for their tracking (particularly obesity, dyslipidemia, and blood pressure) from childhood into adult life [7, 10]. For instance, 2/3 of children obese at age 10 years are at risk of being obese as adults [18]. Not surprisingly, therefore, many features of the metabolic syndrome persist and extend from childhood into adult life [10]. Of particular concern in children is the long length of exposure to risk factors for vascular disease. For example, a prolonged exposure of arteries to the toxic metabolic milieu associated with obesity could explain the greater risk of CVD in those who are obese as children.

The third key mechanism for the early origins of CVD is the environmental equivalent to the thrifty genotype hypothesis, the thrifty phenotype hypothesis [23]. This concept has been recently proposed to explain the epidemiological evidence that factors in utero and in early life program the long-term risk of CVD. The thrifty phenotype hypothesis suggests that resetting of metabolism by early environmental factors affects the long-term phenotype, so that individuals exposed to under-nutrition in early life develop a thrifty phenotype which predisposes them to obesity and its risk factors if exposed to nutrient excess later in life [23]. The hypothesis is part of the broader concept of 'developmental plasticity' [24], shown by many plants and animals, which proposes that organisms are capable of developing in a variety of ways so that they are well adapted to the environment in which they are likely to live. Paradoxically, therefore, the modern epidemic of obesity and CVD may be related to the change in environment that has increased nutrient availability to individuals whose parents and grandparents lived in impoverished conditions.

Overall, it is clear that nutrition is key to most mechanisms for the early development of CVD. Nutrition is the major environmental factor that interacts with genetic predisposition to affect the metabolic syndrome and hence CVD risk. This applies equally to children as it does to adults. Nutrition in fetal life or in infancy is the major factor that programs the later propensity to CVD and, importantly, nutrition may interact with adverse prior programming to affect CVD risk [5]. For instance, the adverse effect of low birth weight on cardiovascular risk is greatest in individuals who become obese as adults [5]. Finally, obesity, itself strongly affected by nutrition, plays a central role in the early development of CVD. Prevention of obesity, along with key nutrition interventions in infancy and childhood are therefore a logical and important focus for the prevention of CVD.

## Nutrition Interventions

Critical to the argument that the primary prevention of CVD should begin in childhood is the observation that in up to 50% of individuals, the first manifestation of CVD is sudden death or myocardial infarction. This makes primary prevention particularly important for population health. Preventative efforts may be especially justified in children because lifestyle risk factors are often adopted in childhood and so, arguably, it is easier to intervene before these habits become established. Dietary and physical activity patterns, for instance, develop in childhood and are known to track into adult life. Risk-taking behaviors that affect CVD, such as smoking, are also often first acquired in childhood or adolescence. Nevertheless, despite the increasing epidemiological evidence, it remains difficult to establish the effectiveness of interventions at a population level using formal randomized trials.

The two main periods for interventions are in infancy and in childhood. However, importantly, there is no evidence to suggest age-related cutoffs that restrict preventative strategies to particular periods.

### Interventions in Infancy

The concept that nutrition in infancy can influence long-term risk factors for CVD first emerged in the 1960s with the pioneering work of McCance. He showed that rats raised in small litters, and therefore overfed early in postnatal life, were programmed for greater body size as adults. Subsequently, rats overfed in the brief suckling period were shown to have permanently higher plasma insulin and cholesterol concentrations while early nutrition in baboons was found to have a major impact on later obesity and atherosclerosis. In baboons, the effects of over-feeding in infancy for obesity emerged only after adolescence, demonstrating the later manifestation of some programming effects [5].

In humans, the major focus of nutritional programming has been the impact of breastfeeding. Breastfed infants have been shown in observational studies to have a lower risk of CVD, obesity, hypercholesterolemia, type-2 diabetes and high blood pressure [5]. These data could be confounded by socioeconomic and demographic differences between breastfed and formula-fed groups. In preterm infants, however, a causal association between breastfeeding and CVD risk was testable using an experimental approach. Infants whose mothers decided not to breastfeed were randomized to breast milk donated by unrelated lactating mothers or to formula milk. Infants assigned randomly to human milk versus formula, for an average of 4 weeks, were found to have marked benefits up to 16 years later for the major components of the metabolic

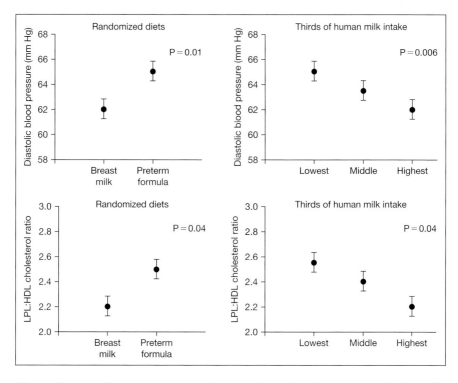

**Fig. 1.** Breast milk consumption in infancy and later blood pressure and lipid profile in adolescents born preterm.

syndrome (blood pressure, leptin 'resistance' suggestive of future obesity, insulin resistance and lipid profile; fig. 1) [5]. As further evidence of causation there were clear dose-response associations between the volume of breast milk intake and later cardiovascular benefit (fig. 1) [5].

The effect size for beast milk feeding on later cardiovascular risk factors is substantial. For blood pressure, for instance, a 3-mm Hg lower diastolic blood pressure in infants given breast milk compared to formula has major public health implications and represents an effect greater than all other non-pharmacological means of reducing blood pressure (such as weight loss, salt restriction, or exercise) [5]. Lowering population-wide diastolic blood pressure by only 2 mm Hg has been estimated to reduce the prevalence of hypertension by 17%, the risk of coronary heart disease by 6% and the risk of stroke/transient ischemic attacks by 15%. Such an intervention would be expected to prevent an estimated 67,000 coronary heart disease events and 34,000 stroke/transient ischemic events annually among those aged 35–64 years, in the USA alone. Similarly, the 10% lowering of the cholesterol concentration with breastfeeding compares favorably with the effects of dietary interventions in adults, which lower cholesterol by only 3–6%. Such an effect on cholesterol concentration would be expected to reduce the incidence of CVD by approximately 25% and mortality by 13–14% [5].

While breastfeeding is advantageous overall for later CVD risk, the optimal duration of breastfeeding remains unknown. In baboons, breastfeeding for the whole of 'infancy' followed by a Western diet increased later dyslipidemia and atherosclerosis compared to those previously fed formula [25]. Similarly, in young adults, breastfeeding beyond 3–4 months was associated with a 'dose-related' decline in vascular distensibility [25]. This study suggested that breastfeeding of longer duration interacted adversely with a subsequent ('unphysiological') Western-style diet, a hypothesis supported by further studies in humans. However, although intriguing, these preliminary and observational data cannot be used to guide public health interventions.

Understanding the mechanisms by which breastfeeding benefits cardio-vascular health is essential in the development of preventative strategies for formula-fed infants. The most common explanation, confounding by socio-biological factors that influence both the mothers' decision to breastfeed and later cardiovascular risk, is unlikely in view of experimental evidence from preterm infants. Other potential explanations include the long-term health benefits of specific nutrients in breast milk, which are absent from some formulas – such as the effect of long-chain polyunsaturated fatty acids in lowering later blood pressure [26]. Most recently, we have suggested that the cardiovascular advantages of breastfeeding may be due to slower growth in breastfed versus formula-fed infants [5].

*The Growth Acceleration Hypothesis*

The postnatal growth acceleration hypothesis suggests that faster growth (upward percentile crossing) particularly in infancy adversely programs the metabolic syndrome [5]. Consistent with this, faster neonatal growth was shown to program insulin resistance and endothelial dysfunction in adolescence. The size of the effect was substantial. Adolescents born preterm with the greatest weight gain had 4% lower flow-mediated dilation of the brachial artery than those with the lowest weight gain, an effect similar to that of insulin-dependent diabetes mellitus (4%) and smoking (6%) in adults [5]. These findings were not confined to infants born prematurely. In an intervention study of infants born full-term but small for gestation, those randomly assigned to a standard formula for the first 9 months had lower blood pressure 6–8 years later than those fed a nutrient-enriched formula that promoted growth (Singhal, unpublished). Further analysis suggested that faster growth explained the adverse effects of a nutrient-enriched formula on later blood pressure.

Data from further studies in both man and animals strongly support this hypothesis. The adverse effects of faster growth are consistent with previous data in animals showing that a higher plane of postnatal nutrition programs the metabolic syndrome. In fact the adverse long-term effects of faster early growth emerge as a fundamental biological phenomenon across animal species [5]. Because growth acceleration is greatest in early infancy, this period may be critical. Consistent with this, faster growth in infancy has been associated with a greater risk of later obesity [5], and, from as early as 2 weeks, with later insulin resistance an endothelial function [5]. Importantly, both infants born prematurely or at term show these effects and, for obesity and endothelial function at least, faster gain in weight and length have both been shown to have adverse long-term effects.

Overall there is now strong evidence to support breastfeeding for the primary prevention of CVD. Whilst, clearly, randomized trials with clinical endpoints to prove efficacy are not possible, and the optimum duration of breastfeeding remains unknown, the effect size is considerable and has major implications for public health.

## Nutritional Interventions in Childhood

*Prevention of Obesity*
Given the strong evidence for the effects of obesity on the early development of atherosclerosis and the metabolic syndrome, there are surprising little data from randomized control trials that support a preventative role for weight loss in children. However, as in adults, weight loss in children is associated with improvements in insulin sensitivity, lipid profile and ultrasound measures of vascular health [27].

Perhaps the most compelling evidence for a cardiovascular benefit of weight loss in children is the effect on endothelial function [28]. In a randomized study, weight loss over only 6 weeks reversed the vascular dysfunction associated with obesity [28]. The addition of exercise training enhanced the beneficial arterial effects, which were sustained when the exercise program was continued for 1 year. These data underscore the importance of diet and exercise in reducing the impact of obesity on vascular disease even from an early age [28].

*Intervention Trials*
Ultimately, to affect public health policy, the efficacy and safety of nutritional interventions have to be demonstrated in large-scale randomized trials based in populations. Such data are difficult and expensive to collect but are now emerging.

For instance, in the Special Turku Coronary Risk Factor intervention project for babies, individual dietary counseling during and after infancy was shown to reduce the fat content of the diet (particularly for saturated fat), and improve the lipid profile up to 10 years later [29]. Similarly, in the dietary intervention study in children with hypercholesterolemia, dietary behavioral intervention reduced fat (and particularly saturated fat) intake, and improved lipid profile at the 1- and 3-year follow-up but not after [30]. Importantly, in both of these studies, there were no adverse effects and the benefits were obtained without affecting growth.

Thus, although further large-scale trials are needed, there is increasing evidence for the efficacy and safety of interventions to reduce cardio-vascular risk factors in childhood. However, the effects of specific therapies (e.g. the use of statins), specific nutrients (e.g. long-chain polyunsaturated fatty acids), or preventing obesity on long-term CVD have been little researched.

## Conclusion

A rapidly increasing prevalence of CVD and its risk factors makes it the most important health issue of the 21st century. The dramatic rise in obesity alone is expected to decrease life expectancy and threatens to reverse the reduction in cardiovascular mortality achieved in the past decades through control of hypertension, hyperlipidemia and smoking. There is now little doubt that the problem has its origins early in life. This has led to a major shift in focus for primary prevention from adults to children. Indeed, it is now reasonable to suggest that lifestyle modification, weight control and specific nutritional interventions (e.g. breastfeeding) in children could help reduce the burden of CVD in populations worldwide.

## References

1 BHF Compendium of annual statistics, 2004. www.heartstats.org
2 Berenson GS, Srinivasan SR, Nicklas TA: Atherosclerosis: a nutritional disease of childhood. Am J Cardiol 1998;82:22T–29T.
3 Klag MJ, Ford DE, Mead LA, et al: Serum cholesterol in young men and subsequent cardio-vascular disease. N Engl J Med 1993;328:313–318.
4 Barker DJ: Fetal origins of coronary heart disease. BMJ 1995;311:171–174.
5 Singhal A, Lucas A: Early origins of cardiovascular disease: is there a unifying hypothesis? Lancet 2004;363:1642–1645.
6 Leeson CPM, Whincup PH, Cook DG, et al: Cholesterol and arterial distensibility in the first decade of life: a population-based study. Circulation 2000;101:1533–1538.
7 Webber LS, Srinivasan SR, Wattigney WA, Berensob GS: Tracking of serum lipids and lipopro-teins from childhood to adulthood: the Bogalusa Heart Study. Am J Epidemiol 1991;133:884–899.
8 Must A, Jacques PF, Dallal GE, et al: Long-term morbidity and mortality of overweight adolescents: a follow-up of the Harvard Growth Study of 1922 to 1935. N Engl J Med 1992;327:1350–1355.
9 Kavey RE, Daniels SR, Lauer RM, et al: American heart association guidelines for primary prevention of atherosclerotic cardiovascular disease beginning in childhood. Circulation 2003;107:1562–1566.
10 Berenson GS: Childhood risk factors predict adult risk associated with sub-clinical cardiovas-cular disease: the Bogalusa Heart Study. Am J Cardiol 2002;90:3L–7L.

11 Berenson GS, Srinavasan SR, Bao W, et al: Association between multiple cardiovascular risk factors and atherosclerosis in children and young adults. N Engl J Med 1998;338:1650–1656.
12 McGill HC Jr, McMahan CA, Herderick EE, et al: Effects of coronary heart disease risk factors on atherosclerosis of selected regions of the aorta and right coronary artery. Arterioscler Thromb Vasc Biol 2000;20:836–845.
13 Tuzcu EM, Kapadia SR, Tutar E, et al: High prevalence of coronary atherosclerosis in asymptomatic teenagers and young adults: evidence from intravascular ultrasound. Circulation 2001;103:2705–2710.
14 Reaven GM: Banting Lecture 1988: role of insulin resistance in human disease. Diabetes 1988;37:1595–1607.
15 Yudkin JS: Adipose tissue, insulin action and vascular disease: inflammatory signals. Int J Obes 2003;27:S25–S28.
16 Weiss R, Dziura J, Burgert TS, et al: Obesity and the metabolic syndrome in children and adolescents. N Engl J Med 2004;350:2362–2374.
17 Manson JE, Willet WC, Stampfer MJ, et al: Body weight and mortality among women. N Engl J Med 1995;333:667–685.
18 Miller J, Rosenbloom A, Silverstein J: Childhood obesity. J Clin Endocrinol Metab 2004;89:4211–4218.
19 Singhal A, Farooqi IS, Cole TJ, et al: Influence of leptin on arterial distensibility: a novel link between obesity and cardiovascular disease. Circulation 2002;106:1919–1924.
20 Neel J: Diabetes mellitus: a 'thrifty' genotype rendered detrimental by 'progress'? Am J Hum Genet 1962;14:353–362.
21 Benjamin EJ, Larson MG, Keyes MJ, et al: Clinical correlates and heritability of flow-mediated dilation in the community: the Framingham Heart Study. Circulation 2004;109:613–619.
22 Yusuf S, Hawken S, Ounpuu S, et al: Effect of potentially modifiable risk factors associated with myocardial infarction in 52 countries (the INTERHEART study): case-control study. Lancet 2004;364:937–952.
23 Hales CN, Barker DJ: Type 2 (non-insulin-dependent) diabetes mellitus: the thrifty phenotype hypothesis. Diabetologia 1992;35:595–601.
24 Bateson P, Barker D, Clutton-Brock T, et al: Developmental plasticity and human health. Nature 2004;430:419–421.
25 Leeson CPM, Kattenhorn M, Deanfield JE, Lucas A: Duration of breast-feeding and arterial distensibility in early adult life: population based study. BMJ 2001;322:643–647.
26 Forsyth JS, Willatts P, Agostoni C, et al: Long chain polyunsaturated fatty acid supplementation in infant formula and blood pressure in later childhood: follow-up of a randomised controlled trial. BMJ 2003;326:953–958.
27 Steinberger J, Daniels SR: Obesity, insulin resistance, diabetes and cardiovascular risk in children. An American Heart Association scientific statement from the Atherosclerosis, Hypertension and Obesity in the Young Committee (Council on Cardiovascular Disease in the Young) and the Diabetes Committee (Council on Nutrition, Physical Activity and Metabolism). Circulation 2003;107:1448–1453.
28 Woo KS, Chook P, Chung W, et al: Effects of diet and exercise on obesity-related vascular disease dysfunction in children. Circulation 2004;109:1981–1986.
29 Lapineleimu H, Viikari J, Jokinen E, et al: Prospective randomized trial in 1062 infants of diet low in saturated fat and cholesterol. Lancet 1995;345:471–476.
30 Lauer RM, Obaranek E, Hunsberger SA, et al: Efficacy and safety of lowering dietary intake of total fat, saturated fat, and cholesterol in children with elevated LDL-cholesterol: the Dietary Intervention Study in Children. Am J Clin Nutr 2000;72:1332S–1342S.

## Discussion

*Dr. Laron:* I have several questions. Is there any new histological or pathological evidence that children who were killed in accidents had developed atherosclerosis? The classical examples are the soldiers killed in Korea. My second question is do you have any data on fatty liver? There are reports that 15% of obese children develop fatty liver. My third question is concerned with increasing growth velocity. Do you think that the new approach of pushing growth hormone in very young children is deleterious?

*Dr. Singhal:* The growth hormone story is very interesting and I think there is some evidence that using growth hormone in children increases the risk of diabetes or insulin resistance [1]. Whether this is reversible when growth hormone is stopped is being investigated. The second question is the fatty liver story. I am not an expert on body composition but fatty liver correlates closely with visceral fat mass. Clearly visceral fat mass is likely to be detrimental for the metabolic syndrome. Regarding postmortem studies, I am not aware of data on atherosclerosis in children who died from accidents. There are certainly data in from heart transplant patients that atherosclerosis is present in adolescence [2].

*Dr. Pereira-da-Silva:* What is your recommendation for neonatologists: (1) to continue providing additional nutrients to premature babies using fortified human milk, preterm formulas and PDF formulas and increase the risk of future morbidity, or to provide a suboptimal diet with the risk of a negative impact on brain structure as shown by Dr. Lucas, and also compromising catch-up growth, and (2) to consider different nutritional interventions for different populations of premature babies, i.e., in the case of being small versus appropriate for gestational age [3, 4], or asymmetrically versus symmetrical intrauterine growth retarded [5]?

*Dr. Singhal:* That is a very interesting question. One of the things that we have talked about is long-term effects and I think it is always important to remember that short-term effects, especially survival in preterm infants, is also important. You need to feed the preterm infant to make the baby strong enough to be extubated and to survive in the first place. So in preterm infants you need good nutrition and growth to make the baby strong enough, and to preserve the brain. I would also recommend that you add as much human milk as possible because of all the benefits with regard to necrotizing enterocolitis and long-term health. I am not aware of data which separate preterm infants into SGA or non-SGA. Our effects on later health were independent of the size at birth, but logically you would expect SGA preterm infants to be at higher risk of malnutrition.

*Dr. Saavedra:* With regard to weight gain, and you nicely showed that there is some evidence for a dose effect from the point of view of exclusive breastfeeding or the amount of breastfeeding versus non-exclusively breast-fed babies, within breast-fed babies and rate of weight gain, or within non-breastfed babies and rate of weight grain. Do you think we still see the kind of effects that you have shown?

*Dr. Singhal:* We do. Everybody would agree that breastfeeding is best, but in Iceland they have shown that faster weight gain in infancy is associated with a greater risk of obesity in breastfed babies. So I think the mechanism is more fundamental. I think breastfeeding works by reducing the growth rate compared to those infants fed formula but I think the growth rate is the important factor.

*Dr. Hanson:* I would like to ask you about the possible role of infections. Firstly, premature babies would have more infections, and secondly some children have repeated infections. In other words would early immunodeficiency be an advantage or not? Also children in poor countries who have lots of infections, what are the long-term effects of that?

*Dr. Singhal:* There is a very interesting paper which showed that in the ALSPAC study children who had more infections, had lower endothelial function [6].

*Dr. Hanson:* I could imagine that there might be a further variation of that based on genetic differences. We are just looking at alleles of cytokine genes, for instance TNF2, the allele of that for TNF-α is presumed to relay to a higher production of TNF-α, and we have seen that the presence of TNF2 relates to poorer outcome, rejection of a transplanted kidney for instance. One could imagine that such genetic variations also may result in variations in the response to infections.

*Dr. Singhal:* I completely agree. The effects have got to be different by different genotype, and the TNF story particularly in intensive care is very interesting.

*Dr. Cohen:* I enjoyed your discussion of leptin and the role of hyperinsulism, obesity and the metabolic syndrome. Is it scientifically plausible that some day either molecular antibodies that would block the leptin receptor or possibly an anti-leptin vaccine that would produce anti-leptin antibodies could be developed as a treatment for obesity?

*Dr. Singhal:* I am not an expert on the role of leptin in the treatment of obesity and I think the anti-leptin story did not work because it is leptin-resistance rather than low leptin levels that are important in obesity. It is interesting that when a paper came out showing that leptin may be a link between obesity and vascular function [7], there was no interest among the pharmaceutical companies to see whether blocking the leptin receptor on endothelial cells could specifically reduce the risk of cardiovascular disease. The effect of obesity on blood levels occurs over many years. So I don't think a simple pharmaceutical bullet to block the actions of leptin on endothelial functions will work.

*Dr. Wang:* In our country, mothers who formula feed their infants normally have some reason for not breastfeeding, such as some form of cardiovascular disease. Do you have any data about family disease history in your studies?

*Dr. Singhal:* I think family history will obviously interact with the effects of early nutrition on long-term cardiovascular health. The advantage of randomized studies is that you remove the effect of the family history because of the randomization procedure. But I do agree that if you are prone to heart disease and have faster growth, this could theoretically make the situation worse. The important point is that we must try to do randomized studies to remove genetic and other confounding effects.

*Dr. Kroke:* I would like to know whether you have calculated the positive predictive value of rapid growth in infancy because I do not think that every child that is growing fast is going to be obese. So what is the quantitative effect?

*Dr. Singhal:* The best data are from Stettler et al. [8] who worked on the effects of faster growth in infancy and long-term risk of obesity. They suggested that the attributable risk of developing obesity or faster growth in infancy is approximately 20%. So there is a huge effect of faster growth in early life on the long-term risk of obesity. We haven't calculated the risk partly because our data are from preterm infants and so there may be other factors involved.

*Dr. Greeff:* With rapid growth is it really in our control to intervene with that? Many of those children will be just as miserable unless we feed them all, and they will have rapid growth whether we like it or not.

*Dr. Singhal:* I think that is a very important point. There is a paper which looked at which factors affect growth acceleration immediately after birth [9]. The most important is genetics, as you would expect, because if the parents are tall the baby is going to try to catch up. But postnatal nutrition also has an effect and this is the one factor that you can manipulate. So in other words if you have a SGA baby you are going to show a catch-up growth immediately after birth, but you don't need to make the situation worse by adding a high nutrient intake.

*Dr. Hursting:* In the cancer story it appears that the obesity cancer link may be driven primarily by insulin resistance, in part independent of the adiposity. I am wondering if a similar story is emerging in cardiovascular disease?

*Dr. Singhal:* I think the story is very similar. The coupling mechanisms between early growth and long-term health are often hormonal. For example faster growth in early life increases the IGF-1 concentration later in life [10], which links the cancer story and the cardiovascular story. So I think that if you set up hormonal systems soon after birth they then go on to effect other systems later in life.

*Dr. Sorensen:* For many years we have considered salt ingestion as a main cause for persistent hypertension and cardiovascular risk. How would you place salt ingestion as a risk factor in the context of these new concepts about increased growth etc., because I think that salt is something that is a lot easier to manage than many of these other factors. I wonder what you think about that?

*Dr. Singhal:* I think you are absolutely right. Nutritional programming effects are not going to work by themselves and the most obvious example of this is that you don't see heart disease in poor communities, regardless of the growth rate in early life. Conventional cardiovascular risk factors such as salt in take and obesity interact with the programming effects much earlier in life.

*Dr. Laron:* After your talk and what Dr. Lucas has said that breastfeeding is so important for the future public health issues, what should the message be from here to the regulatory organizations? We know that postnatal leave differs greatly from country to country, from none to 1 year in Finland, thus I think it would be of interest that something be said by those promoting this important issue.

*Dr. Singhal:* I completely agree. There should be enough time to breastfeed a baby adequately because we now know there are huge short- and long-term effects.

*Dr. Lucas:* I would just add the point that what we still don't know is the optimal duration of breastfeeding to achieve these benefits. There is obviously some concern at the moment that a long period of breastfeeding might actually increase cardiovascular risk. I don't think that that should alter our breastfeeding practices. What it should do is make us to worry about our weaning diet. But nevertheless in the end the amount of maternity leave should logically be based on the optimal duration of breastfeeding to achieve long-term health, and that needs to be resolved.

*Dr. Saavedra:* May I get back to the research related to weight gain and the possible influences it might have. Do we have anything yet to show if it is just weight gain versus changes in body composition for example in relation to adipose tissue in children?

*Dr. Singhal:* This is an area of active research: whether differences in body composition in early life effect the long-term risk. I can point out two studies in which an increase in length gain is associated with long-term cardiovascular risk. One was in preterm infants which showed an effect on endothelial function [11] and another showed an effect on obesity [12].

*Dr. Lake:* In your experimental models, when you provide your extra calories during that programming interval, this is almost always done by increasing the caloric density of the product that is given. Does it matter if the increased calories are provided by allowing a greater volume of intake by the individual during that time?

*Dr. Singhal:* The major, approximately 30%, difference was in the protein content. I think the standard and nutrient-enriched formulas were 68 and 72 kg/cal per 100 ml, respectively, so there wasn't a huge difference in energy. The volume of intake in the preterm infants was determined by the neonatal units and we had no control over this.

*Dr. Hamburger:* Just a comment to emphasize or illustrate the point that Dr. Lucas made a moment ago. I have recently been informed that in later old age lowering cholesterol, which we have all been trying to do, is associated with increased morbidity and mortality. I might agree with the caution not to rush to change practice without good evidence and good data.

*Dr. Singhal:* Sure, I agree with that. At the moment our findings don't change practice because we are encouraging breastfeeding, which is current practice anyway.

*Dr. Klish:* Since we are talking about cholesterol, I also have a question related to one of your early slides where you were talking about carotid artery distensibility and relating it to the cholesterol levels. An obese population has a normal distribution for cholesterol but the normal curve is about 10–15% greater than for a normal weight population. Can your distensibility studies show differences when the cholesterol rises by 10–15%? If so, this could be an important tool to monitor the impact of the increase in cholesterol in obese children.

*Dr. Singhal:* The data that I presented showed that cholesterol was associated with decreased artery distensibility independent of body mass index, not body composition, so I do accept the criticism that obesity may still play a role in association. So certainly there are lots of data now showing that cholesterol concentrations in children influence vascular function.

*Dr. Lucas:* Can I just go back briefly to a point that was made earlier about volume intake. If you increase energy intake in babies they downregulate the volume intake so they control intake and several people have shown that. But if you actually alter protein intake, we have demonstrated that there is no downregulation. So in the studies in which we have measured it, the volume intake is exactly the same in babies on a high- or low-protein diet, so you see the full effect of the intervention. This is an extremely important point if you are influencing growth, then the protein strategy is much more effective.

*Dr. Arvanitakis:* Regarding the endocrine factors of obesity, the leptin data are more or less known. Do we have any evidence on other hormones more recently described such as ghrelin?

*Dr. Singhal:* I am not really the expert on endocrine factors in obesity, I am using the endocrine system as a link between early growth and long-term health.

*Dr. Kroke:* I was wondering whether you have any information about the effects of a woman being obese or having the metabolic syndrome on the composition or the quality of breast milk? Do you think the metabolic profile of the mother is having any effect?

*Dr. Singhal:* Yes it does, and Plagemann et al. [13] published these data showing that the breast milk of gestational diabetic mothers is richer and their babies grow faster and are more prone to obesity and glucose intolerance.

*Dr. Mora:* I wonder if there are any data regarding the use of hydrolyzed formula or amino acid-based formula in premature babies and term babies with regard to cardiovascular disease?

*Dr. Singhal:* I am not aware of anything in that area.

# References

1 Cutfield WS, Jackson WE, Jefferies C, et al: Reduced insulin sensitivity during growth hormone therapy for short children born small for gestational age. J Pediatr 2003;142:113–116.
2 Tuzcu EM, Kapadia SR, Tutar E, et al: High prevalence of coronary atherosclerosis in asymptomatic teenagers and young adults: evidence from intravascular ultrasound. Circulation 2001;103:2705–2710.
3 Godfrey KM, Barker DJ: Fetal nutrition and adult disease. Am J Clin Nutr 2000;71(suppl): 1344S–1352S.
4 Tenhola S, Halonen P, Jaaskelainen J, Voutilainen R: Serum markers of GH and insulin action in 12-year-old children born small for gestational age. Eur J Endocrinol 2005;152:335–340.
5 Law CM, Egger P, Dada O, et al: Body size at birth and blood pressure among children in developing countries. Int J Epidemiol 2001;30:52–57.
6 Charakida M, Donald AE, Terese M, et al, ALSPAC (Avon Longitudinal Study of Parents and Children) Study Team: Endothelial dysfunction in childhood infection. Circulation 2005;111:1660–1665.
7 Singhal A, Farooqi IS, Cole TJ, et al: Influence of leptin on arterial distensibility: a novel link between obesity and cardiovascular disease? Circulation 2002;106:1919–1924.
8 Stettler N, Zemel BS, Kumanyika S, Stallings VA: Infant weight gain and childhood overweight status in a multicenter, cohort study. Pediatrics 2002;109:194–199.

9 Karlberg J, Albertsson-Wikland K: Growth in full-term small-for-gestational-age infants: from birth to final height. Pediatr Res 1995;38:733–739.
10 Cianfarani S, Germani D, Branca F: Low birthweight and adult insulin resistance: the 'catch-up growth' hypothesis. Arch Dis Child Fetal Neonatal Ed 1999;81:F71–F73.
11 Singhal A, Cole TJ, Fewtrell M, et al: Is slower early growth beneficial for long-term cardio-vascular health? Circulation 2004;109:1108–1113.
12 Gunnarsdottir I, Thorsdottir I: Relationship between growth and feeding in infancy and body mass index at the age of 6 years. Int J Obes Relat Metab Disord 2003;27:1523–1527.
13 Plagemann A, Harder T, Franke K, Kohlhoff R: Long-term impact of neonatal breast-feeding on body weight and glucose tolerance in children of diabetic mothers. Diabetes Care 2002;25:16–22.

Lucas A, Sampson HA (eds): Primary Prevention by Nutrition Intervention in Infancy and Childhood.
Nestlé Nutr Workshop Ser Pediatr Program, vol 57, pp 31–50,
Nestec Ltd., Vevey/S. Karger AG, Basel, © 2006.

# Childhood Obesity: Potential Mechanisms for the Development of an Epidemic

*Claudio Maffeis*

Department of Mother and Child, Biology-Genetics, Unit of Pediatrics,
University of Verona, Verona, Italy

## Introduction

By the year 2000, obesity had already spread to such an extent that the World Health Organization defined it the greatest health threat facing the West. Diabetes, the most common metabolic disorder associated with obesity, will shortly occur as a second epidemic. The increasing prevalence of impaired glucose tolerance and type-2 diabetes, also in adolescents and children suffering from obesity, are the first heralds of this epidemic. To arrest this trend, it appears that intervention early in life is the most important step. There are at least four main reasons supporting this claim: (1) the long-term negative effects of early exposure to obesity; (2) the persistence of childhood obesity into adulthood (the higher the age of the obese child the higher the risk; (3) sociopsychological (depression, discrimination), metabolic (impaired glucose tolerance, diabetes, hypertension, dyslipidemia, atherosclerosis) and non-metabolic (respiratory and skin disorders, joint problems, etc.) morbidities associated with obesity, which are already recognizable in childhood, and (4) sensitivity to treatment (higher in children than in adults).

Body weight is determined by the interaction between the genetic makeup of an individual and the environment in which that person lives. Failure to modulate environmental pressures affecting the genetic substrate of an individual is the ultimate cause of the development of obesity in children. There are several control systems that regulate body weight which include signals from the periphery to the hypothalamus, where cognitive and internal signals are integrated. The integration of these signals involves a complex array of neuropeptides, neurotransmitters and structural circuits. These circuits regulate appetite, energy intake and energy expenditure. The system guarantees that energy ingested in excess of requirements is efficiently stored as fat. The efficiency of the energy-storing system was useful in the past, when food deprivation was common, and allowed people to survive during famines. Moreover, chronic famines that accompanied wars and epidemics likely promoted the selection of genes and facilitated a greater resistance to starvation. Therefore, the less severe environmental conditions and unlimited food supplies that characterize our modern lifestyles have likely promoted excess fat accumulation in a large number of subjects that have a genetic predisposition to fat storage, which has eventually led to widespread obesity.

Obesity is a complex condition with multifactor origin. However, incomplete knowledge of the physiopathological mechanisms responsible for excessive fat accumulation limits the efficacy of available treatment and prevention programs. The need to identify more targets for intervention has stimulated basic and clinical research in the field. In this chapter, several genetic and environmental risk factors of childhood obesity will be discussed as well as some potentially relevant metabolic mechanisms involved in the development of childhood obesity. Obesity-related Mendelian disorders (Prader-Willi syndrome, Bardet-Biedl syndrome, Albright hereditary osteodystrophy, etc.) as well as endocrine disorders that cause obesity, which cumulatively are responsible for less than 5% of all the cases of obesity in the population, will not be discussed.

## Genes

The commonly observed coexistence of several obese members within the same family suggests that genetic factors are involved. Family studies have shown that the heritability of body mass index (BMI) is about 25–50%. The correlation coefficient ($r^2$) for BMI in monozygotic twins is 0.70–0.88, among siblings it is 0.24–0.34, and between parents and children it is 0.15–0.24.

There are more than 430 genes, markers and chromosomal regions associated or linked with the human obesity phenotype [5]. Every chromosome, with the exception of chromosome Y, has loci linked with the obesity phenotype. Some extremely rare homozygous monogenic mutations (genes LEP, LEPR, POMC, PCSK1, MC4-R, PPARG, and PPP1R3A) that cause severe obesity have been identified. Subjects affected by these genetic defects are usually recognizable by other phenotypic features (i.e., hypogonadotropic hypogonadism in leptin deficiency, red hair and hypocortisolism in POMC deficiency, etc.) that accompany their obesity. On the contrary, people with heterozygous mutations, carriers of leptin, leptin receptors and POMC genes have a minimal abnormal phenotype; whereas people with heterozygous mutations and carriers of melanocortin (MC) receptor-4 (MC4-R) are severely obese without any other distinctive phenotype characteristic. MC4-R mutations (130 individuals, 42 different mutations of the gene) are by far the most common genetic cause of obesity identified to date. In spite of these encouraging findings, most of the specific genes involved in the development of obesity are as yet unknown.

On the basis of available evidence, childhood obesity is likely a polygenic condition where a number of predisposing alleles confer to increase an individual's risk. Heterogeneity of the complex phenotypes of obesity implies that genetic predisposition may also result from any one of several rare variants in a number of genes. Genetic predisposition to obesity may affect both sides of the energy balance equation (energy intake and energy expenditure) as well as adipogenesis regulation. Examples of genes involved in controlling energy intake are: neuropeptide Y (NPY), proopiomelanocortin (POMC), leptin (LEP) and MC4-R. Other genes involved in controlling energy expenditure, are: uncoupling proteins (UCP)1, UCP2 and UCP3, and adrenoreceptor (ADR)β2 and β3. Interestingly, association studies have shown that a *Trp64Agr* polymorphism of the β3ADR is associated with a higher risk of weight gain in a French population sample, insulin resistance in Finnish subjects, and lower resting energy expenditure in Pima Indians, when compared with a control population. Candidate genes involved in controlling adipogenesis and signaling pathways are: peroxisome proliferator-activated receptor (PPAR)α, PPARγ and PPARδ, fatty acid-binding protein (FABP), etc.

## Central Control of Appetite and Energy Expenditure

Most of the help in understanding the mechanisms that regulate energy balance and body weight has come from studies on animal models. Schematically, there are three main components involved in controlling appetite and satiety [6, 7]: (1) afferent signals to the central nervous system from organs and tissues (stomach, gut, adipose tissue) driven by hormones; (2) a complex neural network in the central nervous system (hypothalamus and brain stem), and (3) efferent signals from the central nervous system to the periphery (sympathetic nervous system, thyroid hormones) (fig. 1).

Several nuclei from the hypothalamus (nucleus arcuatus (ARC), paraventricular nucleus (PVN), nucleus of the solitary tract, etc.) and brain stem are involved. The neurons of these nuclei are provided with receptors for peripheral neurotrophic factors such as ghrelin, peptide YY, cholecystokinin, 5-HT, glucagon-like peptide-1, bombesin, amylin, insulin, cortisol and leptin. Ghrelin, a stomach-secreted hormone stimulates food intake and may influence eating habits; other gut-secreted proteins, such as peptide YY, cholecystokinin, 5-HT, glucagon-like peptide-1, contribute to feeling satiated. Short-term signals that contribute to feeling satiated also include glucose, protein, free fatty acids (FFAs) and insulin. Leptin, a cytokine secreted mainly by adipose tissue, communicates the energy status of the organism (fat mass size) to the brain.

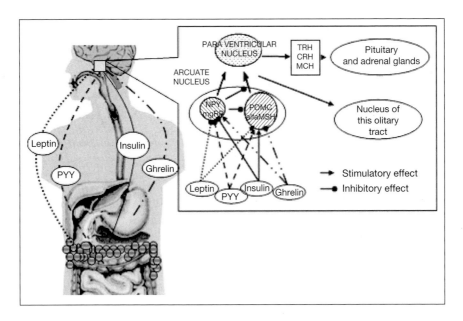

***Fig. 1.*** Hormones from periphery affecting the hypothalamic regulation of food intake and energy expenditure in humans.

Failure of leptin-induced signaling is perceived as starvation, eliciting hunger even in very obese subjects.

Information from the periphery is processed in the hypothalamus. Two types of neurons in the ARC receive the peripheral leptin signal: (1) neurons coexpressing NPY and Agouti-related protein (AgRP), which have projections into the brain stem to the PVN and to the second neurons that receive leptin signals in the ARC, and (2) POMC/cocaine amphetamine-regulated transcript (POMC/CART) neurons that receive projections from neurons in areas of the brain that express serotonin (5-HT) and that have 5-HT receptors on their surfaces. Both POMC/CART and NPY/AgRP neurons project to MC4 receptor (MC4-R)-expressing neurons in the PVN and MC3-R in the ventromedial nucleus. POMC/CART neurons secrete the α-melanocyte-stimulating hormone (α-MSH), an agonist of both MC3-R and MC4-R. NPY/AgRP neurons secrete AgRP, an antagonist of both MC3-R and MC4-R.

*Leptin*

Leptin is the most extensively studied hormone involved in body weight regulation [8]. Studies on animals have shown that leptin stimulation of NPY/AgRP neurons promotes a suppression of NPY and AgRP release as well as a suppression of GABA released into POMC/CART neuron synapses. POMC/CART neurons, under direct leptin stimulation and GABA-mediated disinhibition, stimulate PVN cells expressing MC4-R by releasing α-MSH. The proconvertase-1 enzyme plays a central role in cleaving the POMC molecules, which is necessary for α-MSH secretion. Activation of MC4-R promotes a stimulation of the sympathetic system that releases noradrenalin to peripheral cells expressing β-adrenergic receptors. Thermogenesis increases in the brown adipose tissue of rodents and food intake is inhibited. Consequently, leptin secretion is reduced, NPY/AgRP is stimulated to release NPY and POMC/CART is inhibited. In the MC4-R-positive neurons of the PVN, α-MSH is reduced and AgRP is enhanced. This promotes a reduction in sympathetic nervous system activity, a reduction in energy expenditure and an increase in food intake. Even though a subpopulation of obese individuals are heterozygous for leptin deficiency and are on average more obese than their homozygous wild-type relatives, circulating leptin levels are usually high in obese individuals.

*Endogenous Cannabinoids*

The recent characterization in experimental animals of endogenous ligands for cannabinoid receptors along with their biosynthesis and degradation pathways has allowed researchers to explore the potential role played by the endogenous cannabinoid system in energy balance regulation [9]. Cannabinoids may contribute to central modulation of energy homeostasis via hypothalamic neuropeptides, such as the corticotrophin-releasing hormone, CART, the melanin-concentrating hormone, as well as peripheral regulation by adipose tissue. Cannabinoids, via cannabinoid receptor-1 (CB-1), stimulate appetite and enhance lipogenesis in primary adipocyte cultures. CB-1-selective antagonists have been proposed as potential candidates for the pharmacological treatment of obesity.

*Sympathetic Nervous System*

Most of the energy the body uses daily is to maintain cell function and structure (resting metabolic rate) as well as body movements (energy expenditure for activity). Less than 10% of daily energy expenditure is devoted to food-induced thermogenesis, for example, the energy used to digest food and process and store nutrients, and to thermogenesis induced by drugs or other substances and by exposure to cold (adaptive thermogenesis). Energy-dissipating processes (adaptive thermogenesis) are induced by β-adrenergic receptor stimulation [10]. In brown fat and skeletal muscle, adrenergic signals stimulate the formation of mitochondria and the uncoupling of ATP synthesis from oxidative metabolism. Adrenergic signals, activated by β3ADR, induce PPARγ coactivator-1α (PGC-1α), which enhances the transcription of genes involved in mitochondrial biogenesis and uncoupling. UCP1, UCP2, and UCP3 leak protons and exhaust the electrochemical gradient across the inner mitochondrial membrane, rapidly increasing local heat production and energy dissipation in brown adipose tissue and skeletal muscle. Moreover, β3ADR activation stimulates lipolysis and energy expenditure in white adipose tissue. Activation of the sympathetic nervous system also increases thyroid-stimulating hormone secretion. Sympathetic nervous system activation also increases thyroid-stimulating hormone secretion. The hypothalamic-pituitary-thyroid hormonal axis contributes to regulate UCP expression and increases resting energy expenditure. Finally, activation of the sympathetic nervous system promotes an increase in blood flow to skeletal muscle as well as oxygen consumption in the muscle itself during exercise, to increase voluntary energy expenditure.

The parasympathetic nervous system is also involved in regulating appetite/satiety. In particular, stimulation of the vagus nerve increases energy storage in the form of fat in the adipose tissue via increased glucose-stimulated insulin secretion.

*Adipose Tissue as an Endocrine Organ*

To integrate metabolic, hormonal and neural stimuli, adipocytes respond by releasing hormones. Adipose tissue has an intense endocrine (leptin, adiponectin, resistin, IL-6, etc.) and autocrine or paracrine (TNFα, growth factors, etc.) activity [11]. This activity becomes proportionally more intense as the volume of the adipocyte grows. Leptin secretion is proportionally higher, whereas adiponectin secretion is proportionally lower, with the increasing size of the adipocyte. Moreover, the finding that adipose tissue in obese adults and children shows areas of inflammation with clear macrophage infiltration and that inflammation is associated with insulin resistance suggests that the microenvironment inside the adipose tissue, as well as the secretion activity of the adipocyte, may play an independent role in the development of the metabolic complications of obesity [12].

## Fat Balance

The final common mechanism by which all the different genetic, environmental and psychosocial factors promote obesity is a chronic positive energy balance. Since energy enters the body in the form of nutrients that can be oxidized or stored, the energy balance equation may be considered as the sum of the balance of the three macronutrients: proteins, lipids and carbohydrates. There is consistent evidence that a protein-carbohydrate balance is efficiently self-regulated in humans: protein and carbohydrate intake promotes their oxidation. On the contrary, lipid intake does not promote fat oxidation [13]. Fat balance is affected by the balance of the other two nutrients and depends strictly on them. After ingesting a mixed meal, protein and carbohydrate oxidation increases, whereas fat oxidation decreases; glycogen is synthesized in the liver and muscle and fat are stored in the adipose tissue. In the case of saturated glycogen stores, the conversion of glucose into fat, i.e., de novo lipogenesis, also occurs [14]. This is a high energy-demanding process (~30% of the energy of the substrate to be converted) that occurs in the liver and muscle. The oxidative hierarchy of the body, that prefers the oxidation of carbohydrates and proteins rather than fat, independent of fat intake, suggests a relevant responsibility of fat balance in promoting fat gain [15].

Therefore, in overfeeding conditions (positive energy balance), fat storage is the result of three phenomena that contribute to a positive fat balance: (1) reduction in exogenous fat oxidation (due to the increase in carbohydrate and protein oxidation), with sparing of endogenous fat (fat stored) utilization; (2) storage of fat obtained by carbohydrates (de novo lipogenesis), and (3) storage of exogenous fat (fat ingested with diet).

Fat mass increase is accompanied by an increased triacylglycerol turnover, resulting in increased circulating FFA levels, which favors an increase in resting and daily fat oxidation [16]. Moreover, an increase in the FFA flux to the liver reduces the hepatic clearance of insulin, leading to hyperinsulinemia. Hyperinsulinemia with euglycemia induces an increase in sympathetic nervous system activity, which stimulates thermogenesis and a decrease in energy intake relative to expenditure. All these processes tend to favor a new fat balance equilibrium.

Physical activity is the sole discretional component of the daily energy expenditure of an individual. Skeletal muscle activity causes energy expenditure, but it also increases the fat oxidative potential in skeletal muscle, a contributing factor of fat balance and fat mass regulation. Physically fit people generally display a greater fat cell lipolytic response and lipid utilization than idle subjects. Increased sympathetic nervous system activity, as reflected by an enhanced catecholamine turnover and β-adrenergic stimulation, contributes to explain this finding. These adaptations were also shown to be related to an increase in post-exercise resting energy expenditure and fat oxidation.

**Environment**

Environmental pressure, which affects the behavior of an individual, is able to cause inefficacy in the complex body weight-regulating system, forcing energy intake beyond the required amounts. Environmental risk factors of obesity are potentially sensitive and realistic targets of intervention for the care and prevention of obesity.

*Pregnancy*
The first exposure to the environment is in the uterus. During pregnancy, the active metabolic exchange with the mother affects fetal growth and metabolic maturation with long-term effects, i.e., prenatal programming [17]. Intrauterine exposure to severe malnutrition (second trimester of pregnancy)

or over-nutrition (gestational diabetes mellitus) increases the risk of obesity in childhood and young adulthood. Moreover, a clear association between high birth weight and childhood obesity, independent of the parents' BMI, has been demonstrated [18]. Similarly, low birth weight combined with rapid post-natal growth during early infancy also appears to be associated with glucose tolerance and obesity later in childhood and as an adult.

*First Year of Life*

Eating is the main activity of infants from birth to 6 months of life, when they grow very rapidly: in the first 6 months body weight more than doubles from birth. Nutrition is crucial in this period. Breastfeeding has been shown to have, at least in the short-term, a protective effect on the development of obesity [19]. However, in the long-term, the efficacy of breastfeeding compared to formula feeding in defending the individual from obesity is overwhelmed by the strength of the numerous obesity risk factors encountered by the individual after infancy [20]. Early nutrition may modulate catch-up growth in intrauterine growth-restricted (IUGR) experimental animals, suggesting a potential involvement of early nutrition and timing of IUGR catch-up growth in the programming of orexigenic hormones and obesity. Similarly, in humans, rapid postnatal growth during the first 4 months of life is associated with a higher risk of obesity in young adulthood, independent of other confounders (BMI of the mother, parity, socioeconomic status, etc.) [21]. The type of feeding may play a role in this process, as suggested by the evidence that the speed of growth of breastfed infants is slightly slower than that of formula-fed infants.

Early complementary food introduction (<16 weeks) was associated with greater infant weight gain in a study of 3,768 mother–infant dyads from the Danish National Birth Cohort [22]. However, the timing of complementary food introduction did not increase infant weight gain when breastfeeding lasted 20 or more weeks. Complementary food introduction is associated with an increase in the protein content of an infant's diet and a reduction in the fat/carbohydrate ratio. The role of macronutrient composition of toddlers and young children on the development of overweight and obesity is still a matter of debate. A Danish longitudinal study reported that protein intake at 9 months of age is associated with body size but not with body fat in 10-year-old Danish children [23]. Moreover, animal protein (g/day) and milk intake, but not vegetable protein or meat intake, was positively associated with serum IGF-I concentrations and height in young children. This suggests that cow's milk compounds have a stimulating effect on serum IGF-I concentrations and, thereby, on children's growth. The continuation of a high protein diet later in childhood may increase the risk of excess fat gain as suggested by the results of a follow-up study conducted in France showing that high protein intake at the age of 2 years increases body fatness at 8 years of age [24].

Early experiences with food, the association of food flavors with the context and the consequences of eating may potentially affect food acceptance and food habits of infants and children [25]. Children's eating habits are influenced by the attitudes and behavior of parents, peers, siblings and relatives who live with them. In particular, parents' encouragement to eat usually promotes fat gain in their children.

*Preschool Age and Puberty*
Family lifestyle and eating habits influence a child's food preferences.

Diet Content
An abundance of energy-chocked foods and drinks in the diet leads to a pervasive 'passive over-consumption' of energy in both children and adults. Parents are responsible for food availability and accessibility in the home. Similarities in diet composition may explain, at least in part, familial patterns of adiposity. In fact, parents' adiposity and fat intake have been associated with their children's adiposity and fat intake. Dietary fat is a significant contributor to obesity. A direct relationship between fat content in the diet and adiposity has been shown in children and adolescents in both cross-sectional and longitudinal studies [26].

Consistent evidence is available on the association between the consumption of sugar-sweetened beverages and obesity. Over the past decades children have tended to drink less milk and more sugar-sweetened beverages which contain high amounts of fructose corn syrup [27]. This behavior promoted a reduction in calcium intake and an increase in carbohydrate intake. A decrease in calcium intake has been suggested as a potential cofactor of fat gain, because it increases 1,25-dihydroxyvitamin D in response to low-calcium diets, which stimulates adipocyte $Ca^{2+}$ influx and, consequently, stimulates lipogenesis, suppresses lipolysis, and increases lipid accumulation. A second mechanism by which dietary calcium intake might affect body adiposity is the effect of absorption of triacylglycerol by the gastrointestinal tract. However, some recent findings in animals and in humans suggest that there may be greater effects on body weight from dairy-content foods than might be predicted from their calcium content alone.

Fast Food
'Fast food' has become a prominent portion of the diet of children in the United States and, increasingly, throughout the world. The consumption of fast food among children seems to have had an adverse effect on the quality of their diet in ways that could plausibly increase their risk of becoming obese. Children who eat fast food, compared with those who do not, consume more total energy, more total fat, more total carbohydrates, more added sugars, more sugar-sweetened beverages, less fiber, less milk and fewer fruits and non-starchy vegetables [28]. Overweight adolescents are less likely to

compensate for the extra energy in fast food, by adjusting their energy intake throughout the day, than their lean counterparts. Moreover, children eat more total energy and have poorer diet quality on days when fast food is consumed than on days when it is not. Further longitudinal studies are needed to confirm a causal relationship between fast food consumption in the development of childhood obesity.

Physical Activity

Although a progressive reduction in physical activity by populations in industrialized countries is more than likely, population-level physical activity surveys conducted on children have offered a less clear picture. Children generally perform large volumes of low-intensity activity with short bouts of moderate to vigorous activity. Young children seldom participate in long-sustained moderate or vigorous activities. The mean level of physical activity is higher for boys than for girls; the time devoted to physical activity or sports is dramatically decreasing in girls approaching puberty [29]. Children with parents who regularly perform physical exercise are generally more active than children whose parents get little regular physical exercise.

The Framingham study on children showed that low levels of physical activity during pre-school years affected a change in the level of adiposity of the children [30]. Inactive children accumulated more fat tissue than active children. Moreover, body fat mass at baseline influenced the degree of change: leaner children had a somewhat lower risk of increasing body fatness associated with low activity levels than did heavier children. Thus, inactivity may have a more deleterious effect on pre-school children who already have a greater quantity of body fat. Cross-sectional data showed that obese children spend more time than non-obese youngsters doing sedentary activities and that there is a direct relationship between non-sleeping time devoted to sedentary activities and adiposity [31]. There are several reasons why obese children are less active than their lean peers: lower performance in sports, earlier fatiguing, discrimination and mockery by companions, shame and embarrassment over their physical appearance, etc. Lower performance in sports and earlier fatiguing are absolutely 'physiological' for an obese individual. The greater body weight one has to move in weight-bearing activities causes (1) earlier fatiguing in obese than in non-obese individuals working at the same intensity, and (2) the achievement of maximal aerobic power, an index of cardiorespiratory fitness, at lower exercise intensity in obese than in non-obese individuals. However, when expressed per unit of fat-free mass, the maximal aerobic power of the obese is comparable to that of non-obese individuals, which suggests an apparently normal fitness level in obese subjects [32]. The choice of easy low-cost exercise that does not require particular facilities or equipment, such as walking, may be attractive and acceptable to obese children and adolescents. Low-intensity walking (4 km/h) is a safe aerobic activity able to promote greater fat oxidation than more strenuous exercise and may be performed longer. Further studies are needed to assess the efficacy of a daily walking program in promoting fat loss in obese children [33].

A relevant risk factor for sedentary behavior in children is TV viewing. TV viewing is by far the most common leisure time activity in the USA and in most European countries. A recent meta-analysis of the literature confirmed the relationship between TV viewing and body fatness among children and youths [34]. Children who have a TV set in their bedroom have a 30% greater risk of becoming obese than children who do not. TV viewing and other related media activity such as video games, VCRs, computers and internet use may contribute to obesity through two mechanisms: (1) they reduce energy expenditure during leisure time due to the sedentary nature of the activity, and (2) they increase dietary energy intake both during viewing and as a result of food advertising which tends to promote food consumption. The latter effect seems to be more powerful than the former. Reducing television, videotape and videogame use was suggested as a promising, population-based approach to prevent childhood obesity.

## Psychosocial Factors

The prevalence of obesity is generally higher in children of low-income families that also have a lower educational level. Racial and ethnic minorities have the highest rate of obesity, at least in the USA. Lower awareness as well as access to healthy foods, fitness facilities and health care combined with a particularly susceptible genetic background contribute to explain these findings. Interestingly, the risk of overweight was higher for individuals reared in an area with poor quality housing compared to those from more affluent areas, even when controlling for the effect of parents' education and occupation. Finally, parental neglect during childhood predicts obesity in young adulthood, independent of age and BMI in childhood, gender and social background [35].

TV broadcasting is an important way to advertise food products, but it also provides a variety of models and messages about eating that may affect the food preferences and food selection of children and adults. The ability to recognize food advertisements is higher in obese children and it is significantly correlated with the amount of food eaten after exposure to them. Exposure to food advertisements promotes consumption [36].

## Conclusions

Obesity is the most significant epidemic of the new century in industrialized countries. The sophisticated system that regulates body weight and fat

41

mass is under active investigation. Various signals are carried from the periphery to the hypothalamus where cognitive and internal signals are integrated and appetite, energy intake and expenditure are regulated. The inefficacy of the system to modulate environmental pressures that affect the genetic substrate of the individual causes obesity. Several genes and environmental factors have been identified as those that play a potential role in the processes leading to fat gain. Environmental factors are potentially sensitive to intervention. The mother's nutrition and metabolic state during pregnancy, early infancy nutrition, diet composition (fat intake, energy density and sugar-sweetened beverages) and fast-food consumption are realistic targets for intervention. Moreover, the substitution of sedentary behavior, especially passive viewing activities, with low to moderately intense physical activities seems theoretically promising.

## References

1 Must A, Jacques PF, Dallal GE, et al: Long-term morbidity and mortality of overweight adolescents: a follow-up of the Harvard Growth Study of 1922 to 1935. N Engl J Med 1992;327: 1350–1355.
2 Whitaker RC, Wright JA, Pepe MS, et al: Predicting obesity in young adulthood from childhood and parental obesity. N Engl J Med 1997;337:869–873.
3 Dietz WH: Health consequences of obesity in youth: childhood predictors of adult disease. Pediatrics 1998;101:518–525.
4 Epstein LH, Valoski A, Wing RR, McCurley J: Ten-year follow-up of behavioral, family-based treatment for obese children. JAMA 1990;264:2519–2523.
5 Snyder EE, Walts B, Perusse L, et al: The human obesity gene map: the 2003 update. Obes Res 2004;12:369–439.
6 Korner J, Leibel RL: To eat or not to eat – how the gut talks to the brain. N Engl J Med 2003; 349:926–928.
7 Schwartz MW, Niswender KD: Adiposity signaling and biological defense against weight gain: absence of protection or central hormone resistance? J Clin Endocrinol Metab 2004;89: 5889–5897.
8 Friedman JM, Halaas JL: Leptin and the regulation of body weight in mammals. Nature 1998; 395:763–770.
9 Cota D, Marsicano G, Tschop M, et al: The endogenous cannabinoid system affects energy balance via central orexigenic drive and peripheral lipogenesis. J Clin Invest 2003;112:423–431.
10 Lowell B, Spiegelman B: Towards a molecular understanding of adaptive thermogenesis. Nature 2000;404:652–660.
11 Frayn KN, Karpe F, Fielding BA, et al: Integrative physiology of human adipose tissue. Int J Obes Relat Metab Disord 2003;27:875–888.
12 Sbarbati A, Osculati F, Silvagni D, et al: Obesity and inflammation: evidence of an elementary lesion. Pediatrics 2005, in press.
13 Schutz Y, Flatt JP, Jequier E: Failure of dietary fat intake to promote fat oxidation: a factor favouring the development of obesity. Am J Clin Nutr 1989;50:307–314.
14 Schutz Y: Concept of fat balance in human obesity revisited with particular reference to de novo lipogenesis. Int J Obes 2004;28:S3–S11.
15 Flatt JP: Dietary fat, carbohydrate balance, and weight maintenance: effects of exercise. Am J Clin Nutr 1987;45(suppl):296–306.
16 Maffeis C, Armellini F, Tato L, Schutz Y: Fat oxidation and adiposity in prepubertal children: exogenous versus endogenous fat utilization. J Clin Endocrinol Metab 1999;84:654–658.
17 Godfrey KM, Barker DJ: Fetal nutrition and adult disease. Am J Clin Nutr 2000;71(suppl): 1344S–1352S.

18 Parsons TJ, Power C, Manor O: Fetal and early life growth and body mass index from birth to early adulthood in 1958 British cohort: longitudinal study. BMJ 2001;323:1331–1335.
19 Arenz S, Ruckerl R, Koletzko B, von Kries R: Breast-feeding and childhood obesity – a systematic review. Int J Obes Relat Metab Disord 2004;28:1247–1256.
20 Parsons TJ, Power C, Manor O: Infant feeding and obesity through the lifecourse. Arch Dis Child 2003;88:793–794.
21 Stettler N, Kumanyika SK, Katz SH, et al: Rapid weight gain during infancy and obesity in young adulthood in a cohort of African Americans. Am J Clin Nutr 2003;77:1374–1378.
22 Baker JL, Michaelsen KF, Rasmussen KM, Sorensen TI: Maternal prepregnant body mass index, duration of breastfeeding, and timing of complementary food introduction are associated with infant weight gain. Am J Clin Nutr 2004;80:1579–1588.
23 Hoppe C, Molgaard C, Thomsen BL, et al: Protein intake at 9 mo of age is associated with body size but not with body fat in 10-yr-old Danish children. Am J Clin Nutr 2004;79:494–501.
24 Rolland-Cachera MF, Deheeger M, Akrout M, Bellisle F: Influence of macronutrients on adiposity development: a follow up study of nutrition and growth from 10 months to 8 years of age. Int J Obes Relat Metab Disord 1995;19:573–578.
25 Birch LL, Fisher JO: Development of eating behaviors among children and adolescents. Pediatrics 1998;101:539–549.
26 Maffeis C, Pinelli L, Schutz Y: Fat intake and adiposity in 8 to 11-year-old obese children. Int J Obes Relat Metab Disord 1996;20:170–174.
27 Parikh SJ, Yanovski JA: Calcium intake and adiposity. Am J Clin Nutr 2003;77:281–287.
28 Bowman SA, Gortmaker SL, Ebbeling CB, et al: Effects of fast-food consumption on energy intake and diet quality among children in a national household survey. Pediatrics 2004;113:112–118.
29 Goran MI, Shewchuk R, Gower BA, et al: Longitudinal changes in fatness in white children: no effect of childhood energy expenditure. Am J Clin Nutr 1998;67:309–316.
30 Moore LL, Gao D, Bradlee ML, et al: Does early physical activity predict body fat change throughout childhood? Prev Med 2003;37:10–17.
31 Maffeis C, Zaffanello M, Pinelli L, Schutz Y: Total energy expenditure and patterns of activity in 8–10-year-old obese and nonobese children. J Pediatr Gastroenterol Nutr 1996;23:256–261.
32 Maffeis C, Schena F, Zaffanello M, et al: Maximal aerobic power during running and cycling in obese and non-obese children. Acta Paediatr 1994;83:113–116.
33 Maffeis C, Zaffanello M, Pellegrino M, et al: Nutrient oxidation during moderately intense exercise in obese prepubertal boys. J Clin Endocrinol Metab 2005;90:231–236.
34 Marshall SJ, Biddle SJ, Gorely T, et al: Relationships between media use, body fatness and physical activity in children and youth: a meta-analysis. Int J Obes Relat Metab Disord 2004;28:1238–1246.
35 Lissau I, Sorensen TI: Parental neglect during childhood and increased risk of obesity in young adulthood. Lancet 1994;343:324–327.
36 Halford JC, Gillespie J, Brown V, et al: Effect of television advertisements for foods on food consumption in children. Appetite 2004;42:221–225.

## Discussion

*Dr. Klish:* I have a question regarding inflammation within the adipocyte that you discussed. In steatohepatitis, it has been hypothesized that those individuals who develop inflammation in the liver receive what has been called a second hit. Steatosis of the liver does not always lead to steatohepatitis. One hypothesis that I have heard is that fat itself may be the toxic element in genetically programmed individuals. Do you think that the same hypothesis is true in adipose tissue that becomes inflamed? Is this phenomenon genetically linked or is it a universal?

*Dr. Maffeis:* I have no answer to your question. The number of obese individuals is so high that, in spite of the unequivocal role played by genetic predisposition, a triggering effect of the toxic environment exposition is necessary for obese phenotype expression. With regard to the elementary lesion that we find in adipose tissue, we don't know why it happens.

*Dr. Saavedra:* I have a follow-up to the question that Dr. Klish asked. You were talking about the inflammatory response and the relationships that there are with other things that do happen in other situations where we have adipose tissue accumulation. Chronic inflammatory conditions in general predispose to fat accumulation. Patients with Crohn's disease have increased fat and predominantly patients with hepatitis have increased fat in the liver. We also know that chronic inflammation is associated with increased cardiovascular disease by itself, independent of other markers. We also know that adipocytes are also associated with secretion of tumor necrosis factor and a number of proinflammatory markers. Could it be that, besides the obvious causes of just following the laws of thermodynamics, we are really dealing with more intake and less utilization? Part of the reason why it is hard to deal with the problem once an inflammatory cascade has been set off is that what we really have is an underlying low-grade chronic inflammatory problem that increases fat in the muscle and the liver, and potentially decreases because of the long-term inflammation insulin response at the cellular level. If this is the case, how could the inflammatory component of that potentially be addressed?

*Dr. Maffeis:* Yes I agree with you, certainly the interest here is to understand why inflammation is starting because in children the exposure to overweight is of short duration. However, children have a high level of insulin sensitivity at the beginning of the dynamic phase of obesity. Therefore overnutrition could theoretically promote the increase in size of the adipocytes, but why the child is not so efficient in recruiting new cells and on the contrary is able to produce an elementary lesion in which inflammatory cells are anatomically detected is not known. Research in animals demonstrated that the inflammatory cytokines found in the adipose tissue probably are not just secreted by the adipocytes but also by the macrophages. The reason why macrophages leave the vessels, arrive in the adipose tissue and secrete inflammatory mediators needs to be investigated further.

*Dr. Klish:* It does not appear that inflammation in the liver of children is responsible for recruiting fat. There are many children with steatosis of the liver and no inflammation at all. If we could understand what causes the inflammation we would come a long way in our understanding of the development of steatohepatitis.

*Dr. Lucas:* I have seen some data recently that are rather provocative. You may not have seen them but I wouldn't mind your comment. Jeffery et al. [1] in Britain are doing a very carefully characterized cohort study called the EarlyBird 21 study. They are using accelerometers to measure activity, and have found that children who watch television are no less active than children who don't because they just make up the activity in other periods of their life. They found that children who walk to school have exactly the same activity level as children who are taken to school in a car, and children who go to school where sports are particularly accentuated have exactly the same activity level as children who go to schools that don't encourage sports because they increased their activity elsewhere. So they came to the conclusion that there is an activity stat and that children have a constant level of activity and if you reduce their activity in some places they spontaneously increase it elsewhere. Do you have a comment on that, because this would be very worrying from the public health prevention point of view?

*Dr. Maffeis:* In my opinion, the role of physical activity is crucial for the development and maintenance of obesity. However, the accurate measure of physical activity is very difficult in free-living conditions. Therefore we have to be cautious in evaluating data obtained by accelerometers which offer just a quantitative 'estimation' and not a 'measure' of physical activity. It is likely that in obese children the proportion of energy daily devoted to physical activity is similar, as reported by studies combining total energy expenditure, measured by the doubly labeled water method, and the basal metabolic rate, measured by indirect calorimetry. These studies demonstrated that the gross index of physical activity, obtained by dividing the total energy expenditure by the basal metabolic rate, was similar in obese and non-obese individuals [2, 3]. However, this is not to say that they have the same level of activity. In fact, several other studies demonstrated that the time devoted to sedentary behavior was higher in obese than in non-obese children [4, 5]. The obese children spend less time in moderate or vigorous physical activity but the higher energy expenditure for performing weight-bearing activities tends to compensate, in terms of energy, for this sedentary behavior [6, 7]. The scarce validity of self-reported measures of physical activity was emphasized by the evidence that obese individuals tend to overestimate their physical activity and to underestimate their sedentary behavior or food intake. Moreover, we have to be cautious in evaluating data on physical activity obtained in cross-sectional studies. At the moment, insufficient data are available from longitudinal studies. I totally agree with you that it is very difficult to give a clear definition of the role played by physical activity in the development of obesity independent of food intake. It has been estimated that just a difference of 2% between total energy expenditure is enough, if prolonged for weeks and months, to have relevant weight and fat gain in humans. Unfortunately, available techniques are not sensitive and accurate enough to detect such a small difference in energy balance.

*Dr. Exl-Preysch:* I just wanted to add that there is a very new study from Germany by Diehl [8] with a general overview on the topic 'Is advertising making children fat'. He quantitatively measured the TV consumption of children and compared it with their weight. There was no difference between the hours of TV watching and weight. Several other studies and German ones also looked at the TV consumption, weight and growth development of children from 1991 to 2005 and there was no difference in the hours per day that 3- to 13-year-old children spent watching TV. Only after 14 years of age did the average daily time spent watching TV increase, therefore suggesting that in the younger age the 'so-called increasing TV watching cannot be the true reason for increasing their weight', but in some studies it may be an indicator for another real reason. Another interesting result was the hours children spend watching TV increases with age as a steadily increasing line over time – the younger the child the fewer hours spent watching TV, and then there is a stiff increase per day to 20 years of life, increasing constantly to 65 years and over. So it is rather difficult to get a real causal relationship between TV watching and obesity, and this is being discussed more and more critically.

*Dr. Maffeis:* A meta-analysis was recently published on this topic. The authors found that TV watching is able to predict fat gain but the importance of this variable was very low [9]. However, most of the studies conducted to investigate the association between video exposure and obesity in children used self-reported data and not objective recording methods. Finally, recent data seem to support the hypothesis that TV viewing is a relevant obesity risk factor in young children too [10].

*Dr. Klish:* I find it interesting that in Italy the average amount of time spent watching television was 2.5 h. In the United States, the average number of hours is somewhere in the neighborhood of 4–5. Perhaps television watching is a surrogate for other forms of inactivity and if an individual spends little time watching TV the relationship with obesity is not picked up.

*Dr. Hanson:* If you have inflammatory disease with obesity and it is treated long-term with anti-inflammatory drugs, would that make a difference? I would like to add an observation that could possibly be related to the problem. We are working with something called antisecretory factor (AF) which is induced by certain enterotoxins and certain foods, and we noticed that Swedish mothers do not normally have this factor. When we induced it we could significantly prevent clinical mastitis which is an inflammatory condition (in contrast to breast abscess). Then I wanted to repeat this in Pakistani village women but they did not have mastitis, they did not know what it was, and they all had a high level of AF because they live in an area where it would be induced by exposure to enterotoxins. So then we investigated women in Lahore who went to private hospitals, and they were less exposed to enterotoxin-related infections and had an intermediate level of AF that permitted them to have a low prevalence of mastitis. Now my question is: in women exposed to this factor, which is strongly anti-secretory and anti-inflammatory, would that influence obesity?

*Dr. Maffeis:* To the best of my knowledge, there are no data available to reply to your question.

*Dr. von Berg:* I have a question regarding a possible genetic link between obesity and asthma because of two observations: first, in a large study it was observed that with each BMI point the asthma rate increased significantly in women but not in men, and second, obese tissue actually has a very similar pattern to inflammatory markers as is seen in asthmatics.

*Dr. Maffeis:* I agree, I think that investigating the relationship between these diseases with such a high epidemiological impact may help to better understand some of the mechanisms of their pathogenesis.

*Dr. Hursting:* The discussion about sweeteners in the diet was interesting. I have heard the hypothesis that the diet is now getting sweeter but the type of sweetener is changing, and the potential role that it has metabolically. I wonder if you could comment on that, particularly with regard to corn syrup and soft drinks and so on.

*Dr. Maffeis:* Yes, the type of sugars added to soft drinks, in particular fructose, seems to play a key role in the development of weight gain. There are no receptors for fructose in the brain or in the pancreas, so the organism has no possibility to check the changes in the blood concentration of this carbohydrate as it does for glucose. So we do not have insulin-induced regulation of fructose intake; fructose can be accumulated and can follow metabolic pathways stimulating fat gain.

*Dr. Sorensen:* Are the metabolic and endocrine mechanisms leading to obesity very different depending on the age of the patient? If they are different, what consequences should one draw regarding prevention and intervention mechanisms, let's say in a very young child that is beginning to be overweight versus an older child? Is there a difference and should we draw some consequences from it?

*Dr. Maffeis:* Since obesity risk factors are variously relevant in infants, young children, older children and adolescents, intervention should focus on different potentially sensitive targets of treatment or prevention in the various ages. In the first year of life early feeding (breast versus formula, weaning characteristics and modalities) is crucial and the mother is the principal object of intervention. Further data especially on the relationship between nutrient composition of the weaning diet, early growth, and the risk of obesity are needed. In the young child, the role of the family is absolutely relevant whereas the socio-cultural environment (school, friends, community and media) starts to influence the food and physical activity habits of the child. Food availability in the house, kind of food available, diet composition of the family, portion size, attitude and consideration about the food of the parents and caregivers, patterns of food intake are all potential targets of intervention. Moreover, a reduction in sedentary behavior by increasing the time spent playing with friends and/or outside the house could be helpful. Regular practice of sports and physical activity of the parents are associated with a more active lifestyle of their children. Video exposure is another potentially sensitive target of intervention. In older children and adolescents, the role of the extra-family environment is progressively becoming more important. Therefore, the intervention should be directed toward the family but with active involvement of the social community (school, media, etc.).

*Dr. Zeiger:* Dr. Lucas rather convincingly showed us earlier the power of imprinting and programming on children which lead not to the development of obesity and hypertension early on but later in childhood. The question I have is: are these new lifestyles and the effect of the poor diet really only affecting those children who have been imprinted earlier?

*Dr. Maffeis:* I think that the programming hypothesis is very fascinating but I think that it can only justify part of the epidemic of obesity.

*Dr. Zeiger:* But I meant specifically are the only ones at risk those who were programmed earlier and that those who weren't programmed earlier can eat whatever they want and do whatever they want related to exercise. In other words, if programming imprinting is so powerful that it manifests not early but later, and we now have the change in the food consumption and activity, the question I was trying to raise is, is this adverse diet and activity differentially affecting those who were imprinted early on and not affecting those who were not?

*Dr. Maffeis:* To the best of my knowledge, we have no data to give a definitive reply to your question. Probably Dr. Lucas could give an answer based on his own data.

*Dr. Lucas:* I don't think that programming explains all of adult disease by any means, it is just one important lead into it, but the combination of what happens very early combined with subsequent events has obviously a very powerful influence on cardiovascular risk factors including obesity, but certainly not an exclusive risk, and a large number of other factors need to be brought up. Obviously the really important issue is to identify those factors that you can do something about and programming is an area which lands itself to intervention.

*Dr. Klish:* I might also point out that you said earlier in your lecture that obviously there are many genotypes that cause obesity which give rise to multiple phenotypes which we probably don't all recognize yet. Obesity is not a singular disease, it is a group of diseases, and if we could understand the phenotypes we could begin to focus on individual therapies.

*Dr. Hursting:* We have done macal raise from animal studies of adipose tissue in mice that were made lean by calorie restriction and made obese by high calorie diets and we have seen that the macrophage genes as well as the inflammatory genes are the most differentially expressed in that setting. I think it is consistent with what you are saying, the influx of macs into those inflammatory lesions and even in the children. So my question is why are macs getting in there in adipose tissue, what is driving that process?

*Dr. Maffeis:* I have no answer to this central question. Further studies are needed to obtain potential explanations.

*Dr. Klish:* There are studies that imply that adhesion molecules such as ICAM are altered by obesity, so the migration of inflammatory cells through the epithelium into adipose tissue is enhanced by the presence of obesity.

*Dr. Roma:* Concerning the quality of fat intake, did you find any difference compared to polyunsaturated and monosaturated fatty acids? For example, in Italy as in Greece, we consume more olive oil. Have you found any protective role of monosaturated fat?

*Dr. Maffeis:* Yes, we tried to compare the different kinds of fat in the diets of obese and non-obese children but we did not find any difference. In Italy, the use of olive oil is very common and a difference in fat composition between obese and non-obese children is unlikely. On the contrary, the problem seems to be not just the quality but the quantity of fat ingested.

*Dr. Arvanitakis:* In fact olive oil does not appear to protect Greek children because, besides Eurovision and football, Greece is going to have a price to pay for childhood obesity. We have been studying obese children for many years. We have studied two groups, preadolescents and adolescents, and have found that insulin insensitivity is almost as high in preadolescents as in adolescents. I think this is frightening because we can foresee a generation of fat people with all these problems of the metabolic syndrome. We have to have an intervention in these children who are already adolescents and have insulin resistance. As you said insulin resistance can be a cofactor or stimulating factor for obesity in adulthood. All these adolescents will go into adulthood being obese. We know about diet, we know about the positive effect of exercise. However, we have to find a strategy to intervene, to change the eating behavior of the children and the parents, and even the dog of the family. The most difficult problem is how to change the behavior of these families so that they eat less and exercise more, because so far we cannot change their genes.

*Dr. Maffeis:* I agree with your comments, certainly insulin resistance plays a key role in the development of the metabolic disorders associated with obesity. Physical activity is crucial because exercise is able to reduce insulin levels, blood cholesterol and other cardiovascular risk factors. Exercise or stimulation of physical activity is certainly a good way to work but it is very difficult to change the behavior of the families and the children. We still have to improve the techniques to motivate behavioral changes in our patients.

*Dr. Exl-Preysch:* I think you are right, exercise is very important. In the mean time I have the impression that we are perhaps talking too much about the lack of exercise programs and not enough about nutrition educational programs. These children are growing up in a world with over flow that we cannot change. Therefore they should learn early in life how to have a balanced nutrition. There are some programs: in France there is a very big governmental program going on that has already been validated and has been successful in not further increasing overweight in children. It has been enlarged to a lot of cities in France in the meantime, and further information can be found at www.villesante.com. Another important program for general nutrition education is the so-called Nutrikid Program and further information can be found at www.nutrikid.ch. This concept for children aged 10–12 years of age (until now) has been evaluated, validated and published. It contains a CD-ROM/video, a brochure for the children, a card game, a background information CD for the teacher or parents, and is completely free of any product connections or advertising. It was founded as a separate organization by the Swiss Society of Nutrition, the Nestlé Foundation 'Alimentarium' and Nestlé Switzerland.

*Dr. Maffeis:* Nutrition really plays a key role in the development of obesity in adults and in children as well. However, the only component of energy expenditure which is subjected to voluntary control, the energy expenditure of physical activity, does have some responsibility in the obesity epidemic. In particular a recent study clearly demonstrated that the minimum physical activity level (PAL) to avoid fat gain should be roughly equal to 1.7. Unfortunately, most children and adults living in industrialized countries have a PAL of <1.7. Moreover, objective difficulties encountered in measuring physical activity, using accurate methods, in free-living conditions in a large sample of children are an important barrier to appropriately explore the real role played by physical activity in the development and maintenance of obesity. Theoretically, as I tried to show in my presentation, skeletal muscle activity has an important effect on fat balance regulation in humans as well as in animals and this may justify, together with all the benefits for morbidity and mortality associated with the regular practice of physical activity, the need to reduce sedentary behavior and to promote physical activity especially in children. Therefore I believe that living with a constant exposure to such a 'toxic' environment, we should not push all our efforts on nutrition completely and forget physical activity promotion. But unfortunately there is a combination between unapparent energy intake and fat gain in Mediterranean populations as in other countries. In the USA, an analysis of the variations in energy intake of the population from 1900 to 2000 revealed that starting from 1960 there was a steep increase in energy intake per person. On the contrary, data reported from nutritional surveys did not show this phenomenon. It is likely that conscious and unconscious underreporting of food intake is becoming more frequent in the population in which obesity is much more common and this may potentially affect the information obtained by the surveys. Therefore I do not believe that there is a causal relationship between the Mediterranean diet and obesity, but that obesity in the Mediterranean areas is a result of progressively higher food and energy intake accompanied by increasing sedentary behavior. Moreover, the Mediterranean lifestyle is different now from that in the middle of the last century. Also the typical Mediterranean diet is progressively changing, especially in the young generations, to a more 'international' one.

*Dr. Laron:* Linking the previous lecture with yours, it has been shown in adults that it is the visceral fat which is important for the development of cardiovascular disease. How do you propose to measure visceral fat in children? MRI on a routine basis is certainly not practical.

*Dr. Maffeis:* In my presentation I tried to suggest a method which is very simple, cheap, not invasive, and may be performed in each out- or in-patient clinical setting: waist circumference. Interesting studies have explored the relationship between waist circumference and cardiovascular risk factors in children, independent of body weight or BMI. Obviously, waist circumference is not MRI, but for clinical use it is the best that we have at present.

*Dr. Laron:* Why would skin-folds not be better than body circumferences which in children would not be very exact?

*Dr. Maffeis:* The measure of subcutaneous skin-fold thickness is simple, cheap and not invasive (as waist circumference) but it is open to high inter- and intra-operator variability. Moreover subcutaneous skin-fold thickness is more associated with total fat mass that to visceral fat mass.

*Dr. Singhal:* This is a comment rather than a question regarding the point about visceral fat. I completely agree that cardiovascular risk has to do with visceral fat, and so I think we do need a new technique to try and measure visceral fat in children. This is one of the things that we are trying to do in our group. We are using DEXA in combination with ultrasound and this appears to be a better marker of visceral fat than waist circumference in children.

*Dr. Maffeis:* Absolutely yes, but this is not feasible in out-patient clinical settings, it is just for research.

*Dr. Hamburger:* Is anybody testing or examining the use of anti-inflammatory medications (NSAIDs) in obesity?

*Dr. Maffeis:* Yes, an anti-inflammatory drug, salicylate, was used in obese animals. High doses of salicylate were able to dramatically reduce the insulin resistance associated with obesity [11].

## References

1 Jeffery AN, Voss LD, Metcalf BS, et al: Parents' awareness of overweight in themselves and their children: cross sectional study within a cohort (EarlyBird 21). BMJ 2005;330:23–24.
2 Bandini LG, Schoeller DA, Dietz WH: Energy expenditure in obese and nonobese adolescents. Pediatr Res 1990;27:198–203.
3 Treuth MS, Figueroa-Colon R, Hunter GR, et al: Energy expenditure and physical fitness in overweight vs non-overweight prepubertal girls. Int J Obes Relat Metab Disord 1998;22: 440–447.
4 Rennie KL, Livingstone MB, Wells JC, et al: Association of physical activity with body-composition indexes in children aged 6–8 y at varied risk of obesity. Am J Clin Nutr 2005;82: 13–20.

5 Maffeis C, Zaffanello M, Pinelli L, Schutz Y: Total energy expenditure and patterns of activity in 8–10-year-old obese and nonobese children. J Pediatr Gastroenterol Nutr 1996;23:256–261.
6 Maffeis C, Schutz Y, Schena F, et al: Energy expenditure during walking and running in obese and nonobese prepubertal children. J Pediatr 1993;123:193–199.
7 Ekelund U, Aman J, Yngve A, et al: Physical activity but not energy expenditure is reduced in obese adolescents: a case-control study. Am J Clin Nutr 2002;76:935–941.
8 Diehl JM: Macht Werbung Dick? Einfluss der Lebenmittelwerbung auf Kinder und Jugend-liche. Ernährungsumschau 2005;52:40–46. www.ernährungsumschau.de
9 Marshall SJ, Biddle SJ, Gorely T, et al: Relationships between media use, body fatness and physical activity in children and youth: a meta-analysis. Int J Obes Relat Metab Disord 2004; 28:1238–1246.
10 Jago R, Baranowski T, Baranowski JC, et al: BMI from 3–6 y of age is predicted by TV viewing and physical activity, not diet. Int J Obes Relat Metab Disord 2005;29:557–564.
11 Yuan M, Konstantopoulos N, Lee J, et al: Reversal of obesity- and diet-induced insulin resist-ance with salicylates or targeted disruption of Ikkbeta. Science 2001;293:1673–1677.

Lucas A, Sampson HA (eds): Primary Prevention by Nutrition Intervention in Infancy and Childhood.
Nestlé Nutr Workshop Ser Pediatr Program, vol 57, pp 51–65,
Nestec Ltd., Vevey/S. Karger AG, Basel, © 2006.

# Prenatal and Postnatal Development of Obesity: Primary Prevention Trials and Observational Studies

*Anja Kroke*

Research Institute of Child Nutrition, Rheinische Friedrich-Wilhelms-Universität Bonn,
Dortmund, Germany

## Introduction

Since Barker et al. [1] presented the fetal origins hypothesis in 1989 introducing the concept of the developmental origins of chronic diseases, the interest in this early life period has increased dramatically. What has been observed from developmental biologists for many years became relevant for disease-related research in clinical medicine, epidemiology, pediatrics, and nutrition research. Many scientists began to study the effects of external and internal exposures of the fetus or newborn on later health-related outcomes. Initially, cardiovascular diseases (CVDs) were the main focus of research. Today, a vast amount of studies has documented relations between fetal and/or early life experiences and later risk for CVD, cancer, diabetes and other chronic diseases. As overweight and obesity and their health consequences began to emerge as epidemic-like problems, the spectrum of research was extended to study the potential role of prenatal and early postnatal exposures on these outcomes. Due to unique periods of cellular differentiation and development, the early life period is considered to be particularly vulnerable for obesity development [2]. It has been suggested that developmental plasticity allows the fetus to adjust to environmental influences thereby adapting to the current, but also to the predicted postnatal situation. As elaborated in reviews by Gluckman et al. [3], later disease risk, which also includes the risk of obesity, appears to depend on the degree of match between the environment predicted during the developmental phase and the actual later environment.

Among the potential environmental exposures, nutrition is considered to play the most critical role in influencing placental and fetal growth, including adipose tissue [4]. However, this specific field of obesity development provides comparably little human data, and long-term studies to support the role of nutritional influences in early life on adolescent or adult obesity are scarce. The aim of this presentation is to give a broad overview of the current status of research on the relation between early nutritional exposures and human obesity development as can be derived from studies in humans.

To date, the vast majority of studies on prenatal and early postnatal nutritional factors influencing later obesity are animal experiments, mostly in rats and sheep. These studies have documented that critical periods during fetal and neonatal development exist, when nutritional influences are able to exert long-lasting effects on body weight development [5, 6]. However, the described effects and mechanisms derived from these studies are only to a limited extent applicable to humans. Therefore, studies with human data are necessary to evaluate the relevance of the findings for the human species, and to substantiate the available observational, epidemiological data. Obviously, such studies are difficult to conduct, and ethical and practical restrictions lead to a body of evidence which has to rely mainly on observational studies or on disease-oriented clinical trials.

A further drawback is the very long time needed in human studies to prospectively evaluate the effect of early nutritional exposures on adult overweight or obesity. Therefore, only a few retrospective cohort data exist, characterized by very limited detail on exposure and outcome assessment. Other human studies work with intermediate outcomes such as birth weight or childhood body mass or obesity. Nevertheless, these studies provide useful insights.

Many studies approach the topic of obesity development with samples of small-for-gestational-age children, intrauterine growth retardation, or diabetic mothers. These specific clinical situations make it difficult to judge the impact of nutritional factors on 'normal growth'. Consequently, the impact of nutritional exposures on birth weight and adiposity need to be interpreted with caution. For reasons of clarity and relevance for this overview, studies with children appropriate for gestational age are mainly considered, as well as studies among well-nourished and healthy pregnant women. In order to structure this overview, it appears useful to partition the complex theme into three main topics: (1) birth weight and later weight; (2) prenatal nutritional exposures and later weight, and (3) early postnatal nutrition and later weight.

## Background

Maternal nutrition, and partly influenced by it, the metabolic and hormonal intrauterine environment, may strongly influence the amount, metabolic activity and endocrine sensitivity of adipose tissue in the offspring [2], thereby possibly influencing the development of obesity in childhood and/or adulthood. The fetal supply, which determines fetal growth, results from a complex maternal-fetal supply line. It involves maternal food intake, absorption, metabolism, health and hormonal status, as well as maternal nutrient partitioning and placental functioning. Consequently, maternal nutrition may lead to long-lasting effects via prenatal programming. The term 'programming' subsumes the diverse developmental adaptations to a stress or stimulus in a sensitive period of development evoked by nutritional and/or endocrine influences. This process can lead to permanent changes in organ structure and size, altered cell number, hormonal set points and altered gene expression, among others. These changes may predispose to metabolic and endocrine diseases later in life. Dietary restriction, macronutrient amount and composition, as well as micronutrient intake or status have been considered as potentially relevant prenatal exposures in this context. An important feature of programming is the observation that it may vary depending on the developmental period of the fetus or neonate, and on the species.

In addition to environmental influences, genetic factors are also considered to be important contributors. Studies with monozygotic twins have indicated that intra-pair differences between twins are to some extent influenced by the fetal environment and by birth weight. Body height appears to be influenced more strongly by birth size than adult body mass index (BMI) [7]. However, the relative importance of genetic and environmental factors remains unknown, although it appears to change with age [8].

During recent years, a considerable number of reviews about pre- and postnatal programming have summarized different aspects of maternal nutrition, fetal growth, and body weight. Table 1 presents selected publications for further reading.

## Discussion

### Topic 1: Birth Weight and Later Weight

Birth weight has become the most frequently used indicator of fetal growth in human studies trying to link prenatal influences to later disease-related events including obesity. However, several caveats need to be considered when interpreting these data. Although many prenatal influences are thought to affect fetal size and thereby birth weight, prenatal programming may occur in the absence of changes in fetal size. Different growth patterns may result in the same birth weight, so that the potential effect of intrauterine growth patterns and their respective potential effect on later weight development cannot be accounted for.

Birth weight is related to birth length and gestational age, which in many studies were not taken into account. Parental body size is another important determinant of offspring size, e.g. maternal size is closely linked to birth size for preventing labor obstruction, which is often not considered when data on

***Table 1.*** Selected reviews addressing aspects of pre- and postnatal programming of obesity

| Title | Author, year | Reference number |
|---|---|---|
| Timing of nutrient restriction and programming of fetal adipose tissue development | Symonds et al., 2004 | 2 |
| Life-long echoes – a critical analysis of the developmental origins of disease model | Gluckman et al., 2005 | 3 |
| The influence of birth weight and intrauterine environment on adiposity and fat distribution in later life | Rogers, 2003 | 9 |
| Micronutrients and fetal growth | Fall et al., 2003 | 21 |
| Breast-feeding and childhood obesity – a systematic review | Arenz et al., 2004 | 27 |
| The developmental origins of adult disease | Barker, 2004 | 33 |
| Critical periods in human growth and their relationship to diseases of aging | Cameron and Demerath, 2002 | 34 |
| Fetal origins of obesity | Oken and Gillman, 2003 | 35 |
| Early nutrition and leptin concentrations later in life | Singhal et al., 2002 | 36 |
| Maternal nutrition and fetal development | Wu et al., 2004 | 37 |
| Obesity epidemic in India: intrauterine origins? | Yajnik, 2004 | 38 |
| Early nutrition and later adiposity | Martorell et al., 2001 | 39 |

birth weight are related to adult body mass. Also, other relevant factors such as maternal smoking and socioeconomic status were frequently not taken into account. Furthermore, the relation between birth weight and adult weight is affected by trans-generational effects, as it has been observed that offspring birth weight is related to the mother's birth weight [8]. Finally, birth weight may be differentially related to additional facets of body mass, that is to lean and fat body mass and to body fat distribution.

The relation between birth weight and later BMI was analyzed in numerous studies [for a comprehensive review see, 9], and was described to be linear, j- or u-shaped. Taking the above-mentioned caveats into account, it has to be stated that although a positive association appears to exist, a definitive answer about the shape of that relation as well as the causes remains to be elucidated (fig. 1). Recent data indicate, however, that birth weight displays a more complex relation to adult BMI, body fat distribution and fat mass. For example, low birth weight in combination with rapid infant growth appears to increase the likelihood of obesity and/or central obesity in adulthood. Others suggest that birth weight is related to adult height and weight, but not to adult BMI.

The discussion on this issue would also be advanced by separating both the upper and lower extremes of the birth weight distribution, e.g. low birth

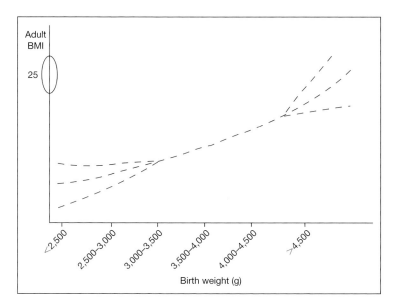

**Fig. 1.** Potential relation between birth weight and adult BMI.

weight (<2,500 g) and macrosomia (>4,000 g) from the rest. In both cases, pathophysiological factors might be operating (e.g. placental dysfunction, diabetes of the mother) which confound the relation birth weight and later weight. The evidence that children born with macrosomia are at increased risk of obesity is much stronger, partly explained by maternal diabetes or impaired glucose tolerance.

Given the previous findings that with increasing birth weight other outcomes such as CVD and diabetes appear to be reduced, this positive relation of birth weight with later weight and obesity status needs to be further elucidated. One school of thought about this paradoxical situation is the suggestion that body composition and/or body fat distribution might mediate this relation. As only very few studies have assessed a more detailed anthropometry beyond weight and height either at birth or later in life, respective data are less abundant. However, the available studies indicate that birth weight is more strongly related to later lean body mass than to fat mass (table 2). Later body fat distribution was also considered in its relation to birth weight. Here, the findings are rather inconsistent, partly due to heterogeneity in applied measures and subjects studied. While several studies observed that birth weight was positively related to waist circumference, no such findings were reported for waist-to-hip ratio or other measures of fat distribution. Overall, the interpretation of findings is hampered by methodological discussions about the pros and cons of controlling for attained BMI in these studies.

**Table 2.** Results of studies relating birth weight to subsequent body lean and fat body mass

| Reference | Age years | Year of birth | n | Study population | Outcome measure | Adjustment for | Results |
|---|---|---|---|---|---|---|---|
| Phillips [10], 1995 | 47–55 | 1935–1943 | 217 | Men and women, UK | BMI Muscle mass | / | Relation to BMI, n.s. Significant positive association with muscle mass |
| Kahn et al. [11], 2000 | 17–22 | | 192 | Men | Thigh muscle+ bone area, thigh subcutaneous fat area | Race, height | Thigh muscle+bone area bone area significantly associated with BW (regression coefficient 0.22, p < 0.01); Thigh subcutaneous fat area not associated with BW (p > 0.05) |
| Gale et al. [12], 2001 | 70–75 | | 143 | Men and women, UK | LBM FBM | Age, sex, height | Positive association, rises from 22.16 kg for BW; 3:3 <3.15–23.14 kg for BW >3.64 kg, p < 0.0001 no association |
| Loos et al. [7], 2002 | 18–34 | 1964–1982 | 415 | Female twins in Belgium (East Flanders) | LBM | GA, body mass | Positive association, increases from 42.4 kg for BW-GA z-score ≤1 to 44.1 kg if BW-GA z-score ≥1 (p < 0.001) |
| Loos et al. [7], 2002 | 18–34 | 1964–1982 | 388 | Male twins in Belgium (East Flanders) | LBM | GA, body mass | LBM increased by 0.64 kg/kg increase in BW (p = 0.01) |
| Singhal et al. [13], 2003 | mean 7.4 | | 86 | Male and female children in UK (Cambridge) | LBM FBM | Age, sex, socio-economic status, Tanner stage, physical activity, height squared | SD increase in BW = 0.9 – 1.4 kg more in fat free mass No association with fat mass |
| Sayer et al. [14], 2004 | mean 64.3 | 1931–1939 | 737 | Men in UK (Hertfordshire) | LBM, FBM BMI | Age, social class, smoking status, alcohol consumption, physical activity | Strong association of BW with LBM (r = 0.27), moderate association with BMI (r = 0.13), weak association with FBM (r = 0.10) |

BMI = Body mass index (kg/m$^2$); BW = birth weight; GA = gestational age; FBM = fat body mass; LBM = lean body mass; n.s. = non-significant. Adapted from Rogers [9].

Associations between the considered measures disappear or change direction depending on whether attained BMI is adjusted for or not.

In summary, the relation between birth weight and adult BMI or obesity status is complex and not entirely understood so far. This complicates the interpretation of studies that use birth weight as a measure of fetal growth and prenatal nutritional influences respectively.

## Topic 2: Prenatal Nutritional Exposures

Most studies on prenatal nutritional exposures examined the effects on birth weight. Only very few data are available on later weight development. As nutritional exposures are a diverse group, they are considered separately.

### Dietary Restriction during Gestation

Numerous animal studies indicate that the timing of maternal nutrient restriction plays a major role in determining fetal adipose tissue mass. Restrictions in early pregnancy (with later adequate intake) tend to increase adipose tissue deposition, whereas later restrictions decrease it [2]. Observational human data come from the Dutch famine of 1944–1945, and appear to confirm these results for humans. In this retrospective cohort study, the effect of the intrauterine exposure to a limited period of famine was assessed. An exposure to maternal malnutrition during early gestation (as compared to exposure in late gestation) was associated with higher BMI at age 19 in men [15], and with higher BMI and waist circumference in women only at age 50 [16]. Exposure to famine during mid and late pregnancy was associated with lower birth weight und birth length. Data from developing countries clearly show that protein/energy malnutrition of the mother is associated with intrauterine growth retardation. Prenatal growth retardation followed by infant catch-up growth was found to increase the risk of obesity. Low birth weight has also been described to be associated with a pattern of central fat accumulation.

An issue of increasing interest in industrialized countries is the dietary management of overweight/obese pregnant women. Three trials on energy/ protein restriction in overweight women were reviewed in a Cochrane review [17]. A significant reduction in gestational weight gain was reported, whereas the results on birth weight were inconclusive, with one study reporting no effect and the other a significant reduction in birth weight. Data on later weight development of the offspring were not available.

With the increasing prevalence of obesity, dietary restraint during pregnancy might become another issue of concern. Restrained eating appears to negatively influence weight gain during pregnancy, however, data on this are scarce.

*Maternal Food Intake*

Very few studies in humans have reported on the effects of specific food items on fetal or postnatal weight development (except for alcohol consumption and abuse, aspects not considered here). Coffee and caffeine consumption were considered in several studies, but significant effects on birth weight, independent of smoking behavior, were not found. Fish intake and/or the intake of n-3 fatty acids were considered in several studies, mainly for their potential protection against preterm delivery. Both observational and experimental studies (with n-3 supplements) reported on fetal growth, as assessed by birth weight. These data partly indicate that with increasing intake of fish or n-3 fatty acids fetal growth increases. However, a very high level of intake was also shown to be associated with decreased birth size. Therefore, the effects of the nutritional factors might depend on the amount consumed.

*Maternal Macronutrient and Energy Intake*

The major focus in the area of macronutrients has been placed on protein intake. Animal studies indicate that high protein intake is associated with low birth weight, but data from human observational studies remain inconclusive [18]. Experimental human studies, summarized in a Cochrane review, were not able to demonstrate significant effects on birth weight or birth length. Considered exposures were advice to increase energy and protein intake, and a balanced energy/protein supplementation [17].

Recently, interest has increased in the role of carbohydrate intake, particularly in the role of the intensely discussed glycemic index. Again, results appear to be conflicting. While some studies found no influence of carbohydrate intake on birth weight, others have found some effects for the glycemic index, indicating that with an increasing glycemic index birth weight tends to increase and vice versa.

In light of the current obesity epidemic, energy intake during pregnancy and the associated pregnancy weight gain are of increasing interest. As in other studies, the relation between dietary energy intake and weight development remains difficult to ascertain. If, however, maternal weight status or pregnancy weight gain are used as indicators for maternal energy balance, more insights can be derived. For example, in a retrospective cohort study maternal obesity significantly increased the risk of obesity in children up to 4 years of age [19]. Maternal overweight was suggested to be the reason of increasing the rates for neonatal macrosomia [20], which is associated with an increased risk of obesity.

*Micronutrients*

A vast number of studies have dealt with the effects of single or combined micronutrient supplementation and a reduction in low birth weight, growth retardation or other adverse pregnancy outcomes, mainly in developing countries. Recent reviews [21, 22] indicate that for some micronutrients evidence was sufficient to assume a positive effect on birth weight or a reduction in low birth weight infants. However, many trials were considered to be of inadequate design, so that final conclusions cannot be drawn at this stage. Only a few studies were dedicated to the effects of micronutrient intake among pregnant women from industrialized countries. In several Cochrane reviews of randomized controlled trials single nutrient supplementation was considered, but parameters of fetal growth were not their main endpoint. The presented results on birth weight did not indicate significant effects, except for calcium supplementation, which was reported to protect against low birth weight [23].

A large prospective cohort study from the UK found only vitamin C intake in early pregnancy to be significantly related to birth weight, but the effect was very small. Maternal circulating nutrient concentrations were also assessed. Unexpectedly, high retinol concentrations were associated with reduced birth weight [24, 25]. A few other observational studies exist, but the sophistication of the dietary intake assessment or of data handling was often rather poor.

## Topic 3: Early Postnatal Nutrition

### Breastfeeding

The first observation indicating that breastfeeding might be related to childhood weight development was made in a case-control study published in 1981 [26]. Since then, numerous studies have investigated this relation, and some but not all of these have confirmed this finding. A recent meta-analysis, based on a systematic literature review, found a small but statistically significant protective effect of breastfeeding [27]. The pooled, adjusted effect estimate derived from 9 studies, including data from more than 69,000 children, indicated a 22% lower risk of childhood obesity among breastfed children compared to formula-fed children (fig. 2). The duration of breastfeeding, however, was not found to have an effect in all studies. Possible mechanistic explanations for the protective effect of breastfeeding include metabolic programming via hormonal and metabolic effects of nutritive and/or non-nutritive compounds in breast milk, energy and protein content, behavioral effects such as self-regulation of energy/food intake, but also residual confounding by parental characteristics [for further details see, 28].

The relation of breastfeeding to adult overweight/obesity was assessed in two prospective studies. A small study with 172 subjects found an increased body mass and fat mass among men (aged 32) who had been breastfed [29]. The much more powerful analysis of data from the British 1958 Birth Cohort, with BMI data from 9,287 subjects at age 33, indicated no significant relation to breastfeeding status when confounding variables were taken into account [30].

Kroke

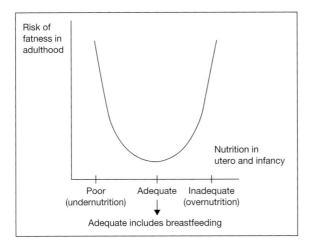

*Fig. 2.* Schematic description of the relation between nutrition in utero and infancy and its relation to the risk of adult body fatness. Adapted from Martorell et al. [39].

*Protein Intake and Energy Intake*

The different anthropometric development of breast- and bottle-fed children could be partly due to their difference in protein content. But also beyond breastfeeding, several studies found a positive association between protein intake in the first year of life and infant weight gain and later body mass development respectively. Others, however, could not support these findings so that an ultimate conclusion cannot be drawn at this stage. Similarly, among the few studies that looked at energy intake some found a positive relation with weight status in childhood [31], whereas other studies did not [32].

**Conclusions**

Because obesity is extremely difficult to treat, prevention is of paramount importance. Therefore, nutritional research is evaluating all critical periods of human obesity development during the life course, including the prenatal period, to identify appropriate and sound nutritional recommendations. Current developments, e.g. an increasing prevalence of overweight and obesity before and during pregnancy, inadequate weight gain in the majority of pregnancies, as well as restrained eating behavior during pregnancy, are additional challenges in this context. Overall, it appears that further data are needed to develop more elaborate recommendations for pregnant women, taking recent research findings into account. Adequate micronutrient intake to reduce low birth weight, and adequate macronutrient and energy intake to avoid macrosomia may have considerable preventive potential (fig. 2). However, so far, no optimal nutritional recommendations can be made with respect to the long-lasting effects of maternal nutrition as a determinant of the developmental origin of obesity [3]. Similarly, nutritional influences during early postnatal life appear to bear some potential for obesity risk reduction, with the most extensive research support for a preventive effect of breast-feeding. For other recommendations, e.g. carbohydrate modification or energy restriction, an adequate data base is lacking.

## References

1 Barker DJ, Winter PD, Osmond C, et al: Weight in infancy and death from ischaemic heart disease. Lancet 1989;ii:577–580.
2 Symonds ME, Pearce S, Bispham J, et al: Timing of nutrient restriction and programming of fetal adipose tissue development. Proc Nutr Soc 2004;63:397–403.
3 Gluckman PD, Hanson MA, Morton SM, Pinal CS: Life-long echoes – a critical analysis of the developmental origins of adult disease model. Biol Neonate 2005;87:127–139.
4 Wu G, Bazer FW, Cudd TA, et al: Maternal nutrition and fetal development. J Nutr 2004;134(9):2169–2172.
5 Waterland RA, Garza C: Potential mechanisms of metabolic imprinting that lead to chronic disease. Am J Clin Nutr 1999;69:179–197.
6 Holemans K, Aerts L, Van Assche FA: Fetal growth restriction and consequences for the offspring in animal models. J Soc Gynecol Investig 2003;10:392–399.
7 Loos RJ, Beunen G, Fagard R, et al: Birth weight and body composition in young women: a prospective twin study. Am J Clin Nutr 2002;75:676–682.
8 Drake AJ, Walker BR: The intergenerational effects of fetal programming: non-genomic mechanisms for the inheritance of low birth weight and cardiovascular risk. J Endocrinol 2004;180:1–16.
9 Rogers I: The influence of birthweight and intrauterine environment on adiposity and fat distribution in later life. Int J Obes Relat Metab Disord 2003;27:755–777.
10 Phillips DI: Relation of fetal growth to adult muscle mass and glucose tolerance. Diabet Med 1995;12:686–690.
11 Kahn HS, Narayan KM, Williamson DF, Valdez R: Relation of birth weight to lean and fat thigh tissue in young men. Int J Obes Relat Metab Disord 2000;24:667–672.
12 Gale CR, Martyn CN, Kellingray S, et al: Intrauterine programming of adult body composition. J Clin Endocrinol Metab 2001;86:267–272.
13 Singhal A, Wells J, Cole TJ, et al: Programming of lean body mass: a link between birth weight, obesity, and cardiovascular disease? Am J Clin Nutr 2003;77:726–730.
14 Sayer AA, Syddall HE, Dennison EM, et al: Birth weight, weight at 1 y of age, and body composition in older men: findings from the Hertfordshire Cohort Study. Am J Clin Nutr 2004;80:199–203.
15 Ravelli GP, Stein ZA, Susser MW: Obesity in young men after famine exposure in utero and early infancy. N Engl J Med 1976;295:349–353.
16 Ravelli AC, van Der Meulen JH, Osmond C, et al: Obesity at the age of 50 y in men and women exposed to famine prenatally. Am J Clin Nutr 1999;70:811–816.
17 Kramer MS, Kakuma R: Energy and protein intake in pregnancy. Cochrane Database Syst Rev 2003(4):CD000032.
18 Metges CC: Does dietary protein in early life affect the development of adiposity in mammals? J Nutr 2001;131:2062–2066.
19 Whitaker RC: Predicting preschooler obesity at birth: the role of maternal obesity in early pregnancy. Pediatrics 2004;114:e29–e36.
20 Bergmann KE, Bergmann RL, von Kries R, et al: Early determinants of childhood overweight and adiposity in a birth cohort study: role of breast-feeding. Int J Obes Relat Metab Disord 2003;27:162–172.

Kroke

21 Ramakrishnan U, Martorell R, Rivera J, et al: Micronutrients and pregnancy outcome: a review of the literature. Nutr Res 1999;19:103–159.
22 Fall CH, Yajnik CS, Rao S, et al: Micronutrients and fetal growth. J Nutr 2003;133(suppl 2): 1747S–1756S.
23 Merialdi M, Carroli G, Villar J, et al: Nutritional interventions during pregnancy for the prevention or treatment of impaired fetal growth: an overview of randomized controlled trials. J Nutr 2003;133(suppl 2):1626S–1631S.
24 Mathews F, Youngman L, Neil A: Maternal circulating nutrient concentrations in pregnancy: implications for birth and placental weights of term infants. Am J Clin Nutr 2004;79:103–110.
25 Mathews F, Yudkin P, Neil A: Influence of maternal nutrition on outcome of pregnancy: prospective cohort study. BMJ 1999;319:339–343.
26 Kramer MS: Do breast-feeding and delayed introduction of solid foods protect against subsequent obesity? J Pediatr 1981;98:883–887.
27 Arenz S, Ruckerl R, Koletzko B, von Kries R: Breast-feeding and childhood obesity – a systematic review. Int J Obes Relat Metab Disord 2004;28:1247–1256.
28 Dietz WH: Breastfeeding may help prevent childhood overweight. JAMA 2001;285: 2506–2507.
29 Marmot MG, Page CM, Atkins E, Douglas JW: Effect of breast-feeding on plasma cholesterol and weight in young adults. J Epidemiol Community Health 1980;34:164–167.
30 Parsons TJ, Power C, Manor O: Infant feeding and obesity through the lifecourse. Arch Dis Child 2003;88:793–794.
31 Stunkard AJ, Berkowitz RI, Schoeller D, et al: Predictors of body size in the first 2 y of life: a high-risk study of human obesity. Int J Obes Relat Metab Disord 2004;28:503–513.
32 Parsons TJ, Power C, Logan S, Summerbell CD: Childhood predictors of adult obesity: a systematic review. Int J Obes 1999;23(suppl 8):S1–S107.
33 Barker DJ: The developmental origins of adult disease. J Am Coll Nutr 2004;23(suppl): 588S–595S.
34 Cameron N, Demerath EW: Critical periods in human growth and their relationship to diseases of aging. Yearbook Phys Anthropol 2002;45:159–184.
35 Oken E, Gillman MW: Fetal origins of obesity. Obes Res 2003;11:496–506.
36 Singhal A, Farooqi IS, O'Rahilly S, et al: Early nutrition and leptin concentrations in later life. Am J Clin Nutr 2002;75:993–999.
37 Wu G, Bazer FW, Cudd TA, et al: Maternal nutrition and fetal development. J Nutr 2004;134: 2169–2172.
38 Yajnik CS: Obesity epidemic in India: intrauterine origins? Proc Nutr Soc 2004;63:387–396.
39 Martorell R, Stein AD, Schroeder DG: Early nutrition and alter adiposity. J Nutr 2001;131: 874S–880S.

## Discussion

*Dr. Singhal:* Do you really think that a 20% reduction in obesity with breastfeeding is a small effect, because I think that is a huge effect.

*Dr. Kroke:* I think it is a huge effect in childhood obesity but the effect on adult obesity remains to be quantified and it is going to be less than that.

*Dr. Singhal:* One of the things about the use of body mass index as an outcome is that it is influenced by both lean and fat mass. For example we have shown that birth weight correlates very closely with lean tissue mass but not with fat mass later in life. Do you think that this could explain some of the confounding factors that you see? Are there any data that have actually looked at lean and fat mass separately?

*Dr. Kroke:* Body mass index is clearly not a perfect indicator of body fatness and some, but few studies indicate that early life factors more strongly influence lean body mass than fat mass.

*Dr. Hanson:* In relation to the possible effect of breastfeeding on obesity I would like to ask you about two papers that seem to be related to this. One very recently was using siblings as controls and they did not see any effect of breastfeeding on obesity, and the other one is a large American study showing that the effect was seen in Whites but not so-called Hispanics or Blacks. Why is that, genetic differences or what?

*Dr. Kroke:* I would argue that risk factors are always acting in concert with other risk factors so their relative importance might change with the presence of other risk factors. Differences between risk of obesity in Blacks and Whites might be present, so the relative importance of breastfeeding might change according to that.

*Dr. Hanson:* Could it be dietary habits between these so-called racial groups that differed or could it be other factors? Could their diets be different to an extent that they made a difference?

*Dr. Kroke:* You mean the maternal diet?

*Dr. Hanson:* The mothers diet, yes.

*Dr. Kroke:* Yes, that could be an explanation.

*Dr. Lucas:* As I mentioned this morning the original animal data on programming had all to do with postnatal nutrition and so did the primate data, and so did the first human data experiments that were started in the early 1980s. A hypothesis to test at that stage, which was raised by the animal data, was that it was postnatal nutrition that influences later obesity. The fetal theory came very much later and as you pointed out it has probably not come to very convincingly related birth weight and maternal nutrition. The real hypothesis to test was the data that came from original studies showing that early nutrition made a major difference to later weight, and the first primate studies which showed the late emergence of a program defect on body fatness. Now this is particularly important in the interpretation of the human data because if we go back to the 20% effects of breastfeeding on later obesity, we shouldn't assume that this is actually going to melt away, this could actually become greater with time, it could amplify in a sense that the primate model, the best animal model we have, showed that the effects of early nutrition didn't actually emerge until adolescence and adult life, most of which has not been covered by the human studies. So I don't think we should necessarily be pessimistic. What we have is a very good story that early growth is highly related to later obesity risk, observationally we know that breastfed babies grow more slowly, we know they have got a 20% increased risk of obesity on a meta-analysis, and we might predict amplification in adolescence and adulthood. So I would be slightly less negative about the field.

*Dr. Kroke:* I didn't mean to be negative, I just wanted to point out that there are so many studies out there which are really difficult to interpret and that do not give us information or answers on this prenatal phase. There are data but still we are lacking studies that really work with adult outcomes so it is rather speculative what we can give at the moment, and I think it is important to have some data with outcomes as a basis for recommendations.

*Dr. Lucas:* I agree we are not ready for that.

*Dr. Cohen:* With respect to the breastfeeding cohort, mothers that breastfeed through the first year of life, what were the differences, if any, in terms of different end points for beginning the introduction of solid foods, for example those mothers that may have started at 3 versus 6 months or later in terms of the breastfeeding children and obesity later in life? Were there any differences?

*Dr. Kroke:* I didn't look at that issue, I don't know.

*Dr. Haschke:* I agree with Dr. Lucas that, when it comes to breastfeeding and later obesity, all studies are observational, and most didn't have the relation between early feeding and later fatness in the primary outcome variable. So the design of those studies which have been analyzed in the meta-analysis differed but none of these studies was really designed to answer the question. The only study which had the goal to look at this was the Eurogrowth study which was done in 12 European cities. It went until 5 years of age, and there was definitely no effect of breastfeeding on body mass index until 5 years of age. However, there was always a significant impact of birth weight or body mass index at birth or 1 month of age, and there was a significant impact of mid-parental body mass index, and once these two variables were in the equation everything else disappeared. The influence of breastfeeding was there until 12–18 months of age and it disappeared. When we analyzed the Eurogrowth study according to developed growth charts for breastfed infants as a subgroup it was only necessary to do this until 18 months of age. Then there was no difference between the two cohorts. At least there were 1,500 infants which were followed up so I would doubt whether the association is so clear.

*Dr. Steenhout:* We know that infants from diabetic or obese mothers or from mothers who develop gestational diabetes are more at risk of developing obesity later in life. Have you found studies showing that, in those circumstances, breastfeeding is also protective? As those groups are at higher risk of developing obesity, probably they are also better subgroups to analyze the potential protective effect of breastfeeding. What is your opinion?

*Dr. Kroke:* I am actually not aware of any study that worked with diabetic mothers and then did a follow-up of breastfeeding or type of feeding later on. I would assume that if there is a potential effect of breastfeeding this also has to be found in children that are born macrosomic or that are born to diabetic mothers.

*Dr. Sorensen:* I really know very little about obesity but there is an anecdotal observation that my specialists tell me. When I ask them can we do something in the first year of life? Can we identify children in the first year of life, regardless of how they are fed, that are on the heavier weight side and will continue into obesity? Their observation is that some of those very chubby children, without any intervention, suddenly by age 1 or 2 become perfectly normal, and that is also a perception in the public and it makes it difficult to tell parents that their 6- or 8-month-old is way overweight. They say well, many children in our family were like this and they are fine. While others never stop being on the heavy side. This is totally anecdotal but I just would like to ask you if there is any basis to having two populations, two different ways of going on from very early onset overweight, some that are seen without any intervention and others that actually become obese children?

*Dr. Kroke:* I think this goes into the discussion that we had before on rapid growth and early childhood. There are children who grow fast in the first 1 or 2 years of life, crossing centiles, and remain like this, but there also seem to be children who are similarly fat but remain within their centiles and never cross the line to obesity. So yes, I think we could call them different populations, we know that the predictive value of this risk factor is never 100% so you have just a relative increase in risk of 30–40%; it never explains the entire observation. I think there are no means at the moment to differentiate population subgroups, let's say those with catch-up growth or rapid growth during childhood plus factor X and X and X, they have almost 90 or 100% probability of developing obesity whereas just having been fat during the period without these additional factors that does not have any effect. It could be a way to proceed and to try to do that.

*Dr. Klish:* Just to follow up your comments. In the 1970s I know of at least one paper that implied that the weight of a child below 12 months of age had no correlation to their weight as an adult. That concept has become fixed in pediatrics for many years. I know there have been studies that have shown that this impact does persist. Have you found recent data that correlate infant weight to the ultimate adult weight?

*Dr. Kroke:* The most reliable data on that issue are weight at age 7 as being most predictive of adult BMI, not earlier weight, because there is so much going on in terms of changes that this does not seem to be as predictive as at age 7. But as I said, birth weight is also related to adult BMI, the question is just how strong that association is.

*Dr. Klish:* I think this comes up frequently as a clinical issue. I tell the parents of infants who are rapidly gaining weight to start dieting or restricting during infancy if the infants are significantly above the 95th percentile for weight for height.

*Dr. Maffeis:* You said that there is a relationship between birth weight and BMI in childhood, but you also said that the BMI of the mother is able to negate the effect of birth weight. However, there are some data in the literature suggesting that the relationship between birth weight is maintained if you adjust for the BMI of the mother. Can you comment on this finding?

*Dr. Kroke:* There was just one study from the UK that said that the relation disappears if you adjust for maternal BMI, just to illustrate that there are many questions around this relation. I am not surprised that somebody else found just the opposite, it is just to make the point that we are clearly in a very vague association here that has been described.

*Dr. Laron:* Could you say something about the correlation between brain growth and body growth during early intervention, because we know that in utero it is the brain which is so sensitive and which is relatively larger than other parts of the body?

*Dr. Kroke:* Actually no, I am not an expert in brain and neural development.

*Dr. Laron:* Do the Cochrane reviews mention the influence of various nutrients on the brain versus other growing parts of the body?

*Dr. Kroke:* These studies mainly assessed pregnancy and birth-related clinical outcomes, so they don't even have something like head circumference available which one could use as a proxy for whatever is going on with the brain. Unfortunately there is nothing available, and in a very few cases only there is a follow-up of these children with this intervention. So I cannot give you an answer to that.

Lucas A, Sampson HA (eds): Primary Prevention by Nutrition Intervention in Infancy and Childhood.
Nestlé Nutr Workshop Ser Pediatr Program, vol 57, pp 67–80,
Nestec Ltd., Vevey/S. Karger AG, Basel, © 2006.

# Childhood Diabetes Mellitus with Emphasis on Perinatal Factors

*Zvi Laron*

Endocrinology and Diabetes Research Unit, Schneider Children's Medical Center,
Petah Tikva, and Sackler School of Medicine, Tel Aviv University, Israel

## Background

Diabetes mellitus (DM) is an ancient syndrome described by Aetios in Greece approximately 500 AD and by Chang Chung-Ching in China around 200 AD. From available information it seems that the incidence of diabetes was low for centuries. In the last half-century technological advances have enabled on one hand a better understanding of the underlying causes but, on the other hand, together with changes in lifestyle there has been a dramatic increase in the incidence of DM [1].

## Definition

Childhood DM is a group of endocrine and metabolic diseases characterized by hyperglycemia resulting from absolute or relative insulin deficiency. Chronic hyperglycemia induces a series of metabolic abnormalities which with time cause various organ failures due to micro- or macrovascular complications and a shortened life span. Improved therapy postpones but cannot prevent these complications and prolongs life.

## Classification

DM can be divided into two great categories: (1) insulin deficiency to absence, and (2) insulin resistance which may lead to β-cell exhaustion and thus both types may need insulin replacement therapy. Table 1 presents an etiologic classification of DM. Some types are very rare in childhood (pancreas

**Table 1.** Etiologic classification of childhood diabetes mellitus (DM)

| | | |
|---|---|---|
| I | Type-1 DM (autoimmune β-cell destruction) | |
| II | Type-2 DM (from insulin resistance to insulin deficiency) | |
| III | Genetic types | |
| | a | Neonatal DM (transient or permanent) |
| | b | MODY types (6 different molecular defects) |
| | c | Mitochondrial DNA |
| | d | Insulin receptor defects (severe insulin resistance) |
| IV | Exocrine pancreas disease (cystic fibrosis, trauma, etc.) | |
| V | Endocrinopathies | |
| | a | Cushing's syndrome |
| | b | Pheochromocytoma |
| | c | Hyperthyroidism |
| VI | Drugs | |
| | a | Glucocorticoids |
| | b | Growth hormone |
| | c | Diazoxide |
| | d | Dilantin |
| VII | Associates with syndromes: | |
| | Wolfram, Down, Klinefelter, Turner's, Prader-Willi, Friedreich's ataxia, Roger, Alstrom, Wolcott-Rallison, etc. | |

**Table 2.** Diabetes mellitus of genetic origin

| | |
|---|---|
| 1 | PDX1 (IPF1) mutation causes pancreas hyperplasia and type-2 DM |
| 2 | HNF-4α (MODY1), chromosome 20 |
| 3 | Glucokinase (MODY2), chromosome 7 |
| 4 | HNF-1α (MODY3), chromosome 12 |
| 5 | Insulin-promoter factor-1 (MODY4), chromosome 12 |
| 6 | HNF-1β (MODY5), chromosome 17 |
| 7 | *NeurDI* (MODY6), chromosome 2 |
| 8 | Mitochondrial DNA |

agenesis; mitochondrial DNA mutations), others are rare at any age (association with chromosomal or rare genetic disorders), or develop the clinical symptoms in adult age despite being of genetic origin (MODY types), gestational diabetes, etc. [2] (table 2). The following is a review of present evidence that environmental factors cause the development of type-1 or type-2 diabetes in the perinatal period.

## Childhood Type-1 Diabetes Mellitus

Childhood type-1 DM (CT1DM) is an autoimmune disease which, if triggered in a genetically susceptible subject, induces a progressive process

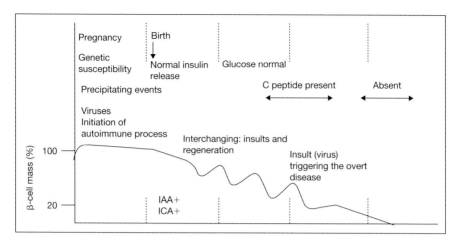

**Fig. 1.** Natural course of autoimmune childhood diabetes mellitus (CT1DM).

which, depending on the frequency and force of subsequent insults, develops into clinical diabetes once 70–80% of the pancreatic β cells are destroyed. This process can last months in babies to years in older children (fig. 1). The exact mechanism of the autoimmune process is not completely known, but in its course results in insulin autoantibodies (IAAs), anti-islet cell antibodies (ICAs) and glutamic acid decarboxylase isoform 65 antibodies (GADs), etc. [3]. Type-1 DM is often associated in the same child with celiac disease (CD; see below), with thyroiditis or Graves disease or even autoimmune gastritis [4]. These autoimmune diseases may appear before or after the clinical diagnosis of diabetes.

*Epidemiology*

Validated registers for childhood diabetes (CT1DM) were started in 1965 in 4 countries (USA, Finland, Japan, Israel) by the Diabetes Epidemiology Research International [2]. When other countries and regions followed, it became evident that there were great differences in incidence between countries and ethnic groups, and that the incidence of CT1DM was progressively increasing. Starting in the 1980s the rise accelerated steeply [2] even in children below age 5. As genetic factors did not change, it was concluded that environmental factors were involved, seemingly connected to changes in lifestyle [3]. Toxic substances (nitrate in water, pesticides used in agriculture) could not be blamed for the worldwide rise. Immunological studies have clearly shown that the autoimmune process and onset of CT1DM can begin early in life. The two most possible culprits for the initiation of this process focused on viral infections and nutrition.

***Table 3.*** Environmental factors involved in the etiology of autoimmune type-1 diabetes mellitus

| Class | Specific agent |
|---|---|
| Viruses | Enteroviruses |
| | Coxsackie B |
| | Rubella (congenital) |
| | Mumps |
| | Rotoviruses |
| | Cytomegalovirus |
| | Echo |
| | Encephalomyocarditis |
| | Epstein-Barr |
| Nutritional | Cow's milk and cow's milk-based infant formulas |
| | Duration of breastfeeding |
| | Nitrates (N-nitroso compounds) |
| | Bafilomycin A1 |
| Life-style | Exposure to β-cell toxins (e.g. Vacor) |

*Evidence for the Viral Etiology of Type-1 Diabetes*

Analyzing the register in Israel, a country with several ethnic groups, we observed that in the Jewish population with a higher incidence of CT1DM the children and adolescents who subsequently developed the disease had a different seasonality in month of birth than the general population [5]. Subsequent studies in several countries and various populations in 4 continents confirmed these observations [6]. The interpretation of these data is that children conceived in the fall or winter during virus epidemics start to develop the anti-β-cell autoimmune process already in utero [7] or perinatally, and subsequently pathogenic agents, causing further damage or enhancing the autoimmune process, lead to the clinical disease [8].

Viruses can cause β-cell damage and HLA alleles which determine the risk for type-1 DM (such as HLA-DR3) modulate the clinical course of many virus infections [9].

The evidence for a link between virus infections and type-1 DM has been obtained from congenital rubella, mumps and enteroviruses, especially coxsackie B outbreaks (table 3). Further examples are the finding of enterovirus RNA in twins who developed CT1DM at age 14 months [10]. Echovirus was also isolated from a child at the onset of diabetes [11] and enterovirus was isolated from the pancreatic islets of some diabetic patients [12].

Mothers with virus infections can transmit the virus to the fetus in utero or by breast milk to the newborn. In case the fetus or baby is genetically susceptible to CT1DM, the pathogenic virus will initiate an autoimmune disease, in this case CT1DM. On the other hand if the mother transmits antiviral antibodies to the susceptible fetus or baby, it will be protected from the pathogenic action of these viruses [13].

Infections and the development of immunization by antibody formation are more common in crowded, non-hygienic conditions, such as more often encountered in lower economic classes. This may possibly explain the lower incidence of CT1DM in underdeveloped countries than in developed ones with a high degree of hygiene [14]. This hypothesis is in line with a recent multi-country study including our group which revealed that a low frequency of enterovirus infections in the background populations would increase the susceptibility of young children to the diabetogenic effect of enteroviruses [15].

*Does Vaccination Affect the Incidence of Type-1 DM?*
On the basis of ecologic evaluations it has been claimed that vaccination as such and its timing are associated with an increased risk of type-1 DM 2–4 years after vaccination [16]. This could not be confirmed [17] but deserves further investigations as vaccinations may be associated with the etiology of autoimmune diseases in general [18, 19].

*Nutritional Risk Factors in the Development of*
*Children with Type-1 DM*
The nutritional risk factors possibly involved with the initiation of type-1 DM has been recently reviewed [20]. A much-discussed issue is that of the role of cow's milk (CM) proteins. Increased concentrations of IgA-class β-lactoglobulin and IgA CM formula antibodies were related to an increased risk of CT1DM [21, 22]. There was also a direct correlation between milk consumption and CM antibodies [22] and risk for CT1DM [23], however these findings remain controversial. To clarify the issue whether indeed CM proteins are a risk factor for type-1 DM in early infancy and whether breast-feeding confers protection [24], an international prospective study was initiated.

*The TRIGR Study*
The TRIGR (Trial to reduce type-1 DM in the genetically at risk) study started October 2001. Inclusion criteria was a first-degree family member with type-1 DM and DR3/4. DQB1*G362, etc., genotype). The plan is to randomize 2,800 of 6,220 infants screened. Source of candidates are medical centers in 15 countries (12 in Europe; main source Finland, Sweden and Poland) and USA (3 centers). The test formulas are casein hydrolysate (Nutramigen[TM], Mead Johnson) not containing antigenic CM protein, or a CM protein formula with a 20% addition of Nutramigen. The intervention is at least age 6 months. If breastfed, 2 additional months of test formula are advised. In addition to the genotyping at birth, serum for ICA, IAA, GAD, CM antibodies and glucose as well as the clinical state are being registered at 3, 6, 9, 12, 18 and 24 months and yearly up to 10 years of age. This study is also expected to provide information on effects of autoreactive T cells and cytokine repertoires related to infant feeding.

The fact that the results of the genetic screening are disclosed to the family is prone to induce long-lasting anxiety, and may have negative effects if leaked to insurance companies, future employers, etc.

## Association between CT1DM and CD

Ziegler et al. [25] from the BABYDIAB study in Germany and Norris et al. [26] from the DAISY (Diabetes Autoimmunity Study of the Young) study in the US present a link between early infant nutrition and the development of autoantibodies against the pancreatic β cells. Both studies suggest that the age at which an infant is fed cereal is important in determining the risk for CT1DM. These studies fail to support the CM hypothesis but associate type-1 DM with CD.

CD is a chronic inflammatory autoimmune disease of the gut induced by gliadin (gluten) or prolamin proteins present in wheat, barley and rye. Upon digestion gliadin is deaminated by transglutaminase [27]. Genetically susceptible subjects develop autoreactive T lymphocytes which cause injury to the small bowel mucosa characterized by crypt hyperplasia and partial or complete atrophy of intestinal villi [28] as well as other organ damage. The frequency of CD in the general population of Europe and North America ranges between 0.4 and 1% [29].

CD and type-1 DM are both autoimmune diseases which share common major histocompatibility antigens (HLA). The association between the two diseases is well established. About 1/20 children with CT1DM have CD and approximately 1/10 express antitransglutaminase autoantibodies and half of these (1/20) have CD proven by biopsy [30]. Of note is that patients with CD who develop T-cell lymphomas express the HLA-DR3/4 genotype [31] so characteristic for CT1DM. The association between CD and CT1DM has both academic and also practical aspects [32]. In most instances the diagnosis of CD is made after the clinical diagnosis of CT1DM [33, 34]. As digestive abnormalities have a negative influence on diabetes control, some clinics propose screening all children with CT1DM for CD (serum for IgA, TG) on a regular basis [35].

Also the inverse procedure has been proposed as in one study 23% of the patients with CD have been found to have GAD and 1A-2 antibodies heralding future type-1 DM [36]. It was also reported that when CD is diagnosed before type-1 DM the clinical onset of the latter is severe with a high prevalence of DKA [37].

In a recent study we found that similar to childhood-onset type-1 DM in homogenous populations [6], subjects with CD have a different seasonality of month of birth than the general population (Lewy et al., submitted) which is again suggestive that the autoimmune onset of disease is during the perinatal period and possibly of viral origin. Considering the high grade associations between the two autoimmune diseases (similarity in genetic background, possible etiologic interrelation, or even a common trigger) led to investigations as to whether a gluten-free diet in infancy can prevent the development of CT1DM [25] as was found to be possible in NOD mice [38]. So far, the experience in humans is not encouraging [39, 40]. Could better results be obtained by starting a gluten-free diet in mothers with type-1 DM before or during pregnancy?

### Possible Role of Vitamin D in the Autoimmune Process

In animal models the active form of vitamin D (1,25-dihydroxyvitamin D) prevents diabetes and other autoimmune diseases [41]. Use of vitamin D supplementation during infancy in a European case-control study (The EURODIAB Study, 1999), and the addition of cod liver oil during the first year of life in Norway, lowered the risk of CT1DM [42], however, augmentation of the vitamin D supplementation to 2,000 IU/day in Finland did not prevent the increase in incidence.

### Attempts to Cure, or Late Prevention Trials of CT1DM

At present there is no cure available or in sight. Trials with tertiary prevention (stopping the disease at clinical diagnosis) including nonspecific immunosuppression with cyclosporine or secondary prevention by nicotinamide (ENDIT trial) and insulin (DPT-1 and 2 trials) have failed [43, 44], so has the trial with DiaPep277 (a synthetic peptide of 65 heat shock protein) which gave negative results in children [45]. This peptide when combined with a hydrolyzed casein diet protected BB rats against type-1 DM [46]. Segmental or pancreatic islet cell transplantation, even if successful, has a time-limited effect and bears serious complications [47] including life-long immunosuppressive therapy. All the above interventions target both the autoreactive T cells as well as the 'good' T cells, which compromise the immune function of the patient. Also new research on stem cell therapy may not necessarily lead to the most suitable tissue for transplantation [48].

### Gene Therapy

Not having found any specific gene linked to type-1 DM, this therapy is at present not feasible. On the other hand, investigations to deliver genes of somatic (non-pancreatic) insulin-secreting cells are being performed [49], but how to control the metabolic responses of transgenic cells is a problem.

## Childhood Type-2 Diabetes Mellitus

Type-2 DM is a complex metabolic-endocrine disorder of heterogeneous etiology with different genetic backgrounds (table 1). Some forms, such as that caused by obesity and insulin resistance or parental diabetes and that linked to perinatal environmental factors have been found to have an increasing prevalence in the last half-century [50]. To adapt to the present symposium only the forms with proven, or suspected in utero, or perinatal etiology will be reviewed.

Numerous studies have reported that the offspring of mothers with type-2 DM are more likely to develop obesity, childhood type-2 DM (CT2DM), or impaired glucose tolerance at an earlier age than the offspring of fathers with diabetes. Studies in Pima Indians suggested that the increase in childhood type-2 DM can be attributed to the diabetic intrauterine environment [51] independent of the genetic predisposition [52]. More subtle is the link between high birth weight and increased risk for future obesity and glucose intolerance [53] in non-diabetic mothers.

The following observations need special attention. In 1992 Hales and Barker [54] proposed the hypothesis that one of the major consequences of poor fetal and early postnatal nutrition is impaired development of the endocrine pancreas and a greatly increased susceptibility to the development of type-2 DM. Series of large studies in the US [55], in Sweden [56] and India [57] show that with a decreasing birth weight, birth length and placental weight there is an increase in future development of type-2 DM.

The mechanisms involved are not completely clear but certainly affect the liver and muscle metabolic disturbances with subsequent slowly progressing development from childhood to adult age of insulin resistance, glucose intolerance, hyperlipidemia and even cardiovascular disease. Of interest also is the observation that children who were born prematurely have an isolated reduction in insulin sensitivity which is a risk factor for type-2 DM [58]. Thus also type-2 DM may be preprogrammed in utero possibly caused by intrauterine malnutrition.

*Prevention of Type-2 DM*

Postnatal nutrition is modifiable by education and so is a change in lifestyle. Both methods could reduce the incidence of obesity, and resulting hyperinsulinism, hyperlipidemia and the development of type-2 DM with its complications. Theoretically this is easy but less so in practice. How to prevent or treat intrauterine growth retardation and/or malnutrition is largely unknown. Improved metabolic control of pregnant mothers with DM may improve, but not abolish the subsequent complications. Better control of in vitro fertilization and a reduction in multiple pregnancies may be a positive measure. But what of the premature infant with appropriate or low weight for gestational age? And what about the malnourished mother due to illness or low economic class? One needs to learn more about the postnatal adaptive mechanisms of intrauterine, metabolic and endocrine restrictions. Is adiponectin the culprit [59]? Only long-term follow-up will demonstrate whether prenatal treatment of intrauterine growth restriction [60] and present neonatal intensive care of premature babies is sufficient to deliver healthy children and healthy adults.

## Conclusions

We are at present confronted with a continuous and worldwide increase in incidence of both CT1DM as well as CT2DM, the first possibly linked to improved hygiene [61, 62] and changes in nutrition acting in the perinatal period. Type-2 DM increases due to intrauterine conditions but mostly due to postnatal changes in lifestyle involving nutrition, and lack of physical exercise leading to obesity, insulin resistance and its exhaustion.

As CT1DM secondary intervention trials have proven to be ineffective [43, 44] only primary prevention is the hope [62]. Is immunization of mothers before or during pregnancy the solution [13]? Immunizations against which virus? Exclusive long-term breastfeeding? Prevention of CT2DM can be envisioned by preventing or early treatment of obesity and increasing energy expenditure. Is this feasible in a modern media-dominated society? New strategies are needed [63]. As animal models do not provide the complete and sometimes not the right answer [64], this is a difficult task.

## References

1 Laron Z: Childhood diabetes towards the 21st century. J Pediatr Endocrinol Metab 1998;11: 387–402.
2 Porter JR, Barrett TG: Acquired non-type 1 diabetes in childhood: subtypes, diagnosis, and management. Arch Dis Child 2004;89:1138–1144.
3 Pietropaolo M, Peakman M, Pietropaolo SL, et al: Combined analysis of GAD65 and ICA512(IA-2) autoantibodies in organ and non-organ-specific autoimmune diseases confers high specificity for insulin-dependent diabetes mellitus. J Autoimmun 1998;11:1–10.
4 Lam-Tse W-K, Batstra MR, Koeleman BPC, et al: The association between autoimmune thyroiditis, autoimmune gastritis and Type 1 diabetes. Pediatr Endocrinol Rev 2003;1:22–36.
5 Laron Z , Shamis I, Nitzan-Kaluski D, Ashkenazi I: Month of birth and subsequent development of type 1 diabetes (IDDM). J Pediatr Endocrinol Metab 1999;12:397–402.
6 Laron Z, Lewy L, Shamis I, et al: Seasonality of month of birth of children and adolescents with type 1 diabetes mellitus in homogenous and heterogenous populations. Isr Med Assoc J 2005; in press.
7 Laron Z: Does childhood diabetes start in utero? Riv Ital Pediatr 2001;27:597.
8 Laron Z: Lessons from recent epidemiological studies in type 1 childhood diabetes. J Pediatr Endocrinol Metab 1999;12(suppl 3):733–736.
9 Hyoty H: Environmental causes: viral causes. Endocrinol Metab Clin North Am 2004;33: 27–44.
10 Smith CP, Clements GB, Riding MH, et al: Simultaneous onset of type 1 diabetes mellitus in identical infant twins with enterovirus infection. Diabet Med 1998;15:515–517.
11 Diaz-Horta O, Bello M, Cabrera-Rode E, et al: Echovirus 4 and type 1 diabetes mellitus. Autoimmunity 2001;34:275–281.
12 Yoon JW, Austin M, Onodera T, Notkins AL: Isolation of a virus from the pancreas of a child with diabetic ketoacidosis. N Engl J Med 1979;300:1173–1179.
13 Vicari M, Dodet B, Englund J: Protection of newborns through maternal immunization. Vaccine 2003;21:3351.
14 Robinson R: The protective effect of childhood infections. BMJ 2001;322:376–377.
15 Viskari H, Ludvigsson J, Uibo R, et al: Relationship between the incidence of type 1 diabetes and maternal enterovirus antibodies – time trends and geographical variation. Diabetologia 2005; in press.

16  Classen B: Clustering of cases of type 1 diabetes mellitus occurring 2–4 years after vaccination is consistent with clustering after infections and progression to type 1 diabetes mellitus in autoantibody positive individuals. J Pediatr Endocrinol Metab 2003;16:495–508.
17  Hviid A, Stellfeld M, Wohlfahrt J, Melbye M: Childhood vaccination and type 1 diabetes. N Engl J Med 2004;350:1398–1404.
18  Wraith DC, Goldman M, Lambert PH: Vaccination and autoimmune disease: what is the evidence? Lancet 2003;362:1659–1666.
19  Tishler M, Shoenfeld Y: Vaccination may be associated with autoimmune diseases. Isr Med Assoc J 2004;6:430–435.
20  Virtanen SM, Knip M: Nutritional risk predictors of β cell autoimmunity and type 1 diabetes at a young age. Am J Clin Nutr 2003;78:1053–1067.
21  Dahlquist G, Savilahti E, Landin-Olsson M: An increased level of antibodies to beta-lactoglobulin is a risk determinant for early-onset type 1 (insulin-dependent) diabetes mellitus independent of islet cell antibodies and early introduction of cow's milk. Diabetologia 1992;35:980–984.
22  Virtanen SM, Saukkonen T, Savilahti E, et al: Diet, cow's milk protein antibodies and the risk of IDDM in Finnish children: Childhood Diabetes in Finland Study Group. Diabetologia 1994;37:381–387.
23  Verge CF, Howard NJ, Irwig L, et al: Environmental factors in childhood IDDM. Diabetes Care 1994;17:1381–1389.
24  Mayer EJ, Hamman RF, Gay EC, et al: Reduced risk of IDDM among breast-fed children: The Colorado IDDM Registry. Diabetes 1988;37:1625–1632.
25  Ziegler AG, Schmid S, Huber D, et al: Early infant feeding and risk of developing type 1 diabetes-associated autoantibodies. JAMA 2003;290:1721–1728.
26  Norris JM, Barriga K, Klingensmith G, et al: Timing of initial cereal exposure in infancy and risk of islet autoimmunity. JAMA 2003;290:1713–1720.
27  Arentz-Hansen H, Korner R, Molberg O, et al: The intestinal T cell response to alpha-gliadin in adult celiac disease is focused on a single deamidated glutamine targeted by tissue transglutaminase. J Exp Med 2000;191:603–612.
28  Marsh MN: Mucosal pathology in gluten sensitivity; in Marsh MN (ed): Coeliac Disease. Oxford, Blackwell, 1992, pp 136–191.
29  Hoffenberg EJ, MacKenzie T, Barriga KJ, et al: A prospective study of the incidence of childhood celiac disease. J Pediatr 2003;143:308–314.
30  Hummel M, Bonifacio E, Stern M, et al: Development of celiac disease-associated antibodies in offspring of parents with Type 1 diabetes. Diabetologia 2000;43:1005–1011.
31  Catassi C, Fabiani E, Corrao G, et al: Italian Working Group on Coeliac Disease and Non-Hodgkin's-Lymphoma: Disease and non-Hodgkin's-lymphoma. Risk of non-Hodgkin lymphoma in celiac disease. JAMA 2002;287:1413–1419.
32  Pocecco M, Ventura A: Coeliac disease and insulin-dependent diabetes mellitus: a causal association? Acta Paediatr 1995;84:1432–1433.
33  Hansen D, Bennedbaek FN, Hansen LK, et al: High prevalence of coeliac disease in Danish children with type I diabetes mellitus. Acta Paediatr 2001;90:1238–1243.
34  Barera G, Bonfanti R, Viscardi M, et al: Occurrence of celiac disease after onset of type 1 diabetes: a 6-year prospective longitudinal study. Pediatrics 2002;109:833–838.
35  Rewers M, Liu E, Simmons J, et al: Celiac disease associated with type 1 diabetes mellitus. Endocrinol Metab Clin N Am 2004;33:197–214.
36  Galli-Tsinopoulou A, Nousia-Arvanitakis S, Dracoulacos D, et al: Autoantibodies predicting diabetes mellitus type I in celiac disease. Horm Res 1999;52:119–124.
37  Valerio G, Maiuri L, Troncone R, et al: Severe clinical onset of diabetes and increased prevalence of other autoimmune diseases in children with coeliac disease diagnosed before diabetes mellitus. Diabetologia 2002;45:1719–1722.
38  Funda DP, Kaas A, Bock T, et al: Gluten-free diet prevents diabetes in NOD mice. Diabetes Metab Res Rev 1999;15:323–327.
39  Hummel M, Bonifacio E, Naserke HE, Ziegler AG: Elimination of dietary gluten does not reduce titers of type 1 diabetes-associated autoantibodies in high-risk subjects. Diabetes Care 2002;25:1111–1116.
40  Pastore MR, Bazzigaluppi E, Belloni C, et al: Six months of gluten-free diet do not influence autoantibody titers, but improve insulin secretion in subjects at high risk for type 1 diabetes. J Clin Endocrinol Metab 2003;88:162–165.

41 Cantorna MT: Vitamin D and autoimmunity: is vitamin D status an environmental factor affecting autoimmune disease prevalence? Proc Soc Exp Biol Med 2000;223:230–233.
42 Stene LC, Joner G, the Norwegian Childhood Diabetes Study Group: Use of cod liver oil during the first year of life is associated with lower risk of childhood-onset type 1 diabetes: a large, population-based, case-control study. Am J Clin Nutr 2003;78:1128–1134.
43 Gale EAM: Can we change the course of beta-cell destruction in type 1 diabetes? N Engl J Med 2002;346:1740–1742.
44 Greenbaum CJ: Type 1 diabetes intervention trials: what have we learned? A critical review of selected intervention trials. Clin Immunol 2002;104:97–104.
45 Cohen I: Peptide therapy for type I diabetes: the immunological homunculus and the rationale for vaccination. Diabetologia 2002;45:1468–1474.
46 Brugman S, Klatter FA, Visser J, et al: Neonatal oral administration of DiaPep277, combined with hydrolysed casein diet, protects against Type 1 diabetes in BB-DP rats: an experimental study. Diabetologia 2004;47:1331–1333.
47 Ryan EA, Lakey JR, Paty BW, et al: Successful islet transplantation: continued insulin reserve provides long-term glycemic control. Diabetes 2002;51:2148–2157.
48 Burns CJ, Persaud SJ, Jones PM: Stem cell therapy for diabetes: do we need to make beta cells? J Endocrinol 2004;183:437–443.
49 Ber I, Shternhall K, Perl S, et al: Functional, persistent, and extended liver to pancreas transdifferentiation. J Biol Chem 2003;278:31950–31957.
50 Hotu S, Carter B, Watson PD, et al: Increasing prevalence of type 2 diabetes in adolescents. J Paediatr Child Health 2004;40:201–204.
51 Dabelea D, Pettitt DJ: Intrauterine diabetic environment confers risks for type 2 diabetes and obesity in the offspring, in addition to genetic susceptibility. J Pediatr Endocrinol Metab 2001;14:1085–1091.
52 Sobngwi E, Boudou P, Mauvais-Jarvis F, et al: Effect of a diabetic environment in utero on predisposition to type 2 diabetes. Lancet 2003;361:1861–1865.
53 Catalano PM, Thomas A, Huston-Presley L, Amini SB: Increased fetal adiposity: a very sensitive marker of abnormal in utero development. Am J Obstet Gynecol 2003;189:1698–1704.
54 Hales CN, Barker JP: Type 2 (non-insulin-dependent) diabetes mellitus: the thrifty phenotype hypothesis. Diabetologia 1992;35:595–601.
55 Rich-Edwards JW, Colditz GA, Stampfer MJ, et al: Birthweight and the risk for type 2 diabetes mellitus in adult women. Ann Intern Med 1999;130:278–284.
56 Iliadou A, Cnattingius S, Lichtenstein P: Low birthweight and Type 2 diabetes: a study on 11 162 Swedish twins. Int J Epidemiol 2004;33:948–953.
57 Yajnik CS: Early life origins of insulin resistance and type 2 diabetes in India and other Asian countries. J Nutr 2004;134:205–210.
58 Hofman PL, Regan F, Jackson WE, et al: Premature birth and later insulin resistance. N Engl J Med 2004;351:2179–2186.
59 Wang H, Zhang H, Jia Y, et al: Adiponectin receptor 1 gene (ADIPOR1) as a candidate for type 2 diabetes and insulin resistance. Diabetes 2004;53:2132–2136.
60 Harding JE, Bloomfield FH: Prenatal treatment of intrauterine growth restriction: lessons from the sheep model. Pediatr Endocrinol Rev 2004;2:182–192.
61 Kolb H, Elliott RB: Increasing incidence of IDDM a consequence of improved hygiene? (Letter). Diabetologia 1994;37:729.
62 Weiss ST: Eat dirt – the hygiene hypothesis and allergic diseases. N Engl J Med 2002;347:930–931.
63 Roep BO, Atkinson M: Animal models have little to teach us about type 1 diabetes: 1. In support of this proposal. Diabetologia 2004;47:1650–1656.
64 Vinicor F, Bowman B, Engelgau M: Diabetes: prevention needed. Lancet 2003;361:544.

## Discussion

*Dr. Björkstén:* I have a comment and a question. I would caution against delayed introduction of a gluten-free diet in infancy. I think we have a scary example from Sweden where the routine was not to introduce gluten until after 6 months of age and we observed an extreme incidence of celiac disease. Then by changing the practice and introducing gluten gradually at an earlier age we got back to normal figures. With that experience it is close to unethical to delay the introduction.

*Dr. Laron:* I have no personal experience other than the knowledge of the relationship between celiac disease and type-1 diabetes. We are looking into further relationships and I can tell you that we are writing a paper showing that also patients with multiple sclerosis (MS) present the same epidemiological changes, i.e. a different seasonality of month of birth than the general population [1]. We are looking into what may be a common denominator linking these diseases, probably viruses, but I don't know whether as you said a gluten-free diet is the reply.

*Dr. Björkstén:* That brings me to my question. There are many similarities in the epidemiology of type-1 diabetes and childhood allergies. You can almost superimpose the increases in diabetes and IgE-mediated allergy on a log scale. So what is known regarding the induction of T-regulatory function in diabetes?

*Dr. Laron:* It is known that we have a change from T cells type 1 and there was the Peptor protein trial to switch T1 over to T2 cells. There is no question that a cytokine process is going on. We are just now starting also to study atopic dermatitis to find out the month of birth epidemiology.

*Dr. Björkstén:* The major driving factor for induction of normal immune regulation is actually the colonization of the gut microbiota, whether that has an impact for diabetes is a hypothesis, however. But I would like to draw your attention to a very interesting study that was done in Melbourne. If you raise mice of a strain that will develop autoimmune disease, as adults under germ-free conditions, they die from fulminant diabetes. The story is similar to what I am going to discuss about allergies. I am therefore wondering whether some of the dietary issues that you brought up are related to the normal colonization of the gut microbiota?

*Dr. Laron:* I think we have to look a little bit further in order find out what the cause is and what the effect is. We really do not know what starts it and at what stage things happen. However there is a relationship, there is no question that type-1 diabetes is an strong ongoing autoimmune process. The late change in this immune process has not succeeded so far, so my idea is that only prevention or very early intervention might be helpful. The allergy process or immune process is perhaps like the kidney stone story, you take it out but it will come again, the 'anlage' is there, and the same thing may happen if we are too late to intervene in the immune process that destroys the β cells and probably also other organs like the thyroid.

*Dr. Klish:* I have also heard similar arguments for inflammatory bowel disease, which has some similarities to all this.

*Dr. Hamburger:* Are you familiar with any studies on probiotics related to the onset of type-1 diabetes?

*Dr. Laron:* No.

*Dr. Björkstén:* Yes, there are ongoing studies both in Finland and Sweden.

*Dr. Laron:* I would appreciate the opinion of the audience as to whether early intervention, meaning during pregnancy in the mother, might influence the perinatal immune process.

*Dr. Björkstén:* We don't know that yet. It has been tried but not systematically and pre- and postnatal interventions haven't been separated properly. There are studies going on in germ-free animals but it is very difficult to answer that question in human studies.

*Dr. Sorensen:* I had a lot of trouble following your hypothesis to explain seasonality because it is very unlikely first of all that they all get the viral infections because they would be protected already, most adults are. Then the transmission of antibodies at best will last 15–16 months after delivery. By then all IgG antibodies that the mother will have transferred transplacentally are completely gone, so the child will be exposed to the development of all those viral infections. So I have trouble understanding how these maternal antibodies could offer a protective effect against virally triggered diabetes.

*Dr. Laron:* First of all one fact has been established, that part of the seasonality of birth of children who develop diabetes, not all, differs from the general population. So it seems to be with celiac disease, also possibly other autoimmune diseases. This is a fact. Now there may be more than one explanation. I think that the antibodies of the mother cross to the fetus during a period where it cannot produce its own antibodies. There is one clear thing which has been demonstrated in animals by Dr. Kolb in Düsseldorf. He took mice which develop spontaneous diabetes, and when they were put in a dirty cage they did not develop diabetes. So there is substantiation that infections may prevent diabetes both in animals as well as in men, not in everybody, depending again on genetic susceptibility or protection by HLA subgroups. It is probably also not one virus. If it were one virus it would be easy to vaccinate. The epidemics in different countries may be caused by different viruses, and this is what we are trying to clarify. In collaboration with Dr. Viskari, we examined several virus antibodies, also polio, and the study showed a correlation between viral antibodies in pregnant mothers and the incidence rate of childhood type-1 diabetes [2].

*Dr. Sorensen:* Is there any seasonality to diabetes itself, because if this is related to a viral infection then you should see seasonality of the onset of diabetes in children.

*Dr. Laron:* We don't know when the onset occurs because the destruction of the β cell is a very slow process and it probably starts already in utero or perinatally. What is known and was described in the UK in 1972 is the diagnosis of clinical diabetes at a stage when 70 or 80% of the β cells have already been destroyed.

*Dr. Klish:* I can't help but ask if there is commonality in the causality between atopic disease and type-1 diabetes mellitus. It should be possible to look at the studies of hydrolyzed protein that have shown a decrease in atopic dermatitis to see if there is also a decrease in diabetes. Dr. Van Berg, is your cohort old enough yet to be able to see this?

*Dr. Laron:* We don't know. There is a hypothesis and more has to be done to prove it. Not only antibodies pass from the mother, viruses pass from the mother, this has been shown with hepatitis virus C.

*Dr. von Berg:* Actually we are just starting to look at type-1 diabetes in our cohort. We haven't done it yet but it is coming.

*Dr. Seidman:* I enjoyed your lecture very much. There are many parallels between celiac disease and type-1 diabetes, but there are also major differences although they both share HLA haplotypes. In fact that only explains perhaps 25% of celiac disease amongst diabetics, and most studies have suggested that it is the diabetes that occurs first and then celiac disease secondarily at some later point, which raises my question. Why do you think that a virus would cause type-1 diabetes, which occurs basically in the first two decades of life, whereas celiac disease, with the same genetic background where the dietary antigen is known, the occurrence which has also been implicated to virus can occur any time in life?

*Dr. Laron:* I don't know. I think perhaps the assembly of gastroenterologists here may have better ideas than me.

*Dr. Seidman:* I think that if we really believe that a virus causes type-1 diabetes then we should think about viruses that only effect people in the first two decades of life, and Epstein-Barr virus would become one of the more likely candidates. Is there an association between Epstein-Barr virus infection and the onset of type-1 diabetes?

*Dr. Laron:* How would you explain the fact that we have data from this country, from the Mayo Clinic, in which we found that patients who develop celiac disease have a different seasonality of month of birth than the general population? How would you explain this?

Laron

*Dr. Seidman:* I haven't seen the data, I can't really comment.

*Dr. Sampson:* One of the ways to look at the possible effect of transmitted maternal antibodies is to look at preterm infants. They don't receive much in the way of antibodies from the mothers. Has anyone looked to see if preterm infants lose the seasonality effect you are talking about?

*Dr. Laron:* Not that I know.

*Dr. Björkstén:* Can you clarify, I was slightly confused from the immunological point of view. You mentioned a score of viruses. The way I understand it, at least some of the literature, is that people are actually discussing molecular mimicry for certain enteroviruses which of course, as you know, is again a very challenged hypothesis from the immunological point of view. But how would you reconcile this? You are mentioning numerous viruses and under those circumstances molecular mimicry or that sort of attack on the islet cells would certainly not be relevant.

*Dr. Laron:* The idea of mimicry was put up by Trucco in Pittsburgh, and at the beginning had quite a few adherents, but in the last few years virologists in Calgary do not speak of that. I am not an immunologist to really give you a scientific answer.

## References

1 Laron Z, Weinberger D: Diabetic retinopathy, nephropathy and cardiovascular disease in a patient with GH-N gene deletion (abstract P-74). 31st Annual Meeting of the International Society for Pediatric and Adolescent Diabetes, Krakow. Pediatr Diabetes 2005; 6(suppl 1): 53–54.
2 Viskari H, Ludvigsson J, Uibo R, et al: Relationship between the incidence of type 1 diabetes and maternal enterovirus antibodies: time trends and geographical variation. Diabetologia 2005;48:1280–1287.

Lucas A, Sampson HA (eds): Primary Prevention by Nutrition Intervention in Infancy and Childhood.
Nestlé Nutr Workshop Ser Pediatr Program, vol 57, pp 81–92,
Nestec Ltd., Vevey/S. Karger AG, Basel, © 2006.

# The Gut Microbiota and Potential Health Effects of Intervention

*Bengt Björkstén*

Centre for Allergy Research and Institute of Environmental Medicine,
Karolinska Institutet, Stockholm, Sweden

## Introduction

The biological and medical communities increasingly realize that the microbiota of the large gut may play important roles in both human health and disease. The perspective of the human colon in health and disease is by no means a new concept, as already a century ago the Russian scientist, Elia Metchnikoff, indicated the clinical importance of the host colonic microbiota. He also suggested that certain live micro-organisms might promote health. Despite this, for many years there was modest interest in this concept among researchers and it is only over the last 10 years that microbial ecology has again become a major research area. It is now generally accepted that the bacterial microbiota of the human gut is an integral component of the host defense system. This has generated considerable interest in the functional food/nutraceutical industry.

It has been suggested that modern living is associated with too little microbial stimulation early in life and that allergic disease and autoimmune disease could be regarded as a consequence of a 'microbial deprivation syndrome' [1]. According to this hypothesis, microbes are essential for the development of a normal immune regulation. In this chapter, the possible role of the gut microbiota in the modulation of immune responses to allergens, autoantigens and foods and microbes in the gut is discussed. The potential for preventing or modulating immunologically mediated diseases by pre- and probiotics, as well as their potential role in infections will be discussed.

### The Intestinal Microbiota

The intestinal tract performs many different functions. In addition to absorption and digestion, it is also the body's largest organ of host defense.

Part of the intestinal mucosal barrier function is formed by a common mucosal immune system, which provides communication between the different mucosal surfaces of the body [2]. The total mucosal surface area of the adult human gastrointestinal tract is up to $300\,m^2$, making it the largest body area interacting with the environment. It is colonized with over $10^{14}$ micro-organisms, weighing over 1 kg, and corresponding to more than 10 times the total number of cells in the body.

The gastrointestinal tract of the newborn baby is sterile. Soon after birth, however, it is colonized by numerous types of micro-organisms. Colonization is complete after approximately 1 week but the numbers and species of bacteria fluctuate markedly during the first 3 months of life. There is a continuous interaction between the microbial flora and the host, comprising a dynamic ecosystem that, once established, is surprisingly stable under normal conditions. Environmental changes, e.g. a treatment period with antibiotics, only temporarily change the composition of the microbiota.

The gut microbiota are thus the quantitatively most important source of microbial stimulation and may provide a primary signal for driving the postnatal maturation of the immune system and the development of a balanced immunity [2]. Thus, there is mounting evidence that commensal microbes acquired during the early postnatal period are required for the development of tolerance, not only to themselves, but also to other antigens. For example, Th2-mediated immune responses are not susceptible to oral tolerance induction in germ-free mice [3]. Oral tolerance was only induced after the introduction of components of the normal microbiota.

It is also recognized that interaction with microbes, especially the normal microbial flora of the gastrointestinal tract, is the principal environmental signal for postnatal maturation of T-cell function (in particular the Th1 component) [4].

Rook and Stanford [1] suggested two major syndromes that could be the result of inadequate microbial stimulation early in life. One was inadequate priming of T-helper cells, leading to an incorrect cytokine balance. The second suggestion was a failure to fine-tune the T-cell repertoire in relation to epitopes that are cross-reactive between self and micro-organisms. The authors coined the expressions 'input deprivation syndrome' and 'uneducated T-cell regulation syndrome'. This hypothesis could be supported by comparative global studies showing that not only allergy, but also type-1 diabetes and celiac disease are associated with a 'Western life style' [5].

If indeed microbes were essential for normal development of immunity, what microbes would be expected to be essential for this process? It would seem unlikely that the postnatal maturation of a balanced immune system would be driven primarily by pathogens, i.e. by stimuli that are potentially harmful to the host. From an evolutionary point of view it is more likely that non-pathogenic micro-organisms that have been present through the evolution

**Table 1.** Definitions

| Probiotic | A live microbial food ingredient that is beneficial to health beyond its nutritional properties |
| --- | --- |
| Prebiotic | A compound that promotes a microbiota that is beneficial to health |

**Table 2.** Suggested beneficial effects of probiotics in infants and young children

| Infectious diarrhea | Confirmed effect |
| --- | --- |
| Antibiotic-associated diarrhea | Likely preventive effect |
| | Unconfirmed therapeutic effect |
| Lactose intolerance | Confirmed effect |
| Inflammatory bowel disease | Possible effect |
| Urogenital infections | Possible effect |
| Allergy | Possible preventive effect of infant eczema |
| | Possible therapeutic effect on infant eczema |
| Type-1 diabetes | Under study |

of our immune system drive the process. The gut microbiota is an obvious place to search for such micro-organisms.

## Probiotics and Prebiotics

Probiotics are non-pathogenic micro-organisms which, when ingested, exert a positive influence on the health or physiology of the host beyond their nutritional value (table 1). The term 'prebiotic' is used for eaten compounds that promote a microbiota that is beneficial to health. Although used for many years, it is only recently that the mechanisms of action and effects of pre- and probiotics have begun to be studied using the same pharmacological approach as for drugs. They have, however, been tried in a wide range of clinical situations, including prevention or treatment of antibiotic-associated disorders, infectious gastroenteritis and diarrhea, lactose intolerance, intestinal infections and colonization by pathogenic bacteria, traveler's diarrhea, irritable bowel syndrome, inflammatory bowel disease, colonic cancer, urogenital infections and tumors, allergy, responses to vaccination, and reduction of serum cholesterol levels (table 2). Only some of the studies for a limit number of disorders have been performed in children. Unfortunately, most of the studies comprise only small study groups and have flaws in their design.

In the search for probiotic bacteria, the industry has mainly focused on various strains of lactobacilli, bifidobacteria and other lactic acid-producing microorganisms. There is so far no conclusive evidence that a certain strain would be superior to other strains, as most studies so far have been limited to comparing a single strain with placebo or with dead micro-organisms, rather than with other live bacteria.

Lactobacilli and bifidobacteria and other lactic acid producers are commensal bacteria common to the gut of all mammals, as well a various non-mammalian vertebrates. The safety in infants, including newborn babies, and in healthy and immunocompromised people is verified by numerous clinical studies, in which up to $10^{11}$ were given [6]. However, rare cases of septicemia and endocarditis have been reported caused by some probiotic bacteria, including *Lactobacillus rhamnosus, L. casei, L. paracasei* and *L. plantarum*.

## Protection against Diarrhea

Diarrhea is common among children and contributes to pediatric morbidity and mortality worldwide. In developing countries it also contributes to malnutrition. Metchnikoff already suggested that live bacterial cultures, such as those found in yoghurt, might help treat and prevent diarrhea. Three recent meta-analyses concluded that lactobacillus therapy for acute infectious diarrhea in children is safe and effective as a treatment for children with acute infectious diarrhea [7–9]. In one of the studies, the initial search yielded 26 studies of which 9 published met defined quality criteria and were included in the analysis. Strains that had been evaluated in at least one of the double-blinded, placebo-controlled studies included strains of *L. acidophilus, L. reuteri* and *L. rhamnosus,* with doses ranging from $10^9$ to $10^{11}$ bacteria. The former figure corresponds roughly to the number of micro-organisms in a regular portion of yoghurt. Summary point estimates indicated a reduction in diarrhea duration of 0.7 days (95% confidence interval 0.3–1.2 days) in the participants who received lactobacillus as compared with those who received placebo. There was also suggestion of a dose-effect relationship.

In the second meta-analysis 18 studies were included [8]. The analysis suggested that administration of probiotics with standard rehydration therapy reduces the duration of acute diarrhea by approximately 1 day.

A Cochrane Database Systematic Review of probiotics for treating infectious diarrhea, 23 studies with a total of 1,917 participants were analyzed. It was concluded that probiotics reduced the mean duration of diarrhea by 30.5 h [9].

Diarrhea associated with antibiotic intake has also been the subject of several clinical studies. Such studies are logical as it is well known that antibiotic treatment affects the composition of the gut microbiota. The efficacy of probiotics in the prevention and treatment of diarrhea associated with the use of antibiotics was recently assessed in a meta-analysis [10]. Nine randomized double-blind, placebo-controlled studies were recovered, two of which included children. The odds ration in favor of active treatment over placebo in preventing diarrhea associated with the antibiotic treatment was 0.37 (95%

confidence interval 0.26–0.53, p < 0.001). It was also concluded, however, that the efficacy of probiotics in treating antibiotic-associated diarrhea remains to be proven.

## Microbiota and Allergy

The wide variations in allergy prevalence between different countries, the fact that the prevalence has increased considerably over the last 40–50 years and the role of the microbiota for the development of immunity in infants, have led to the suggestion that variations in patterns of microbial colonization of the gastrointestinal tract, linked with lifestyle and/or geographic factors, may be important determinants of the heterogeneity in allergy prevalence throughout the world [4]. Over the past few years, differences have been documented in the composition of the intestinal microbiota between healthy infants in countries with a low and a high prevalence of allergy [11] and between allergic and non-allergic infants in both environments [12–15]. The studies indicate an imbalance in the gut flora of allergic infants and could suggest that differences in the indigenous intestinal flora might affect the development and priming of the immune system in early childhood and that the observed differences between allergic and non-allergic children are not secondary phenomena.

Italian studies in military personnel have lent support to a possible role of the intestinal microbiota in the pathogenesis of allergic disease. Matricardi et al. [16] studied the prevalence of allergic disease and sensitization to inhalant allergens among military personnel in relation to serological markers of previous infections. Interestingly, there was an inverse relationship between respiratory allergy and the presence of antibodies against infections transmitted through the oro-fecal route, such as toxoplasmosis, hepatitis A and *Helicobacter pylori*, but no relationship with antibodies against agents transmitted through the respiratory tract, i.e. measles, mumps, rubella, chickenpox, cytomegalovirus, and herpes simplex virus.

There are at least four recent studies in which differences in the composition of the gut flora were observed between allergic and non-allergic infants. In one study, the counts of *Staphylococcus aureus* were higher and the prevalence of *Bacteroides* and *Bifidobacteria* were lower in allergic children at 2 years [12]. A higher prevalence of colonization with *Clostridium difficile* in allergic infants at 12 months was suggested in a considerably larger study, using an indirect method [13]. In that study, various microbial metabolic products were determined in stool specimens from healthy and allergic infants. The advantage with this approach over conventional bacteriological methods is that information is obtained about microbial metabolism and ecology. When analyzing the levels of short-chain fatty acids, which are products of microbial metabolism, isocaproic acid was only detected in stool samples from allergic infants, while the levels of isobutyric acid were higher in healthy children. The former fatty acid strongly indicates colonization with C. difficile and the later findings indicate the presence of a lactic acid-producing gut flora.

These studies were cross-sectional and did not address the issue whether the differences were primary or secondary to disease. In two prospective studies, however, less bifidobacteria were detected already during the first weeks of life in babies who developed allergy during infancy [17, 18]. These studies demonstrate that differences in the composition in the intestinal flora between allergic and non-allergic infants are present already before any manifestations of disease. Thus, the studies indicate a primary imbalance in the gut flora of infants who develop allergic manifestations.

Observed differences in the composition of the gut flora between allergic and healthy infants are not limited to species. The strains of *Bifidobacterium* [14] and *Lactobacillus* [19] also differ between the 2 groups. Although the significance of these differences is unknown, they are interesting as these species are consistently linked to probiotic properties and differences in the presence and type of *Bifidobacterium* between allergic and non-allergic infants is the only consistent finding in all clinical studies so far.

Recently, it was shown in a population-based cohort comprising 3,000 children and their mothers that vaginal colonization with staphylococci during mid-pregnancy was associated with asthma during the 5th year of life in the children (OR 2.2; 95% CI 1.4–3.4) [20]. Staphylococci are not part of the normal vaginal flora, which is normally dominated by lactic acid bacteria. This is interesting, since the maternal vaginal microbiota is an obvious source of colonization of the infant during the birth process.

The composition of gut microbiota may also be relevant for the controversy regarding breastfeeding and the development of asthma and allergy. While a protective effect was reported in several earlier studies published in the 1970s and 1980s, most recent studies have reported no effects of breastfeeding on allergic diseases, although it does reduce wheezing in infants, which is a symptom caused by infections and not allergy. Previously there were pronounced differences in the composition of the gut microbiota between breastfed and formula-fed infants [21]. These differences are not nearly as prominent with the use of modern humanized infant formulae [11]. Thus, any protective effect of breastfeeding in the past may have been a consequence of an ecological effect on the gut microbial flora.

As the differences in the composition in the intestinal flora between allergic and non-allergic infants were present already before any manifestations of disease, perhaps even in the microenvironment during birth, the studies indicate that they are primary. Although all the studies conducted so far confirm differences in the composition of the gut microbiota, no particular protective or potentially harmful bacterial species can yet be identified. This is not surprising, given the enormous number of microbial strains and the complicated ecology in the gut.

## Probiotics and Allergy

The first double-blind placebo-controlled study of infants with atopic eczema given probiotics showed a modest reduction of skin symptoms after 1 month of treatment with a strain of *L. rhamnosus* [22]. Since then, at least 4 small studies have been conducted with this and other [23] strains. Unfortunately, none of the studies are conclusive, but taken together they suggest that there may be a modest effect on eczema, but only so in infants and young children. None of the studies support any effect on IgE-mediated disease, however.

The potentially allergy-preventive effects of probiotics was assessed in a double-blind, placebo-controlled study comprising 132 infants with a family history of allergy [24]. Mothers were given lactobacilli or placebo, starting before birth and the treatment was then continued to the mothers while breastfeeding and to the babies when weaned. The cumulative incidence of atopic dermatitis was reduced by about 50% in the treatment group, although there was no effect on sensitization. Despite that, the authors concluded that the treatment prevented early 'atopic disease'. Indeed, the 4-year follow-up even suggested a higher incidence of IgE-mediated respiratory symptoms [25].

Although there is yet little documentation of the superiority of certain strains of lactic acid bacteria that are marketed as probiotics over other similar wild strains, it seems reasonable to assume that live micro-organisms are more effective than killed bacteria of the same species. The efficacy of oral supplementation of viable and heat-inactivated probiotic bacteria in the management of atopic disease and their effects on the composition of the gut microbiota was studied in 35 infants with atopic eczema and allergy to cow's milk, who received extensively hydrolyzed whey formula with or without viable or heat-inactivated lactobacilli [26]. The treatment with heat-inactivated lactobacilli was associated with adverse gastrointestinal symptoms and diarrhea, while the decrease in the symptom scores among infants treated with viable lactobacilli tended to be greater than within the placebo group, although not significantly so.

The hitherto published studies on lactic acid bacteria in the treatment and prevention of allergy have yielded inconclusive results, although they are encouraging. In a position paper issued by the European Academy of Allergy and Clinical Immunology, it was concluded that evidence supporting the use of probiotics in the prevention or treatment of allergy is still preliminary [27]. Several ongoing studies will hopefully better define the potential of currently marketed lactic acid bacteria in the treatment or prevention of asthma and allergy. If the efficacy is confirmed, it is reasonable to suspect that this may be more obvious in, or even limited to infancy and early childhood, i.e. before the immune responses to allergens and immune regulatory networks have been established.

Björkstén

## Other Conditions

It is established clinical experience that many individuals with lactose intolerance can tolerate at least limited amounts of fermented milk products, despite them having a high lactose content. Although not extensively studied in controlled trials, it is reasonable to conclude that probiotics may reduce symptoms of intolerance.

There are also indications that certain strains of lactobacilli and bifidobacteria may possible in the future find a role in pediatric urology, as decreased risk of infection has been reported [28]. This and other claimed positive effects, such as managing inflammatory bowel disease in children [29], remain rather speculative, however.

## Concluding Remarks

Although it is still unknown what environmental factors in modern industrialized societies are responsible for the high and increasing prevalence of allergic and autoimmune diseases, epidemiological, clinical and experimental research indicates an important, or even critical role of the intestinal microbiota. Lactic acid-producing bacteria have a confirmed effect on infantile infectious diarrhea but it is still too early to recommend them for allergy treatment or prevention, as the published studies are inconclusive. Thus, the results of the clinical studies so far need to be confirmed and extended.

## References

1 Rook GA, Stanford JL: Give us this day our daily germs. Immunol Today 1998;19:113–116.
2 Hooper L, Gordon J: Commensal host-bacterial relationships in the gut. Science 2001;292: 1115–1118.
3 Sudo N, Sawamura S, Tanaka K, et al: The requirement of intestinal bacterial flora for the development of an IgE production system fully susceptible to oral tolerance induction. J Immunol 1997;159:1739–1745.
4 Holt PG, Sly PD, Björkstén B: Atopic versus infectious diseases in childhood: a question of balance? Pediatr Allergy Immunol 1997;8:53–58.
5 Stene LC, Nafstad P: Relation between occurrence of type 1 diabetes and asthma. Lancet 2001;357:607–608.
6 Borriello SP, Hammes WP, Holzapfel W, et al: Safety of probiotics that contain lactobacilli or bifidobacteria. Clin Infect Dis 2003;36:775–780.
7 Huang JS, Bousvaros A, Lee JW, et al: Efficacy of probiotic use in acute diarrhea in children: a meta-analysis. Dig Dis Sci 2002;47:2625–2634.
8 Van Niel C, Feudtner C, Garrison M, Christakis D: *Lactobacillus* therapy for acute infectious diarrhea in children: a meta-analysis. Pediatrics 2002;109:678–684.
9 Allen SJ, Okoko B, Martinez E, et al: Probiotics for treating infectious diarrhoea. Cochrane Database Syst Rev 2004;CD003048.
10 D'Souza AL, Rajkumar C, Cooke J, Bulpitt CJ: Probiotics in prevention of antibiotic associated diarrhoea: meta-analysis. BMJ 2002;324:1361.
11 Sepp E, Julge K, Vasar M, et al: Intestinal microflora of Estonian and Swedish infants. Acta Paediatr 1997;86:956–961.

12  Björkstén B, Naaber P, Sepp E, Mikelsaar M: The intestinal microbiota in allergic Estonian and Swedish 2-year-old children. Clin Exp Allergy 1999;29:342–346.
13  Böttchers MF, Nordin EK, Sandin A, et al: Microbiota-associated characteristics in faeces from allergic and nonallergic infants. Clin Exp Allergy 2000;30:1590–1596.
14  Ouwhand AC, Isolauri E, He F, et al: Differences in Bifidobacterium flora composition in allergic and healthy infants. J Allergy Clin Immunol 2001;108:144–145.
15  Kirjavainen PV, Arvola T, Salminen SJ, Isolauri E: Aberrant composition of gut microbiota of allergic infants: a target of bifidobacterial therapy at weaning? Gut 2002;51:51–55.
16  Matricardi PM, Rosmini F, Panetta V, et al: Hay fever and asthma in relation to markers of infection in the United States. J Allergy Clin Immunol 2002;110:381–387.
17  Björkstén B, Sepp E, Julge K, et al: Allergy development and the intestinal microbiota during the first year of life. J Allergy Clin Immunol 2001;108:516–520.
18  Kalliomäki M, Kirjavainen P, Eerola E, et al: Distinct patterns of neonatal gut microbiota in infants in whom atopy was and was not developing. J Allergy Clin Immunol 2001;107:129–134.
19  Mikelsaar M, Annuk H, Stsepetova J, et al: Intestinal lactoflora of Estonian and Swedish children. Microbiol Ecol Health Dis 2002;14:75–80.
20  Benn CS, Thorsen P, Jensen JS, et al: Maternal vaginal microflora during pregnancy and the risk of asthma hospitalization and use of antiasthma medication in early childhood. J Allergy Clin Immunol 2002;110:72–77.
21  Bullen CL, Tearle PV, Stewart MG: The effect of 'humanised' milks and supplemented breast feeding on the faecal flora of infants. J Med Microbiol 1977;10:403–413.
22  Majamaa H, Isolauri E: Probiotics: a novel approach in the management of food allergy. J Allergy Clin Immunol 1997;99:179–185.
23  Rosenfeldt V, Benfeldt E, Nielsen SD, et al: Effect of probiotic Lactobacillus strains in children with atopic dermatitis. J Allergy Clin Immunol 2003;111:389–395.
24  Kalliomäki M, Salminen S, Arvilommi H, et al: Probiotics in primary prevention of atopic disease: a randomised placebo-controlled trial. Lancet 2001;357:1076–1079.
25  Kalliomäki M, Salminen S, Poussa T, et al: Probiotics and prevention of atopic disease: 4-year follow-up of a randomised placebo-controlled trial. Lancet 2003;361:1869–1871.
26  Kirjavainen PV, Salminen SJ, Isolauri E: Probiotic bacteria in the management of atopic disease: underscoring the importance of viability. J Pediatr Gastroenterol Nutr 2003;36:223–227.
27  Matricardi P, Björkstén B, Bonini S, et al: Microbial products in allergy prevention and therapy. Allergy 2003;58:461–471.
28  Reid G: The potential role of probiotics in pediatric urology. J Urol 2002;168:1512–1517.
29  Guandalini S: Use of Lactobacillus-GG in paediatric Crohn's disease. Dig Liver Dis 2002; 34(suppl 2):S63–S65.

## Discussion

*Dr. Sorensen:* Thank you very much for a very nice review. Do you think that the microbiota can influence the response to vaccines given subcutaneously? Let me preface my question with an explanation. In the United States in our clinics for current infections, we are seeing many children who simply fail to respond to lipopolysaccharides, but we also have a large collection of children who have completely failed to respond to four doses of the conjugated vaccine, and they are indistinguishable from children who have never had a vaccine. The reason for my question is that in studies in Brazil, Chile and Columbia no such unresponsiveness is seen, and I always thought that the use of antibiotics could make a big difference because many of the children that we see have been on multiple courses of broad-spectrum antibiotics. So that is why I wonder if antibiotics are having and influence.

*Dr. Björkstén:* The answer to that is in principle yes, the gut microbiota do modulate systemic immune responses. To answer your question specifically I obviously can't tell you.

*Dr. Saavedra:* I am fascinated as we look more into the differences in what we call the microbiota which is basically a stool, in other words the distal colonic content, that we still see the kinds of differences that you are showing. Ultimately that stool is the equilibrium which that particular host reached with whatever bacterial stimulus and food and mucin and everything they produced. When we talk about the approaches that we are taking, as you say not to go back to infecting everybody but potentially stimulating them, one of the big differences, and I speak as a gastroenterologist where we typically say that anything in the small bowel that is above $10^5$ or $10^6$ constitutes bacterial overgrowth which we actually treat when we deal with patients with this motility, etc. If they have this amount of bacteria we treat them because we think that leads to an inflammatory response which sometimes explains some other symptoms that those patients may have. When we give probiotics, for example, hypothetically if that is going to have an effect, what we are really doing is creating an artificial bacterial overgrowth on a regular basis with low-dose amounts, probably we get to $10^4$, $10^6$ bacteria, some are lost in the small bowel. Do you think that we may be missing something by not trying better to look at the differential inflammatory immunologic response between the small bowel which is 'sterile' in our modern society versus the colon which has never been sterile?

*Dr. Björkstén:* Let me just say one thing first. Modern society is not sterile. The difference versus traditional society is the speed by which colonization takes place, and the fact that after the initial colonization there is less exchange with the environment. There was a study from Göteborg some years ago [1] where they compared Pakistani and Swedish infants with sequential analysis of *Escherichia coli* strains and, in the Pakistani infants it was found that, each time a new sample is taken from the baby, the dominating or common strains have changed, while in Sweden once a coli was found, this strain tended to remain. So that is why I don't like the words 'hygiene hypothesis' and 'sterility'. The other point you are raising is important. Stool cultures are probably relevant for what bacteria are present in the colon as you pointed out, while much of the immune system is really in the small intestine. Preferentially the ecology should be studied in the gut just as you indicated. This is why I am interested in microflora-associated characteristics and not only bacterial cultures. On the other hand I would caution against a reductionist approach because it is clearly an interplay between many microbes. But you are right, we may be looking under the lamp where the light is better.

*Dr. Klish:* I was fascinated by your discussion on the colonization of the intestine between individuals with atopy and normal individuals. Are the differences there because the atopic individual has an upregulated immune system and selects against bacteria or because the bacteria colonize early, downregulate the immune system, and therefore prevent allergy?

*Dr. Björkstén:* It is the chicken and egg situation. I can say that it is probably not an upregulated or a different immune system in their future allergies because as far as we know there are no such differences at birth. However your point is well taken because my arguments could be turned around by saying that there is a difference in the gut of potentially atopic individuals, some are prone to a certain type of colonization. The only way to prove this is of course in the prospective studies we are doing. We have just completed a 2-year follow-up prospective study comparing 189 newborns whose mothers received lactobacillus or placebo 4 weeks before term, and then the baby for 1 year. We have the immunology and we have the stool samples so we will be able to answer your question. I think though that it is reasonable to suggest that the microbiota are the primary issue.

*Dr. Lucas:* Just to get that topic that you got near to. One of the major changes in the last century was an order of magnitude increase in the number of cesarean sections so that the babies were born into a sterile rather than in a dirty environment, and of course cesarean section itself is correlated with certain categories of babies, like premature babies, who may have different immunity-related risks. Has this ever been studied?

*Dr. Björkstén:* Yes, it has. There are several studies showing that cesarean section is associated with an increased risk of allergy development, which would fit into this hypothesis. To answer the question whether the increase in cesarean sections could explain the increase globally, the answer is clearly, no, there is not enough increase to explain this.

*Dr. Hanson:* You referred to our studies comparing Swedish and Pakistani babies and I think that is very relevant. I would like to add that it is very difficult to colonize an individual with a number of coli or what have you. They may just pass and you never see them or they may be around for a day or two. But the difference I think for a child in Pakistan, for example, is that there is very heavy exposure. They get very large doses and then the bugs can remain and influence the immune system. I think that could be part of the difference with regard to exposure.

*Dr. Björkstén:* You are right, that is true. On the other hand, Estonia is not a poor hygiene country. Just as I did not grow up under poor hygienic conditions as a child. So this is a relative term. The size of the inoculum matters and in Estonia they had traditional big baby wards rather than the very strict rooming as in Sweden. I should also say that the consistent finding when comparing non-allergic and allergic children, anthroposophic and conventional children, Estonian and Swedish children, is that the diversity of the gut microbiota is larger in the former. They may have the same bacteria as I showed here, but the diversity, the number of strains that you find is larger. And this raises the point that it is the number of hits on the developing immune system rather than any one given bacteria. It is the sort of intensity of the stimulation.

*Dr. Laron:* Do the gut microbiota influence gastric physiology, and how?

*Dr. Björkstén:* It is not my field so I can't answer but I think it is well established that it does.

*Dr. Laron:* I am asking because the majority of gastrointestinal hormones are actually secreted in the stomach.

*Dr. Björkstén:* That is a very interesting thought, I have no idea.

*Dr. Seidman:* I was very interested in your parallels with inflammatory bowel disease, and it is interesting that cesarean section has never been shown to be a risk factor for the development of inflammatory bowel disease despite the paradigm of the importance of the gut microbiota in the first trimester of life. As Dr. Lucas mentioned yesterday observational studies may often be due to confounding factors and we have been very interested in looking at the gene environmental reactions and predisposing children to develop inflammatory bowel disease. The story that hepatitis A virus is a marker for a lack of sanitary conditions is probably due to a confounder. Now the polymorphism for the hepatitis A virus, genes have been discovered and people who have polymorphisms for the gene that allow the hepatitis A virus to infect the person are those that are susceptible to atopic disease. It is not because they have been exposed or not exposed to environmental pollutants or to bacterial and viral infections. So hepatitis A is very interesting in that regard and it probably has nothing to do with sanitation but it is due to genetic a factor.

*Dr. Björkstén:* You are right and that was precisely the point of my slide.

*Dr. Wang:* Sometimes we suggest that the patients use probiotics, but normally we do not find it very effective for atopic disease in infants. My question is whether probiotics can upregulate the T-regulatory cells? Are there any clinical trials for probiotics in the treatment of asthma? Can the results of your review be explained in that probiotics induce the immune response by blocking the allergen to be absorbed into the body, but the probiotics do not directly regulate the immune response?

*Dr. Björkstén:* I think that probiotics are probably not going to be the panacea for prevention and the reason is the complexity of the microbiotic interaction. Having said that, to my knowledge there are no studies showing any efficacy of probiotics in the treatment of asthma. The positive results relate to infantile atopic dermatitis.

Björkstén

*Dr. Hamburger:* To get back to Dr. Seidman's point, how important is the genetics of IgE and allergy in terms of overriding these minute differences that you are attributing to the bacterial flora?

*Dr. Björkstén:* The genetics is probably trivial in this context and the good news is that not everybody becomes allergic; the bad news it seems that at least 50% of the population has the genetic potential to become allergic. So obviously we have not been able to study the genetics here. I don't think genetics will be very rewarding nor of much interest because what we are looking for in this global epidemiology of immune diseases is clearly not a change in genetic composition of man in one generation. There is clearly an environmental factor operating.

## Reference

1 Carlsson B, Ahlstedt S, Hanson LA, et al: *Escherichia coli* O antibody content in milk from healthy Swedish mothers and mothers from a very low socio-economic group of a developing country. Acta Paediatr Scand 1976;65:417–423.

Lucas A, Sampson HA (eds): Primary Prevention by Nutrition Intervention in Infancy and Childhood.
Nestlé Nutr Workshop Ser Pediatr Program, vol 57, pp 93–108,
Nestec Ltd., Vevey/S. Karger AG, Basel, © 2006.

# The Relationship of Breastfeeding to the Development of Atopic Disorders

*Robert S. Zeiger, Noah J. Friedman*

Department of Allergy, Kaiser Permanente Medical Center, and Department of Pediatrics,
University of California, San Diego, Calif., USA

## Introduction

Allergy prevention efforts must be instituted early in life since there appears to be a critical period for sensitization to food allergens shortly after birth. Some atopic risk factors susceptible to modulation include: (1) intact protein formula feeding; (2) early introduction of allergenic foods, and (3) environmental tobacco smoke. Since Grulee and Sanford [1] reported in 1939 a significant 7-fold reduction in eczema in infants who were breastfed, much uncertainly has surrounded this potential benefit of breastfeeding. Methodological differences and design limitations were observed among studies. However, the complex immunological characteristics of breast milk and maternal–infant interactions may also be at play. Do genetic differences in infant/mother pairs affect the composition of breast milk and influence the modulating effect of breast milk on emerging allergic disorders? Are the nanogram concentrations of food allergens found in breast milk sensitizing or protective?

What is not controversial is that breast milk is the preferred infant nutrition with rare exception (maternal HIV infection) owing to its nutritional, immunological, and psychological benefits. It is included as an important element in allergy prevention guidelines [2, 3]. Since breastfeeding is the recommended infant feeding method, it is more appropriate to examine breastfeeding in the light of 'what may be lost by *not* breastfeeding?' rather than in its allergy-preventive attributes. From the evidence that will be presented here and that we reported in more detail elsewhere [4], one can expect a higher incidence of eczema and wheezing illnesses in early childhood in high-risk infants fed intact formula to the exclusion of breast milk.

Zeiger/Friedman

**Table 1.** Factors in breast milk that are currently being evaluated as either inducing or protecting against food allergies

| Constituents | Inducing | Protective |
|---|---|---|
| Food allergens | Sensitizing | Tolerizing |
| Cytokines | IL-4 | TGF-β |
| | IL-5 | s-CD14 |
| | IL-13 | IL-10 |
| Immunoglobulins | | s-IgA |
| Polyunsaturated | Arachidonic acid | Eicosapentaenoic acid |
| fatty acids (PUFA) | C22:4n-6 | Docosapentaenoic acid |
| | C22:5n-6 | Docosatetraenoic acid |
| | | n-3 PUFA |
| Chemokines | RANTES | |
| | IL-8 | |
| Eosinophil-derived | Eosinophil cationic protein | |
| granular proteins | | |
| Prebiotic oligosaccharides | | Bifidobacteria, lactobacilli |

Transforming growth factor-β (TGF-β), regulated on activation, normal T-cell expressed (RANTES).

Revised and reprinted with permission from Leung et al: Pediatric Allergy, Principles and Practice. St Louis, Mosby, 2003, p 496.

## Immunologic Complexity of Breast Milk

The complexity of the interaction between breast milk and an infant's intestinal milieu and immune system has only recently received attention. Diverse immunological and nutritional factors in breast milk may have pro- or anti-inflammatory functions and as such may exert opposing effects on the development of allergy (table 1).

The increase in food antigen absorption which occurs early postnatally in animals is inhibited by breast milk. While colostrum and breast milk secretory-IgA is passed to the infant from the mother, it is unclear whether low levels of non- or specific secretory-IgA predispose to cow's milk allergy (CMA) in infants as reported by some but not by other prospective studies. Immune factors in milk including IgE antibodies and cytokines involved in IgE synthesis (IL-4 and IL-13) and eosinophil induction (IL-5) are at higher levels in breast milk from atopic than non-atopic mothers, but do not seem to affect the development of allergy.

Breast milk may support Th1 responses that suppress a Th2 bias associated with atopy by supplying IL-1, TNF-α, nucleotides, oligosaccharides, CD14 for bacteria recognition and functional T cells that induce interferon-γ. Transforming growth factor-β (TGF-β) is the dominant cytokine in human

94

breast milk. It may promote specific-IgA to foods and at high levels in breast milk was associated with a lower prevalence of infantile wheeze [5].

It is unclear whether a high arachidonic acid to eicosapentaenoic acid ratio in breast milk is associated with a higher risk of atopy. Spermine and spermidine in breast milk may act immunoprotectively by reducing intestinal permeability. Recently eosinophil cationic protein at higher levels in breast milk was associated with a higher incidence of CMA and atopic dermatitis in infants. It will require future study to determine the real effect of the complex interaction of these immunomodulatory factors in breast milk between the mother and infant in the development of allergic disease.

## Role of Infection

Early childhood infection may have a dual effect on allergy and asthma development that is modulated by breast milk. Anti-viral antibodies and other factors supplied by breast milk may reduce respiratory syncytial virus and other viral infections that predispose susceptible infants in early childhood to wheezing episodes. Other infections by stimulating Th1 immunity may protect against allergy development. The 'hygiene hypothesis' proposes that in the high risk, exposure to the 'right' infections may preferentially induce a Th1-predominant immune system, thereby decreasing allergy risk. In support of this potential dual role, attendance at daycare or the presence of older siblings in the house was associated with lower rates of asthma after age 6 years, but higher incidences of early onset wheezing in infancy [6]. Intracellular organisms may play a role by inducing a polarized Th1 response causing long-term immunity. Breast milk may protect against allergy by a Th1 mechanism by promoting intestinal colonization of lactobacilli and bifidobacteria. The favorable effect of breastfeeding on respiratory and gastrointestinal infections in infancy and their sequelae, including wheezing illnesses, must be interpreted in the context of the complex immunomodulatory role of early infections on the development of allergic diseases.

## Allergens in Breast Milk

Major food allergens from cow's milk, egg, wheat, and peanut can be detected immunochemically in nanogram concentrations in the breast milk of about 50% of the mothers. As reviewed recently, these allergens appear in 1–6 h after ingestion of 120 ml of milk, 1 raw egg, 1 slice of bread, 50 g of peanut [7]. It is unclear, however, whether food allergens in breast milk promote sensitization or tolerance to foods in non-sensitized infants. We do know that atopic infants already sensitized to these foods may experience disease exacerbation after ingesting breast milk containing these allergens and with maternal avoidance of these foods experience disease amelioration.

Zeiger/Friedman

## Studies Evaluating the Role of Breastfeeding in the Development of Atopy

In evaluating these studies, one needs to understand their design: are the cohorts unselected or at high risk, are the studies observation or intervention, are the groups self-selected or randomized. The only randomized prospective study evaluating the role of human milk in the development of atopic dermatitis was done on an unselected cohort of premature infants (n = 446) who were randomized to receive either preterm cow's milk formula or banked human breast milk [8]. In the cohort as a whole, no difference in the development of atopic dermatitis was observed. However, in subgroup analysis of only infants with a positive family history of allergy, preterm formula compared to banked breast milk use early in infancy was associated with an increased incidence of atopic dermatitis by 18 months (odds ratio 3.6; 95% CI 1.2–11, $p < 0.05$). These findings are of particular interest given the delayed gut maturity in premature infants. Unfortunately, immunological analyses were not performed.

In addition, the extent of breastfeeding exposure (never versus ever or exclusive versus partial) and the duration of breastfeeding between different studies need to be known. A detailed description of the atopic outcome must be defined precisely including disorder (specific disorders such as atopic dermatitis (eczema), food allergy, recurrent wheezing versus asthma, allergic rhinitis or any of the above atopic manifestations) or sensitization (skin test or in vitro testing for specific IgE). Finally the period (infancy, early childhood, adolescence/adulthood) at which outcomes are determined must be considered as differential effects by age have been reported. The ideal intervention design will randomize study groups to enhance comparability and minimize bias. Randomization is nearly impossible in studies of breastfeeding versus formula feeding due to ethical considerations. As such, methodological differences are common between studies, as are limitations in study design, making it challenging to compare different studies. Many older studies were hampered by small sample size, brief duration of breastfeeding, lack of immunologic confirmation and insufficient blinding during evaluation [9]. Findings from these studies taken as a whole favored the protective effect of breast compared to intact formula feeding on some aspects of atopy; however, some studies also reported either no effect or a tendency for enhancing atopy.

## Critical Evaluations and Meta-Analyses of Published Data

To better evaluate the scientific strength of the thousands of breastfeeding observation studies, Kramer [9] proposed criteria to assess their adequacy (table 2). Considering these criteria, a European expert panel critically analyzed the pertinent literature from 1966 to 2001 of over 4,000 publications

**Table 2.** Kramer's criteria for assessing adequacy of cohort observational studies examining the association of breastfeeding (BF) and development of allergic disorders [9]

| | |
|---|---|
| Exposure | |
| 1 | No late mom recall |
| 2 | Blind feeding history ascertainment |
| 3 | Sufficient duration of BF |
| 4 | Sufficient exclusivity of BF |
| Outcome | |
| 5 | Strict diagnostic criteria |
| 6 | Blind outcome assessment |
| 7 | Consider outcome severity |
| 8 | Consider onset of outcome |
| Statistics | |
| 9 | Control for confounding factors |
| 10 | Assessment of dose-response effects |
| 11 | Assessment of effects in high-risk |
| 12 | Adequate power |

pertaining to breastfeeding and allergic disease [10]. Only 56 (1.3%) of the prospective and retrospective studies merited review by established criteria. The panel concluded that exclusive breastfeeding was associated with a reduced risk of asthma in childhood, and that any breastfeeding reduced recurrent wheeze for at least the first decade in all children, regardless of atopic risk. Benefit appeared to increase with increasing duration of breast-feeding up to 4 months. Atopic dermatitis in infancy, but not atopy in later life, was favorably affected by breastfeeding. Some evidence suggested a higher risk of CMA when intact cow's milk formula in lieu of breast milk was fed in the first days of life, regardless of risk. The protective effect of breastfeeding on these outcomes was even greater in children at high risk of atopy [10].

The critical assessment of studies published between 1966 and 2000 was advanced by the strength of meta-analysis. The criteria presented in table 2 were defined further. Accepted studies met the following criteria: (1) blinded maternal feeding history recall of less than 12 months; (2) at least 3 months of any or exclusive breastfeeding; (3) strict diagnostic outcomes; (4) blinded assessments; (5) onset of disease recorded, and (6) controlled for confounding factors and high-risk children [11, 12]. Only prospective studies in developed countries were included in these meta-analyses. Eighteen studies with more than 4,000 subjects followed for 4.5 (range 1–5) years were accepted for the analysis of atopic dermatitis [11]. Twelve studies with more than 8,000 children followed for 4.1 (range 1–8.4) years were evaluated for the analysis of asthma [12]. A significant protective effect of exclusive breastfeeding for at least 3 months was reported for the development of atopic dermatitis in the cohort as a whole, particularly in children at high risk of atopy, but not in

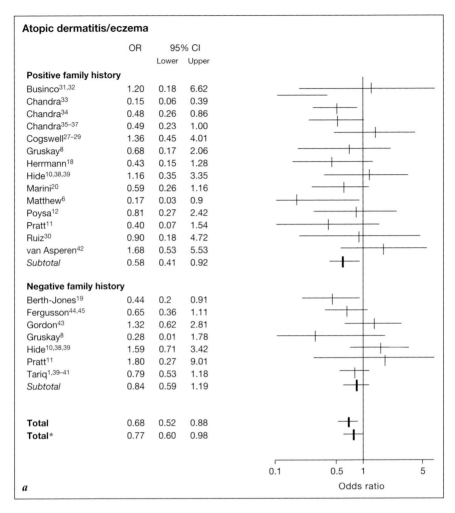

**Atopic dermatitis/eczema**

| | OR | 95% CI Lower | Upper |
|---|---|---|---|
| **Positive family history** | | | |
| Businco[31,32] | 1.20 | 0.18 | 6.62 |
| Chandra[33] | 0.15 | 0.06 | 0.39 |
| Chandra[34] | 0.48 | 0.26 | 0.86 |
| Chandra[35–37] | 0.49 | 0.23 | 1.00 |
| Cogswell[27–29] | 1.36 | 0.45 | 4.01 |
| Gruskay[8] | 0.68 | 0.17 | 2.06 |
| Herrmann[18] | 0.43 | 0.15 | 1.28 |
| Hide[10,38,39] | 1.16 | 0.35 | 3.35 |
| Marini[20] | 0.59 | 0.26 | 1.16 |
| Matthew[6] | 0.17 | 0.03 | 0.9 |
| Poysa[12] | 0.81 | 0.27 | 2.42 |
| Pratt[11] | 0.40 | 0.07 | 1.54 |
| Ruiz[30] | 0.90 | 0.18 | 4.72 |
| van Asperen[42] | 1.68 | 0.53 | 5.53 |
| *Subtotal* | 0.58 | 0.41 | 0.92 |
| **Negative family history** | | | |
| Berth-Jones[19] | 0.44 | 0.2 | 0.91 |
| Fergusson[44,45] | 0.65 | 0.36 | 1.11 |
| Gordon[43] | 1.32 | 0.62 | 2.81 |
| Gruskay[8] | 0.28 | 0.01 | 1.78 |
| Hide[10,38,39] | 1.59 | 0.71 | 3.42 |
| Pratt[11] | 1.80 | 0.27 | 9.01 |
| Tariq[1,39–41] | 0.79 | 0.53 | 1.18 |
| *Subtotal* | 0.84 | 0.59 | 1.19 |
| **Total** | 0.68 | 0.52 | 0.88 |
| **Total*** | 0.77 | 0.60 | 0.98 |

0.1    0.5    1    5

Odds ratio

*a*

**Fig. 1.** Meta-analyses of studies demonstrating a protective effect of at least 3 months of exclusive breastfeeding compared to cow's milk feeding on the development in infants with a family history of atopy of atopic dermatitis/eczema (*a*) and asthma/wheezing (*b*). *Analyses after exclusion of studies with non-blinded outcomes. Numbers next to authors refer to references in the original article. *a* Reprinted with permission from the American Academy of Dermatology, Inc. and Gdalevich et al. [11]. *b* Reprinted with permission from Mosby, Inc. and Gdalevich et al. [12].

children at low risk (fig. 1a) [11]. In addition, exclusive breastfeeding for 3 months protected against the development of early childhood asthma-like symptoms in those children at high risk of atopy, but not in those at low risk (fig. 1b) [12]. In contrast, a meta-analysis examining exclusive breastfeeding for at least 3 months did not note a significant protection on the development

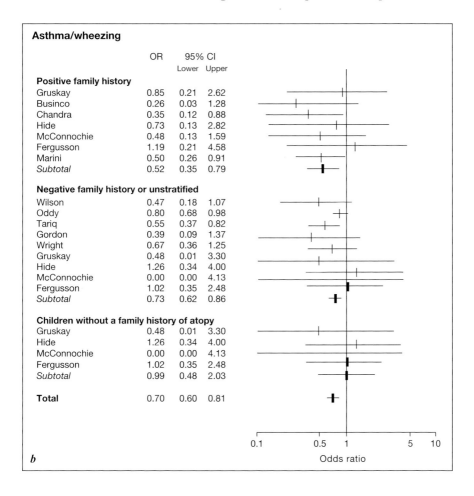

**Asthma/wheezing**

| | OR | 95% CI Lower | 95% CI Upper |
|---|---|---|---|
| **Positive family history** | | | |
| Gruskay | 0.85 | 0.21 | 2.62 |
| Businco | 0.26 | 0.03 | 1.28 |
| Chandra | 0.35 | 0.12 | 0.88 |
| Hide | 0.73 | 0.13 | 2.82 |
| McConnochie | 0.48 | 0.13 | 1.59 |
| Fergusson | 1.19 | 0.21 | 4.58 |
| Marini | 0.50 | 0.26 | 0.91 |
| *Subtotal* | 0.52 | 0.35 | 0.79 |
| **Negative family history or unstratified** | | | |
| Wilson | 0.47 | 0.18 | 1.07 |
| Oddy | 0.80 | 0.68 | 0.98 |
| Tariq | 0.55 | 0.37 | 0.82 |
| Gordon | 0.39 | 0.09 | 1.37 |
| Wright | 0.67 | 0.36 | 1.25 |
| Gruskay | 0.48 | 0.01 | 3.30 |
| Hide | 1.26 | 0.34 | 4.00 |
| McConnochie | 0.00 | 0.00 | 4.13 |
| Fergusson | 1.02 | 0.35 | 2.48 |
| *Subtotal* | 0.73 | 0.62 | 0.86 |
| **Children without a family history of atopy** | | | |
| Gruskay | 0.48 | 0.01 | 3.30 |
| Hide | 1.26 | 0.34 | 4.00 |
| McConnochie | 0.00 | 0.00 | 4.13 |
| Fergusson | 1.02 | 0.35 | 2.48 |
| *Subtotal* | 0.99 | 0.48 | 2.03 |
| **Total** | 0.70 | 0.60 | 0.81 |

*b*

of allergic rhinitis [13]. The latter finding was not unexpected given the imprecise diagnostic criteria used in these studies, the young age of the children (mean age of 2.4 years follow-up) and the usual onset of allergic rhinitis after age 3.

## Recent Prospective Observational and Interventional Studies Supporting a Protective Role of Breastfeeding

Several recent well-designed prospective intervention studies that fulfill Kramer's criteria have confirmed the above meta-analyses and are summarized in table 3 [14–19]. In high-risk infants participating in an intervention study comparing hydrolyzed formulas to cow's milk formula, exclusive

**Table 3.** Recent prospective birth cohort studies on effect of BF on atopy

| Study | Birth cohorts | Comparison | Outcome, OR (95% CI) |
|---|---|---|---|
| Kramer et al. [14] (Belarus) | Unselected RC (n = 16,491) | BF support/promotion group vs. controls 43% of intervention group was exclusively BF at 3 months | 1 year AD: 0.54 (0.31–0.95): |
| Kull et al. [15, 16] (Sweden) | Observational (n = 773 vs. 3,013) | Sole BF ≥4 vs. <4 months | (a) 2 years AD: 0.85 (0.7–1) (b) 2 years asthma, cumulative prevalence 0.7 (0.5–0.8) (c) 4 years asthma, period prevalence 0.72 (0.53–0.97) |
| Oddy et al. [28] (Australia) | Observational (n = 2,602) | Predominant BF ≥4 vs. <4 months | 1 year wheeze and ≥2 acute visits: 0.6 (0.4–0.8) |
| Kerkoff et al. [18] (Netherlands) | High-risk RC (n = 708) | Sole BF ≥3 vs. <3 months | 1 year AD: 0.4 (0.2–1.0) |
| Laubereau et al. [19] (Germany) | High-risk RC (n = 2,030 vs. 522) | Sole BF ≥4 months vs. CMF | AD in 1st 3 years: 0.64 (0.45–0.90) |

OR = Odds ratio; RC = randomized controlled study; BF = breastfeeding; CMF = cow's milk formula; AD = atopic dermatitis. Revised and reprinted with permission from Friedman and Zeiger [4, table 2] and Mosby, St Louis., Mo.

breastfeeding compared to cow's milk had a significant protective effect on the development of atopic dermatitis in the first 3 years of life [19]. Similar protective effects on the incidence of atopic dermatitis by age 1 [14, 18] and 2 years [15] were seen with exclusive breastfeeding for at least 3 or 4 months compared to lesser periods. Specifically a 46% reduction in the incidence of atopic dermatitis was seen in infants whose mothers participated in a program designed to facilitate breastfeeding compared to infants whose mothers were not provided such support [14]. A lower risk of asthma-like symptoms from 1 to 6 years of age was seen in infants breastfed exclusively for 4 months in observational studies from Sweden [16] and Australia [17, 20].

## Duration of Exclusive Breastfeeding

Given that *not* breastfeeding may be associated with an increase in eczema and wheezing disorders in early childhood, how long should intact protein formulas be avoided?

A Swedish prospective, observational, birth cohort study demonstrated significant decreases with effect estimates from 20 to 34% in wheezing, asthma diagnosis, atopic dermatitis, and multiple allergic manifestations in infants breast-fed for ≥4 months [16]. An additive protective effect was observed in high-risk infants' breastfed for 6 months. In agreement, an Australian birth cohort study of 2,187 children found that exclusive breast-feeding for at least 4 months was associated with a reduced risk of asthma and atopy at 6 years. Benefits reported included: (1) a longer time to first wheeze and physician-diagnosed asthma; (2) a lower incidence of recurrent wheezing after age 1 year; (3) less sleep disturbance from asthma within the past year, and (4) a lower incidence of at least 1 positive aeroallergen skin test [20]. Evidence was presented that supported the age of introduction of intact protein formula more than the duration of exclusive breastfeeding as responsible for the above effect, but the strong correlation between the two prevents rejection of the possible role of breastfeeding.

## Breastfeeding by Asthmatic Mothers

Recently, concern regarding the potential adverse consequences associated with breastfeeding by atopic or asthmatic mothers has been voiced due to the fear of transfer of higher levels of pro-Th2 cytokines or n-6/n-3 polyunsaturated fatty acids from their breast milk to their infants as discussed earlier.

Wright et al. [21] first raised this concern after reporting a higher rate of asthma in atopic children of asthmatic mothers starting at age 6 years in the Tucson Children's Respiratory Study, a prospective longitudinal observational study of 1,246 newborns. This finding was in contrast to a significantly lower rate of wheezing, regardless of maternal asthma, up to age 3 years.

In contrast to the above study, an observational birth cohort study of 2,602 Australian children [17] found no interaction between maternal asthma and the lower rate of physician-diagnosed asthma and active wheeze at 6 years in infants exclusively breastfed for at least 4 months. Since both studies demonstrated an overall protective effect of breastfeeding on wheezing illness in early childhood, even the asthmatic mother should still be encouraged to breastfeed. Further studies are needed to determine which one of the above findings in school-age children is correct.

## Recent Prospective Observational Studies not Supporting a Protective Role of Breastfeeding

A few recent studies not included in the above meta-analyses have reported an adverse association of breastfeeding on atopy development. Table 4 highlights these studies and comments upon their potential methodological limitations. A long-term observational birth cohort of more than 1,300 German children, the important Multicenter Atopy Study (MAS), examined

**Table 4.** Selected studies reporting an increase in atopy with breastfeeding

| Study | Cohort | Finding | Comment |
|---|---|---|---|
| Kaplan and Mascie-Taylor [29] | 14,000 British 7-year-olds | Any BF: increased asthma at 7 years | Recall bias FH not controlled |
| Rusconi et al. [30] | 16,333 Italian 6- to 7-year-olds | BF ≥6 months: increased transient asthma; decreased late-onset asthma; no change in persistent asthma | Recall bias No control FH atopy |
| Wright et al. [21] | 1,246 Tucson birth cohort: birth–13 years | BF ≥4 months: increased recurrent wheeze at age ≥6 years | BF recall at 2 years Questionnaires |
| Bergmann et al. [31] | 1,314 German children: birth–7 years | >BF >AD to age 7 years: OR 1.03 (1.00–1.06) | Parent AD >factor Nursery CM common |
| Sears et al. [22] | 1,037 New Zealand; birth cohort: 3–26 years | BF 4 weeks or longer: increased current asthma 9–26 years; + skin tests at 13 years | Recall bias; lack of dose response |

BF = Breastfeeding; AD = atopic dermatitis; CM = cow's milk; FM = family history. Revised and reprinted with permission from Friedman and Zeiger [4, table 3] and Mosby, Inc. St Louis., Mo.

the role of breastfeeding in the development of allergic disease. After adjusting for potential confounding, MAS reported that breastfeeding was associated with an increased risk of atopic dermatitis from birth to age 7 years (p = 0.034). Breastfeeding for at least 1 month was associated with this adverse effect which could mean that an important maternal–infant interaction occurred early postnatally. It is possible that a confounding factor not addressed or inadequately adjusted for in the multivariate analysis might be responsible for these divergent findings. One such factor was the longer duration of breastfeeding by mothers who themselves or their spouses had atopic dermatitis. Adjustments were attempted but may have been inadequate to account for this important maternal behavior/practice. Supportive of the MAS study is an observational study from New Zealand [22]. This study enrolled patients at age 3 years from a cohort previously taking part in a separate earlier neonatal study. In all, 62.5% (n = 1,037) of the original birth cohort was enrolled in this latter study. Breastfeeding for 4 weeks or longer was associated with a significantly increased risk of asthma at ages 9–26 years (OR 1.8, 95% CI 1.4–2.5, p < 0.0001) and sensitization to aeroallergens at age 13 years (OR 1.9, 95% CI 1.4–2.6). Design limitations were raised [23]: (1) frequent intact cow's milk ingestion in the nursery and therefore infrequent exclusive breast-feeding; (2) no effect of atopic family history; (3) no dose response, and (4) biased early recall of feeding patterns in infancy since the cohort was enrolled at age 3 years. Evaluating only 60% of the original cohort may also be a factor. Though Sears et al. [24] did not refute the first 3 criticisms, they noted that maternal recall was corroborated with nurse home-visit records obtained in the earlier neonatal study about 98% of the time. Notwithstanding these criticisms, the study raises potentially important issues that can only be resolved with long-term follow-up of the studies listed table 3.

## Maternal Food Allergen Avoidance Diets during Lactation

One of the factors raised to help explain the differences in study outcomes may relate to the variability of food allergens in breast milk that is dependent on maternal eating habits. In addition, breast milk food allergens have been blamed for the development of atopic disease and sensitization in approximately 6% of exclusively breastfed infants. As noted above, exposure to food allergens through breast milk might either sensitize or tolerize.

A Cochrane meta-analysis evaluated the maternal lactation diet issue and reported a small positive effect of maternal elimination diets on the development of atopic dermatitis during the first 12–18 months of life [25]. However, the report noted that the number of studies was limited, most of the effect was due to 1 study [26], and the number of patients was small. As such, they concluded that more studies are necessary to generalize these findings.

It is possible that a route other than breast milk, such as dermal food exposure, may be responsible for the sensitization of exclusively breastfed infants. A murine food allergy model provided proof of principle of primary IgE food sensitization through dermal food exposure. Evidence that a similar mechanism may be functional in humans is supported by the findings of the Avon longitudinal study of nearly 16,000 children. In this study peanut allergy was independently associated with the presence of eczematous skin and use of skin care products containing peanut oil, but not with maternal ingestion of peanut products during lactation [27]. These findings raise the real possibility that sensitization may more readily occur through skin absorption than through direct ingestion of peanut protein through breast milk.

## Conclusions

We have examined the possible atopic consequences of *not* breastfeeding. Meta-analyses of older studies and recent well-designed birth cohort studies both provide reasonable evidence that exclusive breastfeeding for at least 4 months is associated with a reduction in atopic dermatitis and wheezing illnesses up to age 6 years. There is weaker evidence to suggest that CMA and atopic sensitization may also be reduced. A few observational studies question these conclusions, particularly in older children, but there is sufficient definitive evidence to discount these findings at least in early childhood. The effect of exclusive breastfeeding on atopy and asthma beyond age 6 years lacks sufficient study to make any reasonable conclusions. In addition, allergen avoidance diets during lactation should remain investigational. Finally, exclusive breastfeeding for at least 4 months should be a keystone of allergy-prevention efforts for both high- and low-risk infants as recommended by the AAP [2] and ESPACI/ESPGHAN [3] and supported by the evidence presented here and elsewhere [4]. Such recommendations are consistent with the principles of not interfering with Mother Nature or prematurely instituting unproven or burdensome interventions (lactation diets). Furthermore, the presence of maternal asthma should not deter from following these recommendations.

## References

1 Grulee CG, Sanford HN: The influence of breast and artificial feeding on infantile eczema. J Pediatr 1930;9:223–225.
2 American Academy of Pediatrics: Committee on Nutrition. Hypoallergenic infant formulas. Pediatrics 2000;106:346–349.
3 Host A, Koletzko B, Dreborg S, et al: Dietary products used in infants for treatment and prevention of food allergy. Joint Statement of the European Society for Paediatric Allergology and Clinical Immunology (ESPACI) Committee on Hypoallergenic Formulas and the European Society for Paediatric Gastroenterology, Hepatology and Nutrition (ESPGHAN) Committee on Nutrition. Arch Dis Child 1999;81:80–84.
4 Friedman N, Zeiger R: The role of breast-feeding in the development of allergies and asthma. J Allergy Clin Immunol 2005;115:1238–1248.
5 Oddy WH, Halonen M, Martinez FD, et al: TGF-beta in human milk is associated with wheeze in infancy. J Allergy Clin Immunol 2003;112:723–728.
6 Ball TM, Castro-Rodriguez JA, Griffith KA, et al: Siblings, day-care attendance, and the risk of asthma and wheezing during childhood. N Engl J Med 2000;343:538–543.
7 Vadas P, Wai Y, Burks W, Perelman B: Detection of peanut allergens in breast milk of lactating women. JAMA 2001;285:1746–1748.
8 Lucas A, Brooke OG, Morley R, et al: Early diet of preterm infants and development of allergic or atopic disease: randomised prospective study. BMJ 1990;300:837–840.
9 Kramer MS: Does breast feeding help protect against atopic disease? Biology, methodology, and a golden jubilee of controversy. J Pediatr 1988;112:181–190.
10 van Odijk J, Kull I, Borres MP, et al: Breastfeeding and allergic disease: a multidisciplinary review of the literature (1966–2001) on the mode of early feeding in infancy and its impact on later atopic manifestations. Allergy 2003;58:833–843.
11 Gdalevich M, Mimouni D, David M, Mimouni M: Breast-feeding and the onset of atopic dermatitis in childhood: a systematic review and meta-analysis of prospective studies. J Am Acad Dermatol 2001;45:520–527.
12 Gdalevich M, Mimouni D, Mimouni M: Breast-feeding and the risk of bronchial asthma in childhood: a systematic review with meta-analysis of prospective studies. J Pediatr 2001;139: 261–266.
13 Mimouni BA, Mimouni D, Mimouni M, Gdalevich M: Does breastfeeding protect against allergic rhinitis during childhood? A meta-analysis of prospective studies. Acta Paediatr 2002;91: 275–279.
14 Kramer MS, Chalmers B, Hodnett ED, et al: Promotion of Breastfeeding Intervention Trial (PROBIT): a randomized trial in the Republic of Belarus. JAMA 2001;285:413–420.

15 Kull I, Wickman M, Lilja G, et al: Breast feeding and allergic diseases in infants-a prospective birth cohort study. Arch Dis Child 2002;87:478–481.
16 Kull I, Almqvist C, Lilja G, et al: Breast-feeding reduces the risk of asthma during the first 4 years of life. J Allergy Clin Immunol 2004;114:755–760.
17 Oddy WH, Peat JK, de Klerk NH: Maternal asthma, infant feeding, and the risk of asthma in childhood. J Allergy Clin Immunol 2002;110:65–67.
18 Kerkhof M, Koopman LP, van Strien RT, et al: Risk factors for atopic dermatitis in infants at high risk of allergy: the PIAMA study. Clin Exp Allergy 2003;33:1336–1341.
19 Laubereau B, Brockow I, Zirngibl A, et al: Effect of breast-feeding on the development of atopic dermatitis during the first 3 years of life–results from the GINI-birth cohort study. J Pediatr 2004;144:602–607.
20 Oddy WH, Holt PG, Sly PD, et al: Association between breast feeding and asthma in 6 year old children: findings of a prospective birth cohort study. BMJ 1999;319:815–819.
21 Wright AL, Holberg CJ, Taussig LM, Martinez FD: Factors influencing the relation of infant feeding to asthma and recurrent wheeze in childhood. Thorax 2001;56:192–197.
22 Sears MR, Greene JM, Willan AR, et al: Long-term relation between breastfeeding and development of atopy and asthma in children and young adults: a longitudinal study. Lancet 2002;360:901–907.
23 Peat JK, Allen J, Oddy W, Webb K: Breastfeeding and asthma: appraising the controversy. Pediatr Pulmonol 2003;35:331–334.
24 Sears MR, Taylor DR, Poulton R: Breastfeeding and asthma: appraising the controversy – a rebuttal. Pediatr Pulmonol 2003;36:366–368.
25 Kramer MS: Maternal antigen avoidance during lactation for preventing atopic disease in infants of women at high risk. Cochrane Database Syst Rev 2000;2:CD000132.
26 Chandra RK, Puri S, Hamed A: Influence of maternal diet during lactation and use of formula feeds on development of atopic eczema in high risk infants. BMJ 1989;299:228–230.
27 Lack G, Fox D, Northstone K, Golding J: Factors associated with the development of peanut allergy in childhood. N Engl J Med 2003;348:977–985.
28 Oddy WH, Sly PD, de Klerk NH, et al: Breast feeding and respiratory morbidity in infancy: a birth cohort study. Arch Dis Child 2003;88:224–228.
29 Kaplan BA, Mascie-Taylor CG: Biosocial factors in the epidemiology of childhood asthma in a British national sample. J Epidemiol Community Health 1985;39:152–156.
30 Rusconi F, Galassi C, Corbo GM, et al: Risk factors for early, persistent, and late-onset wheezing in young children. SIDRIA Collaborative Group. Am J Respir Crit Care Med 1999;160:1617–1622.
31 Bergmann RL, Diepgen TL, Kuss O, et al: Breastfeeding duration is a risk factor for atopic eczema. Clin Exp Allergy 2002;32:205–209.

## Discussion

*Dr. Lucas:* Just to clarify our trial here. There was no effect of breastfeeding; there was only an effect when a subgroup analysis was done, and then it was found that the group with the positive family history had an effect but the group with the negative family history was, if anything, the other way around giving advantage to the cow's milk group. It was not quite significant but in fact in another trial comparing a high-protein with a low-protein formula, in the negative family history group the high-protein formula was associated with low atopic disease, suggesting that it was good if you had a negative family history to have cow's milk protein. So my point here is that you obviously recognize that there are many other reasons for maintaining breastfeeding but, based on atopy alone, this would not be the case even from the data that you presented showing that there is not a case for recommending breastfeeding if there is a negative family history of atopy, and that is the majority of infants.

*Dr. Zeiger:* I would agree. With an effect size of up to 30% reported by mainly observational studies for breastfeeding on the reduction of atopic disorders in early childhood in high-risk newborns, one should recommend breastfeeding in non-high-risk infants for its nutritional, physiological, immunological, and psychological benefits and not for its potential properties to reduce wheezing and atopic dermatitis in early childhood.

*Dr. Björkstén:* The bulk of the evidence is that breastfed babies are less prone to wheezing, and I would suggest that this is because breastfeeding clearly protects against infections. In addition, you do have at most a modest effect on dermatitis. But if you go into allergy prevention, I am less convinced. The Finnish study was started in the early 1970s and breastfeeding was not compared with modern infant formula. The recent Kramer study as I see it is irrelevant to Western Europe as it was done in the Republic of Belarus where the gut microbiota are different. So in summary, what you should say is that breastfeeding protects against infant wheezing of infectious origin, but you may not have an allergy protection.

*Dr. Zeiger:* I would agree. We probably should not be looking upon breastfeeding as allergy-preventive in the sense of preventing IgE-mediated disease. There are only one or two studies to suggest that specific IgE sensitization can be affected by breastfeeding and no study to show such an effect on allergic asthma. However, meta-analyses of multiple studies conclude that breastfeeding is associated with a significant reduction in episodes of wheezing within the first 2 years of life. We should recommend breastfeeding for its proven nutritional, immunological and physiological benefits. Breastfeeding may in addition reduce some aspects of wheezing and eczema early in childhood in high-risk children. As you suggest we should not promote breastfeeding in a way that would engender guilt in a mother who does not breastfeed for whatever reason.

*Dr. Sampson:* I have two questions that are a little bit unrelated. The first related to the study by Oddy et al. [1] and looking at whether or not it mattered if the mother was atopic. I can't remember the exact article, but there was a study from Finland that suggested there was a difference if the mother had active disease at the time of breastfeeding as opposed to just having a history of atopic disease. I wonder if you would comment on that. The second question is related to maternal avoidance diets while breastfeeding. One of the things we struggle with, and I am sure you do as well, is when mothers come with one child in the family having peanut allergy and then wondering should they be avoiding peanuts while breastfeeding. I guess the thing I struggle with is whether or not peanut is really different from the other food allergens because when we look at a registry of over 5,000 peanut-allergic patients almost 90% of those children were breastfed and 80% of those children reacted on the first known exposure to peanut, suggesting that somewhere they had been sensitized. We know that the peanut protein is present in breast milk, we also know that dry roasting a peanut makes a more allergenic and much hardier protein. When AraH1 has been dry-roasted, it forms a very robust trimer that it is very difficult to break down. So do you think that peanuts may be different?

*Dr. Zeiger:* The relationship of active atopic disease in a mother and the development of wheezing illnesses in her child has been examined in only a few studies. The Australian studies of Oddy et al. [1] specifically looked upon active asthma in mothers and the development of asthma in their children. There was no interaction between the mother's active asthma and the protective effect of breastfeeding on wheezing illnesses. The Tucson Children's Respiratory Study analyzed the effect of a mother's history of wheezing, not active disease, on the development of wheezing in their probands [2]. This study reported an increased risk for recurrent wheeze starting at about 6 years in allergic sensitized children whose mothers had a history of asthma. I am not familiar with the Finnish study. There are enough disparate data on this issue to suggest that we do not alter our recommendations regarding breastfeeding based on these data. With respect to lactation diets and avoidance of peanut, my take on this issue is the following: I think there is more evidence perhaps for the food allergens in breast milk to be tolerizing than sensitizing. The concentration of milk allergen within breast milk is comparative to the concentration of milk protein in Nutramigen. These milk protein levels are from a hundred thousand to a million lower than in cow's milk. There is no evidence to suggest that peanut protein concentrations in breast milk would be too different from cow's milk protein levels. Relative to exposure of an infant to peanut, excluding infant ingestion, one would expect a greater burden imposed by direct contact of the infant with peanut protein on the body or clothing of caregivers or home surfaces than from lactation. Peanut sensitization through abraded skin has been proposed as a potential non-ingestion mechanism for peanut sensitization as suggested by Lack et al. [3]. In addition, proof of principle for food sensitization by the dermal group was recently reported in a murine model of food allergy [4]. As such, one may need to be more concerned with reducing peanut contact than interfering with lactation diets.

*Dr. Lake:* Would you comment on whether or not peanut restriction plays a role in utero, in other words changing the maternal diet before the child is born?

*Dr. Zeiger:* The epidemiologic studies have not been convincing. Prospective randomized clinical control trials that were done by Dr. Björkstén's group were not able to demonstrate any benefit from the avoidance of milk and egg during the last trimester of pregnancy in the development of atopic disease from birth to 5 years of life. They did not study peanut avoidance. We should not be modifying pregnancy diets until there is evidence to show benefit from such modifications.

*Dr. Björkstén:* It is not only that the study was negative, all 5 of the 200 children who, by the age of 6 years, kept egg allergy were in the maternal avoidance group. As I mentioned yesterday when in Sweden we delayed the introduction of gluten until after the age of 6 months, we got an increase in celiac disease, and going back to gradually introducing glutens while breastfeeding we immediately went back to the normal incidence. So I am suggesting a word of caution.

*Dr. Zeiger:* I think a good deal of caution. We should not begin to interfere with Mother Nature unless we know definitively that it will be beneficial.

*Dr. Chad:* Do you think we should be looking at studies giving mothers who are pregnant and/or lactating more allergen to see if we can induce tolerance in the babies? I know that it is fooling with Mother Nature again, but it is going to the other extreme. We looked at avoiding and found no improvement.

*Dr. Zeiger:* We don't know enough about it. There are very few animal studies to begin with and I think we need to do more animal studies to see whether there is a dose response that occurs with increasing tolerance.

*Dr. Hamburger:* I would certainly agree with your last statement, and I wonder about this whole business of obstetricians and gynecologists recommending that the mother drink a liter or two of milk a day in order to protect her teeth and bones as being bad advice as well.

*Dr. Zeiger:* Yes, that amount of milk daily might be considered excessive.

*Dr. Roma:* During the last years we have noticed an increase in allergic colitis in exclusively breastfed infants. Have you had the same experience and if so, have you got an explanation for that?

*Dr. Zeiger:* In my health plan membership of about 4,500 births yearly, as allergists, we have not been aware of an increase in allergic colitis in exclusively breastfed infants. Perhaps Dr. Lake might be able to give some overview related to colitis.

*Dr. Lake:* As gastroenterologists, we are recognizing more breastfed babies with eosinophilic proctitis in the first 2–6 months of life. More than 90% are non-IgE-mediated, so we are avoiding the term 'allergic colitis' [5]. A more dramatic increase in eosinophilic esophagitis and gastritis has been noted in infants presenting as eosinophic reflux, poorly responsive to acid reduction and featuring food refusal as a prominent symptom. Confirming a specific dietary protein-induced etiology has been difficult [6].

107

*Dr. Laron:* What is known about the genes involved in atopy? We have a Jewish population coming from Iraq. Their children have a high incidence of asthma and a high incidence of G6PD deficiency.

*Dr. Zeiger:* There have been several hundred genes identified that relate to the causation of atopic disease, including asthma and atopic dermatitis. It is reasonable to expect that gene polymorphisms will be found that identify children at high risk for specific atopic disorders and even responsiveness to specific therapies. The practical use of these findings will be one of the major future challenges of allergy prevention.

## References

1  Oddy WH, Peat JK, de Klerk NH: Maternal asthma, infant feeding, and the risk of asthma in childhood. J Allergy Clin Immunol 2002;110:65–67.
2  Wright AL, Holberg CJ, Taussig LM, Martinez FD: Factors influencing the relation of infant feeding to asthma and recurrent wheeze in childhood. Thorax 2001;56:192–197.
3  Lack G, Fox D, Northstone K, et al: Factors associated with the development of peanut allergy in childhood. N Engl J Med 2003;348:977–985.
4  Hsieh KY, Tsai CC, Wu CH, Lin RH: Epicutaneous exposure to protein antigen and food allergy. Clin Exp Allergy 2003;33:1067–1075.
5  Lake AM: Food-induced eosinophilic proctocolitis. J Pediatr Gastroenterol Nutr 2000;30: S58–S60.
6  Furuta GT: Eosinophilic esophagitis: an emerging clinicopathologic entity. Curr Allergy Asthma Rep 2002;2:67–72.

Lucas A, Sampson HA (eds): Primary Prevention by Nutrition Intervention in Infancy and Childhood.
Nestlé Nutr Workshop Ser Pediatr Program, vol 57, pp 109–123,
Nestec Ltd., Vevey/S. Karger AG, Basel, © 2006.

# Prevention of Atopy and Allergic Disease: Type of Infant Formula

*Hugh A. Sampson*

Pediatric Allergy and Immunology, Elliot and Roslyn Jaffe Food Allergy Institute,
Mount Sinai School of Medicine, New York, N.Y., USA

## Introduction

The prevalence of allergy and atopic disorders has been increasing over
the past several decades [1] and consequently investigators have sought to
understand the reason for this increase and to develop strategies to reverse
this trend. A great deal of attention has been focused on early intervention
since most children afflicted with atopic disorders first develop symptoms
during infancy and subsequently develop other atopic symptoms, i.e. the
'atopic march' [2]. About 70 years ago an article was published suggesting that
breastfeeding could prevent eczema [3], and since then many studies have
both supported and refuted this claim. Unfortunately, as discussed elsewhere
in this symposium, most of these studies have serious methodological flaws
making the arrival at firm conclusions impossible. Nevertheless, two recent
meta-analyses of studies published between 1966 and 2000 indicate that
exclusive breastfeeding in the first 4 months of life can reduce the prevalence
of atopic dermatitis (AD) [4] and asthma [5] in children at risk of developing
atopy, i.e. offspring of atopic parents. Given that not all women can or will
breastfeed, alternative infant formulas also have been evaluated for their
protective effect. On the basis of a retrospective study over 50 years ago [6],
it has been suggested that soy-based formulas provide protection against
allergic disease compared to milk-based formulas. However, a recent meta-
analysis of studies done since the 1960s clearly demonstrated that soy- and
milk-based formulas are no different in their ability to prevent food allergy or
atopic disorders [7].

Sampson

**Table 1.** Hydrolyzed protein- and amino acid-based infant formulas

'Non-allergenic' infant formulas – amino acid-derived
  Neocate, Neocate 1[a,b]
  EleCare[a]
  Nutri-Junior
Extensively hydrolyzed bovine casein-based formulas
  Nutramigen[a]
  Pregestimil[a]
  Alimentum[a]
Extensively hydrolyzed bovine whey-based formulas
  Alfa-Re
  Profylac[b]
  Pepti-Junior
  Nutrion Pepti
  Peptidi-Tutteli
Partially hydrolyzed whey-based formula
  Nan HA/Bebe HA/Good Start/Nidina HA
Extensively hydrolyzed soy-based formula
  Pregomin

[a]Available in the United States and fulfill the AAP 'hypoallergenic for treatment' criteria.
[b]Not available in the United States but fulfills the AAP 'hypoallergenic for treatment' criteria.

## Hydrolyzed Infants Formulas

The first extensively hydrolyzed milk-based formula (Nutramigen®) was developed over 60 years ago for use in infants with cow's milk allergy or intolerance. Since then a number of extensively and partially hydrolyzed infant formulas, and more recently amino acid-based formulas, have become available (table 1). These extensively hydrolyzed formulas became know as 'hypoallergenic' since most infants and young children with cow's milk allergy could tolerate these formulas without apparent symptoms. However, since the term 'hypoallergenic' was never clearly defined and in essence simply means 'less allergenic', a partially hydrolyzed formula was introduced in the United States in the late 1980s and was labeled 'hypoallergenic' (Goodstart HA®), which led to confusion among consumers and resulted in a number of severe reactions in cow's milk-allergic infants [8]. Consequently the Committee on Nutrition of the American Academy of Pediatrics established a subcommittee which was asked to develop criteria for the labeling of infant formula as 'hypoallergenic' [9]. The subcommittee recommended that in order to label a formula 'hypoallergenic for the *treatment* of cow's milk-allergic infants', the formula must fulfill a series of pre-clinical and clinical requirements, including the use of double-blind placebo-controlled oral food

110

challenges and subsequent open feeding for at least 7 days to demonstrate (with ≥95% confidence) that at least 90% of cow's milk-allergic children could ingest the formula without developing allergic symptoms. In addition, the subcommittee recommended criteria for labeling a formula 'hypoallergenic for the *prevention* of allergic disorders'. Prospective clinical trials were necessary to demonstrate that significantly fewer children at risk of allergy (based on family history), and given the study formula exclusively for at least the first 6 months of life, would experience significantly fewer allergic symptoms at 18 months or later compared to similar infants receiving a standard cow's milk formula. If any allergic symptoms were reported due to either formula, they had to be confirmed by blinded oral food challenge. These recommendations were accepted by the American Academy of Pediatrics and reaffirmed more recently in an Academy position statement [10]. While several extensively hydrolyzed and amino acid-based formulas have fulfilled the American Academy of Pediatrics' criteria 'hypoallergenic for treatment' of IgE-mediated cow's milk allergy [11–13], no formula has been established as 'hypoallergenic for prevention'.

## Hydrolyzed Formulas for the Prevention of Atopic Disease and Allergy

The rationale for utilizing extensively hydrolyzed infant formulas for the prevention of milk allergy and atopic disease is based on the fact that these formulas are hypoimmunogenic as demonstrated in animal models as well as man, hypoallergenic for the treatment of milk allergy, and contain levels of milk proteins (β-lactoglobulin) [14] comparable to what is found in human breast milk. In the past 3 decades, at least 90 studies have been published comparing the utility of 'hypoallergenic' infant formulas to standard infant formulas for the prevention of allergy and atopic disease. However, as indicated in a recent meta-analysis [15], only 18 of these studies had <80% dropouts and fulfilled the Cochrane Neonatal Review Groups criteria for inclusion [16–33]. Studies were excluded from the analysis primarily because they had greater than a 20% dropout rate and/or lacked adequate randomization and allocation concealment, blinding of parents or caretakers and assessors to the intervention, and completeness of assessment in all randomized study subjects. In this review, a number of subgroup analyses were performed comparing the types of milk used in the control group, the length of supplementary feeding, the presence of co-interventions, the type of subject enrolled (high vs. low risk for atopic disease), the type of hydrolyzed formula used, and whether clinical allergy was confirmed by allergy testing.

Primarily for ethical reasons, no randomized study has been conducted comparing the prolonged use of hydrolyzed infant formula to exclusive breastfeeding. Two studies evaluated short-term supplemental feeding (3 and

4 days) with extensively hydrolyzed formula and donor breast milk and found no difference between the two regimens [22, 27]. In addition, short-term feeding of hydrolyzed and standardized formulas followed by breastfeeding were compared and no significant differences were found. No study has compared the allergy-preventative effect of prolonged feedings with hydrolyzed formulas to standard infant formulas in children at low atopic risk. In the Cochrane Report [15], 12 studies compared prolonged hydrolyzed formula feeding to standard cow's milk formula, but only seven of these studies did not incorporate other preventative interventions. Meta-analysis of seven studies, five of which included other interventions, found a significant reduction in 'any allergic manifestations' in infancy, and in 3 studies that evaluated a total of 333 children for a more prolonged period of time, a significant reduction in childhood allergy was also reported in infants who had received hydrolyzed formulas. Nine studies evaluated the development of AD in a total of 870 infants. Meta-analysis of these 9 studies revealed a significant reduction in AD during infancy in the infants receiving hydrolyzed formula (RR = 0.59; 95% CI = 0.40, 0.86). Similar findings were reported for 2 studies following a total of 198 children through early childhood [16, 24], and one study following 135 children through 5 years of age [19]. Six studies evaluated the incidence of asthma and meta-analysis of the six studies incorporating 945 infants found a significant reduction in asthma in those receiving the hydrolyzed formula (RR = 0.59; 95% CI = 0.40, 0.86). When meta-analyses were performed on the seven studies incorporating no co-interventions, infants receiving hydrolyzed formulas had reduced allergic symptoms (RR = 0.63; 95% CI = 0.47, 0.85) and AD (RR = 0.48; 95% CI = 0.34, 0.66) in infancy compared to infants receiving standard infant formulas. However, no difference was seen in the incidence of wheezing or asthma.

In the Cochrane Report [15], seven studies were analyzed that compared prolonged feeding of partially hydrolyzed formulas to standard cow's milk formulas with no other preventative measures. Six of these seven studies were supported by industry. Meta-analysis of four studies containing 386 high-risk infants found a significant reduction in allergic manifestations in infancy (RR = 0.63; 95% CI = 0.47, 0.85) and meta-analysis of three studies with a total of 230 infants found a significant reduction in eczema in infancy (RR = 0.64; 95% CI = 0.42, 0.98). No significant difference in asthma symptoms in infancy was noted. Three studies compared the supplemental use of extensively hydrolyzed versus partially hydrolyzed formula in infants at high risk of atopic disease. Meta-analyses failed to demonstrate any significant difference in food allergy, any allergic manifestations, eczema or asthma between the two groups. One study compared the prophylactic effect of prolonged feeding with hydrolyzed soy formula to standard infant formula in high-risk infants, although other preventative interventions were employed [16]. While the authors found a significant difference in the incidence of infant (RR = 0.50; 95% CI = 0.32, 0.79) and childhood allergy (RR = 0.60;

95% CI = 0.39, 0.92), there was no significant difference in the incidence of infant or childhood eczema, asthma, rhinitis or food allergy.

Overall the authors of the Cochrane Report on the use of hydrolyzed formulas for the prevention of allergy [15] concluded that there is no evidence to support the use of hydrolyzed infant formulas in place of exclusive breast-feeding in the prevention of allergic disease. However, in infants who are unable to receive exclusive breastfeeding for at least the first 4 months of life, use of hydrolyzed formulas can reduce the incidence of allergy, especially atopic eczema, through the first 5 years of life, but further studies are necessary to determine whether the benefit persists beyond this age. While the use of meta-analysis provides a powerful tool to assess the validity of clinical trials addressing a similar medical question, its outcomes remain subject to a number of limitations including publication bias, inconsistent quality of trial design, and potential inconsistency of study conduct.

In the late 1990s, a government-sponsored multicenter study was initiated in Germany to compare the efficacy of three hydrolyzed infant formulas to standard cow's milk formula in the prevention of milk allergy and atopic disorders [34]. Between 1995 and 1998, 2,252 infants at high risk of developing atopic disease were enrolled in a multicenter, prospective, randomized, double-blind interventional trial to compare the efficacy of three different hydrolyzed infant formulas to standard cow's milk formula for the prevention of milk allergy and atopic disorders (German Infant Nutritional Intervention Study – GINI Study). To be included in the study, infants had to be healthy, ≥2.5 kg at birth, ≥ than 37 weeks gestation and born to a family with at least one atopic family member (mother, father, and/or sibling). At the time of enrollment, infants were randomized to one of four study formulas, standard cow's milk-based formula (CMF; Nutrilon Premium®, Nutricia/Numico), partially hydrolyzed whey formula (p-HWF; Beba HA®, Nestlé), extensively hydrolyzed whey formula (e-HWF; Hipp HA®, Hipp/NutrilonPepti®, Nutricia/Numico) or extensively hydrolyzed casein formula (e-HCF; Nutramigen®, Mead Johnson), and stratified by an independent person for single or double parental history of atopy and region. All mothers were encouraged to breastfeed exclusively for at least 4 months, and preferably 6 months. However, if this was not possible, supplementation or exclusive use of the study formula was initiated and continued through the first 6 months of life. Solid foods were excluded for the first 6 months of life and then added in a standardized fashion. Parents were asked to record the type of feeding (breast milk or study formula), the time of first introduction of study drug, kind of solid foods introduced, health problems, and any 'allergic manifestation,' e.g. AD, allergic urticaria, food allergy with manifestation in the gastrointestinal tract, or asthma.

A total of 1,249 infants received study formula and, as shown in table 2, similar numbers of infants received each of the study formulas. A total of 304 infants dropped out or were excluded, so 945 of 1,249 (76%) infants receiving formula were evaluable at 12 months. Of note, significantly more infants

Sampson

**Table 2.** Distribution of 2,232 infants to formula feeding groups in GINI study

| | Number enrolled | | | | |
|---|---|---|---|---|---|
| | CMF | p-HWF | e-HWF | e-HCF | Breast milk |
| Initial assignment | 556 | 557 | 559 | 580 | – |
| Received study formula | 328 | 315 | 302 | 304 | 889 |
| Compliant: 12-month follow-up | 256 | 241 | 238 | 210 | 865 |
| Evaluated at 3 years | 245 | 229 | 230 | 200 | 543 |

dropped out or had to be excluded for 'non-compliance' from the e-HCF group (18%) than from the other study formula groups (10–12%). At the 1-year evaluation, the incidence of 'allergic manifestations' in each group was the following: CMF = 16%; p-HWF = 11%; e-HWF = 14%; e-HCF = 9%, and BF = 11%. Only infants fed the e-HCF had significantly less 'allergic manifestations' at 1 year compared to infants receiving the standard milk formula (adjusted for AD in family history, sex, and maternal smoking (adj) OR = 0.51 (0.28–0.92)). The incidence of 'AD' in each group was the following: CMF = 15%; p-HWF = 9%; e-HWF = 13%; e-HCF = 7%, and BF = 9.5%. Infants fed the e-HCF and p-HWF had significantly less 'AD' at 1 year compared to infants receiving the standard milk formula (adj OR = 0.42 (0.22–0.79) and adj OR = 0.56 (0.32–0.99), respectively) [34]. The cumulative incidence of 'allergic manifestations' at 3-year follow-up was the following: CMF = 31.4%; p-HWF = 25.8%; e-HWF = 32.2%, and e-HCF = 26.5%. There was no significant reduction in 'allergic manifestations' in infants receiving hydrolyzed formula compared to standard milk formula. As depicted in table 3, the cumulative incidence of AD at 3 years was the following: CMF = 22.5%; p-HWF = 14.9%; e-HWF = 20.9%; e-HCF = 14.0%, and BF = 19.2%. Only infants receiving p-HWF or e-HCF had significantly less AD over the 3-year period and at the 3rd year evaluation, i.e. period prevalence. No difference in the incidence of asthma was noted during the first 3 years of evaluation. Interestingly, the p-HWF appeared to be more protective for AD in infants who came from families without a history of AD while e-HCF appeared more protective for infants from families with a history of AD. Since the BF infants were not randomized to treatment and therefore represent an observational cohort, their incidence of atopic disorders cannot accurately be compared to that of the formula-fed groups.

**Recommendations**

A number of other large prospective studies not fulfilling the Cochrane Report inclusion criteria for evaluation of hydrolyzed formulas also suggest a

**Table 3.** Cumulative incidence and period prevalence of AD and asthma in the first 3 years according to study formula and adjusted odds ratios (OR)[*] in comparison to cow's milk feeding (assigned OR = 1)

| | | CMF (n = 245) | p-HWF (n = 229) | e-HWF (n = 230) | e-HCF (n = 200) |
|---|---|---|---|---|---|
| Cumulative incidence of AD in the 1st 3 years | Cases, n OR (95% CI) | 55 (22.5%) 1 | 34 (14.9%) 0.60 (0.37–0.97) | 48 (20.9%) 0.87 (0.56–1.4) | 28 (14.0%) 0.53 (0.32–0.88) |
| No AD in FH | | 32/158 1 | 0.45 (0.24–0.87) | 0.63 (0.34–1.18) | 0.60 (0.32–1.13) |
| AD in FA | | 23/87 1 | 0.88 (0.43–1.81) | 1.26 (0.66–2.42) | 0.44 (0.19–1.01) |
| Contribution to incidence in 2nd and 3rd years | Cases, n OR (95% CI) | 17 (6.9%) 1 | 15 (6.6%) 0.95 (0.46–2.0) | 17 (7.4%) 1.1 (0.52–2.1) | 16 (8.0%) 1.1 (0.53–2.2) |
| Contribution to incidence in the 1st year | Cases, n OR (95% CI) | 38 (15.5%) 1 | 19 (8.3%) 0.49 (0.27–0.88) | 31 (13.5%) 0.81 (0.48–1.4) | 12 (6.0%) 0.33 (0.17–0.66) |
| Period prevalence of AD in 2nd year | Cases, n OR (95% CI) | 27 (11.0%) 1 | 16 (7.0%) 0.62 (0.32–1.2) | 24 (10.4%) 0.88 (0.49–1.69) | 11 (5.5%) 0.44 (0.21–0.91) |
| Period prevalence of AD in 3rd year | Cases, n OR (95% CI) | 29 (11.8%) 1 | 13 (5.7%) 0.46 (0.23–0.90) | 20 (8.7%) 0.68 (0.37–1.2) | 12 (6.0%) 0.46 (0.23–0.93) |
| Cumulative incidence of 'asthma' in 3rd year | Cases, n Crude OR (95% CI) | 25 (10.2%) 1 | 28 (12.2%) 1.2 (0.69–2.2) | 29 (12.6%) 1.3 (0.72–2.2) | 19 (89.5%) 0.92 (0.49–1.7) |

[*] Adjusted for gender, maternal smoking in the first year, family history of AD.
Adapted from von Berg et al. for the GINI Study Group, with permission.
Significant effects are underlined.

protective effect of e-HCF for the prevention of AD in infants up to the 4th year of life [35–38]. While the ideal study to evaluate the protective effects of hydrolyzed formulas is yet to be performed (i.e. a randomized trial comparing exclusive breastfeeding to exclusive use of hydrolyzed infant formula for at least the first 4 months of life, and therefore a trial that is very unlikely to be performed for ethical reasons), the weight of the evidence appears to support a number of conclusions. First, there is no evidence to support the use of any hydrolyzed infant formula over exclusive breastfeeding for the prevention of atopic disorders. At this time there is no evidence that breastfeeding beyond 4–6 months provides further benefit with respect to prevention of atopic disease. Second, if exclusive breastfeeding is not possible, infants from 'high-risk' families, i.e. those with one or two parents and/or a sibling with food allergy, AD, asthma or allergic rhinitis, should be given a p-HWF or e-HCF for the first 6 months of life. Evidence from one large, prospective multicenter trial (GINI Study) suggests that infants from atopic families without a history of AD in a primary relative will receive the protective effect from the less expensive partial whey hydrolysate formula whereas those infants

Sampson

who have first-degree relatives with AD should receive the e-HCF. Third, while some studies suggest that the use of hydrolyzed infant formulas in high-risk infants also may prevent the development of allergic rhinitis or asthma [19, 29, 33], there are insufficient data at this time to demonstrate any prophylactic benefit. Finally, there are no data to demonstrate that the use of hydrolyzed formulas in the first 4–6 months of life will prevent atopic disease in infants from low-risk families. Given that the majority of children diagnosed with atopic disease come from 'low-risk' families, it may be beneficial to evaluate the effect of partial hydrolysate formulas, which are palatable and no more expensive than standard cow's milk infant formulas (in the US), for their potential prophylactic effect on the development of atopy in this population.

## References

1 Wahn U, von Mutius E: Childhood risk factors for atopy and the importance of early intervention. J Allergy Clin Immunol 2001;107:567–574.
2 Liu A, Martinez FD, Taussig LM: Natural history of allergic diseases and asthma; in Leung DYM, Sampson HA, Geha RS, Szefler SJ (eds): Pediatric Allergy: Principles and Practice. St. Louis, Mosby, 2003, pp 10–22.
3 Grulee CG, Sanford HN: The influence of breast feeding and artificial feeding in infantile eczema. J Pediatr 1936;9:223–225.
4 Gdalevich M, Mimouni D, David M, Mimouni M: Breast-feeding and the onset of atopic dermatitis in childhood: a systematic review and meta-analysis of prospective studies. J Am Acad Dermatol 2001;45:520–527.
5 Gdalevich M, Mimouni D, Mimouni M: Breast-feeding and the risk of bronchial asthma in childhood: a systematic review with meta-analysis of prospective studies. J Pediatr 2001;139: 261–266.
6 Johnstone D, Glaser J: Use of soybean milk as an aid in prophylaxis of allergic disease in children. J Allergy 1953;24:434–436.
7 Osborn DA, Sinn J: Soy formula for prevention of allergy and food intolerance in infants. The Cochrane Database of Systematic Reviews CD003741. Cochrane Rev 2004;3:1–33.
8 Ellis MH, Short JA, Heiner DC: Anaphylaxis after ingestion of a recently introduced hydrolyzed whey protein formula. J Pediatr 1991;118:74–77.
9 Kleinman RE, Bahna SL, Powell GK, Sampson HA: Use of infant formulas in infants with cow milk allergy. Pediatr Allergy Immunol 1991;4:146–155.
10 American Academy of Pediatrics. Committee on Nutrition. Hypoallergenic infant formulas. Pediatrics 2000;111:346–349.
11 Sampson HA, Bernhisel-Broadbent J, Yang E, Scanlon SM: Safety of casein hydrolysate formulae in children with cow milk allergy. J Pediatr 1991;118:520–525.
12 Sampson HA, James JM, Bernhisel-Broadbent J: Safety of an amino acid-derived infant formula in children allergic to cow milk. Pediatrics 1992;90:463–465.
13 Halken S, Host A, Hansen LG, Osterballe O: Safety of a new, ultrafiltrated whey hydrolysate formula in children with cow milk allergy: a clinical investigation. Pediatr Allergy Immunol 1993;4:53–59.
14 Rosendal A, Barkholt V: Detection of potentially allergenic material in 12 hydrolyzed milk formulas. J Dairy Sci 2000;83:2200–2210.
15 Osborn DA, Sinn J: Formulas continuing hydrolysed protein for prevention of allergy and food intolerance in infants. The Cochrane Database of Systematic Reviews CD003664[4]. Cochrane Rev 2003;5:1–59.
16 Arshad S, Matthews S, Gant C, Hide D: Effect of allergen avoidance on development of allergic disorders in infancy. Lancet 1992;339:1493–1497.

17  Chan-Yeung M, Manfreda J, Dimich-Ward H, et al: A randomized controlled study on the effectiveness of a multifaceted intervention program in the primary prevention of asthma in high-risk infants. Arch Pediatr Adolesc Med 2000;154:203–204.
18  Chandra R, Shakuntla P, Hamed A: Influence of maternal diet during lactation and use of formula feeds on development of atopic eczema in high risk infants. BMJ 1989;299:228–230.
19  Chandra R: Five-year follow-up of high-risk infants with family history of allergy who were exclusively breast-fed or fed partial whey hydrolysate, soy, and conventional cow's milk formulas. J Pediatr Gastroenterol Nutr 1997;24:380–388.
20  Chirico G, Gasparoni A, Ciardelli L, et al: Immunogenicity and antigenicity of a partially hydrolyzed cow's milk infant formula. Allergy 1997;52:82–88.
21  Halken S, Hansen KS, Jacobsen HP, et al: Comparison of a partially hydrolyzed infant formula with two extensively hydrolyzed formulas for allergy prevention: a prospective, randomized study. Pediatr Allergy Immunol 2000;11:149–161.
22  Juvonen P, Mansson M, Andersson C, Jakobsson I: Allergy development and macromolecular absorption in infants with different feeding regimens during the first three days of life. A three-year prospective follow-up. Acta Paediatr 1996;85:1047–1052.
23  Mallet E, Henocq A: Long-term prevention of allergic diseases by using protein hydrolysate formula in at-risk infants. J Pediatr 1992;121:S95–S100.
24  Marini A, Agosti M, Motta G, Mosca F: Effects of a dietary and environmental prevention programme on the incidence of allergic symptoms in high atopic risk infants: three years' follow-up. Acta Paediatr Suppl 1996;414:1–21.
25  Nentwich I, Michiva E, Nevoral J, et al: Cow's milk-specific cellular and humoral immune responses and atopy skin symptoms in infants from atopic families fed a partially (pHF) or extensively (eHF) hydrolyzed infant formula. Allergy 2001;56:1144–1156.
26  Oldaeus G, Anjou K, Bjorksten B, et al: Extensively and partially hydrolysed infant formulas for allergy prophylaxis. Arch Dis Child 1997;77:4–10.
27  Saarinen KM, Juntunen-Backman K, Jarvenpaa AL, et al: Supplementary feeding in maternity hospitals and the risk of cow's milk allergy: A prospective study of 6209 infants. J Allergy Clin Immunol 1999;104:457–461.
28  Szajewska H, Albrecht P, Stoinska B, et al: Extensive and partial protein hydrolysate preterm formulas: the effect on growth rate, protein metabolism indices, and plasma amino acid concentrations. J Pediatr Gastroenterol Nutr 2001;32:303–309.
29  Tsai M, Chou CC, Hsieh KH: The effect of hypoallergenic formula on the occurrence of allergic diseases in high risk infants. Acta Paediatr Sin 2001;32:137–144.
30  Vandenplas Y, Hauser B, Blecker U, et al: The nutritional value of a whey hydrolysate formula compared with a whey-predominant formula in healthy infants. J Pediatr Gastroenterol Nutr 1993;17:92–96.
31  Vandenplas Y, Hauser B, Van den BC, et al: Effect of a whey hydrolysate prophylaxis of atopic disease. Ann Allergy 1992;68:419–424.
32  Willems R, Duchateau J, Magrez P, et al: Influence of hypoallergenic milk formula on the incidence of early allergic manifestations in infants predisposed to atopic diseases. Ann Allergy 1993;71:192–193.
33  de Seta L, Siani P, Cirillo G, et al: The prevention of allergic diseases with a hypoallergenic formula: a follow-up at 24 months. The preliminary results. Pediatr Med Chir 1994;16:251–254.
34  von Berg A, Koletzko S, Grubl A, et al: The effect of hydrolyzed cow's milk formula for allergy prevention in the first year of life: the German Infant Nutritional Intervention Study, a randomized double-blind trial. J Allergy Clin Immunol 2003;111:533–540.
35  Zeiger R, Heller S, Mellon M, et al: Genetic and environmental factors affecting the development of atopy through age 4 in children of atopic parents: a prospective randomized study of food allergen avoidance. Pediatr Allergy Immunol 1992;3:110–127.
36  Halken S, Host A, Hansen LG, Osterballe O: Preventive effect of feeding high-risk infants a casein hydrolysate formula or an ultrafiltrated whey hydrolysate formula. A prospective, randomized, comparative clinical study. Pediatr Allergy Immunol 1993;4:173–181.
37  Host A, Halken S: Hypoallergenic formulas – when, to whom and how long: after more than 15 years we know the right indication! Allergy 2004;59:45–52.
38  Muraro A, Dreborg S, Host A, et al: Dietary prevention of allergic diseases in infants and small children. Part III: Critical review of published peer-reviewed observational and interventional studies and final recommendations. Pediatr Allergy Immunol 2004;15:291–307.

## Discussion

*Dr. Chad:* As you all know soy and peanut are both in the legume families and to a certain degree do share some antigens. I was wondering if early use of soy formula can actually be a sensitizer for the development of peanut allergy later on? In other words is that the hidden exposure we are looking for in some of these children?

*Dr. Sampson:* That is a very good question. Certainly the study published by Lack et al. [1] in the *New England Journal of Medicine* a couple of years ago looked at the utilization of soy formula in those infants who did develop peanut allergy and found a correlation between soy formula ingestion and the development of peanut allergy. I think the problem that we have again, it being an observational study, is possible sampling bias. We know that if you have a child who develops milk allergy or is suspected of having milk allergy, one of the first formulas these infants go onto is going to be a soy-based formula. The other thing we know is that if you look at an infant who has cow's milk allergy and also has atopic dermatitis, which many of them do, a higher rate of those children will go on to develop peanut allergy and that may be as high as 25%. So I am not sure whether the association that Lack et al. saw in their study was more related to the fact that these are children who are at high risk of developing food allergy and were given soy. Also, it is not clear how long these infants received soy, so whether or not it would really have a particularly sensitizing effect is not known. On the other hand, when we look at the actual allergenic epitope recognition, or where the IgE binds the peanut compared to where IgE binds the soy, the places where children who are peanut-allergic generate IgE antibody to epitopes that are in areas which are different than those on the soy protein. In other words, the areas that are non-homologous or non-identical are the areas that seem to distinguish those children who develop peanut allergy from those who develop soy allergy, and we know that about 90% of peanut-allergic children eat soy without any problem. Whether or not there still could be some potential T-cell cross-reactivity and T-cell promotion, we don't know, but my feeling is that we don't have the evidence to say that the ingestion of soy promotes the development of peanut allergy at this point.

*Dr. Kerner:* I have a couple of clarifications and questions and these relate to the pediatricians who are attempting to get family history for allergy. The first question is if you have a history, I mean you define very clearly what atopic history should be, but if you have a history for example of an allergic colitis which is supposed to be a non-IgE-mediated reaction, would you classify that as an allergic; is that part of the family history of allergy or not?

*Dr. Sampson:* No, I would not classify that as atopic. Most of the studies that have been done, especially those that have evaluated hydrolyzed formulas, such as the GINI study, would not consider that as an atopy.

*Dr. Kerner:* Because when a history of bleeding is found in allergic colitis some pediatricians may think that. This may be more controversial, when families are screened and an allergic reaction to a drug is found, should that be considered as part of the family history of allergy?

*Dr. Sampson:* No, I would not consider that either.

*Dr. Cohen:* As a pediatrician I was wondering if there is a potential future rapid diagnostic test in the newborn period, other than cord blood IgE, that might help us identify those children that might be predisposed to atopy?

*Dr. Sampson:* I am sure we would all like to develop one but right now I am not aware of any. At the moment, family history is still our best indicator of those at high risk. But as I said, we are still going to miss at least half of the children that develop atopic disease because that history is not going to be present.

*Dr. Bowen:* Given that no difference has yet been shown in the outcome of rhinitis or asthma, is there any reason to suspect we shouldn't wait for the development of atopic dermatitis first and then switch to a fully hydrolyzed formula? Would that have any different outcome from fully hydrolyzed from day 1?

*Dr. Sampson:* Number one, I don't know the answer to that because I am not aware of anybody who has looked at that question. I think the biggest problem though is that we don't have long enough observation studies to really make any comment on what the effect is on allergic rhinitis or asthma. If we are in some way altering the atopic predisposition, which is demonstrated by a decrease in atopic dermatitis early on, there is a potential that it may have some beneficial effect, but at this point in time, I don't think anybody has really adequately followed these patients long enough to be able to tell us that.

*Dr. Moukarzel:* Can you speculate on why hydrolyzed casein will not work but hydrolyzed whey protein will work? Is it because the hydrolyzation process is different?

*Dr. Sampson:* It is actually the other way around. It was the extensively hydrolyzed whey formula that didn't work whereas the extensively hydrolyzed casein did. One of the things that I think we have to be aware of is that there are significant differences in the outcome of different hydrolysate processes. We have evaluated a number of hydrolyzed formulas for use in the treatment of children who have cow's milk allergy, and I was quite surprised by the number that didn't work, i.e., were not hypoallergenic. Yet when you looked at their preclinical profile, they actually looked to be comparable to what we saw in Nutramigen and Alimentum. I think the difference reflects where exactly these breaks in the protein took place relative to the relevant epitopes that account for the generation of sensitization or to reactivity. So all hydrolysates are not going to be comparable and I think that each hydrolysate is going to have to be looked at individually to really know whether or not it is going to have the beneficial effect that we want, and I think that is going to be especially true in the partial hydrolysates.

*Dr. Greeff:* The role of the hydrolyzed formulas in the over 6-month-old infants, could you comment on that, please?

*Dr. Sampson:* As far as prevention I don't think we have any good data. The AAP recommends that we continue these hydrolyzed formulas for the first year of life but I am not aware of any data to support that practice. As far as the infants who have cow's milk allergy, we either have to put them on a different type of protein so that they are not going to react to or continue to keep them on hydrolyzed formula.

*Dr. Hamburger:* Were there any other restraints in the GINI study and in the German study that you reported that might be relevant to the results that we saw?

*Dr. Sampson:* I am not sure what you mean by restraints.

*Dr. Hamburger:* Dietary restrictions, changes in the home environment, anything at all, were there instructions given that I don't know about?

*Dr. Sampson:* Dr. von Berg will comment on that.

*Dr. von Berg:* Yes, I think I should comment on that. First of all we gave the advice to avoid solid foods for the first 4 months and thereafter to avoid certain foods, but asked the parents to record all solids that the child was given in diaries. We looked at that and I am going to talk about it afterwards. In addition we had questionnaires about almost everything. So we looked at houses and pets and other environmental factors and adjusted for them in the analysis.

*Dr. Zeiger:* You or Dr. von Berg could also speculate on the potential reasons for the differential effect of the hydrolysates on the development of atopic dermatitis with respect to a family history of atopic dermatitis?

*Dr. Sampson:* That is a great question. I would speculate that we are seeing a genetically different population and consequently the response to the size of the protein or the particular protein presented is going to be different. In those individuals with atopic dermatitis in the family, you might say they have a more robust atopic

119

predisposition and therefore are going to require a greater alteration of the protein to be able to have a protective effect.

*Dr. Zeiger:* When you examine the GINI data at both 1 and 3 years, one observes that extensive casein hydrolysates reduced atopic dermatitis more than the partial whey hydrolysate regardless of stratification by family history of atopic dermatitis.

*Dr. Sampson:* I think that when we look at these atopic individuals, we are going to have to subdivide patients into different populations, e.g., there is a population that has a more severe, more persistent atopic predisposition compared to those individuals that are going to have a transient predisposition. Certainly in food allergy, we see the majority of children who react to milk and egg have a transient effect, and it doesn't seem to matter too much how we do the initial feeding, whereas with those individuals that have this more persistent form, again whether they were breastfed or whether they got formula, it doesn't seem to alter the fact that they are going to stay sensitized. For example, most of the children who develop milk or egg allergy while they are being breastfed are the ones who almost never tend to outgrow their allergy.

*Dr. Zeiger:* In clarification to the question that was asked relative to hydrolysates and weaning, there was one study that looked at a weaning diet at about 6 months with hydrolysates, and no difference in the subsequent development of atopic disease was found when such feedings were started after weaning [2].

*Dr. Saavedra:* A question with regard to the population study. You pointed out very well that, as might be expected, most of the studies that show these differences are in at-risk populations and, as discussed earlier, each one of those studies identified risk in their own particular way. In many instances, as far as we know there is no true standardized way of getting a family history, and in real practice pediatricians don't go through an extensive questionnaire before making decisions on the kind of feeding recommendations. How good are the tools that we currently use to identify a family history, if any, and what would you recommend from a practical point of view?

*Dr. Sampson:* To begin with, I am not aware of any validated history for diagnosing atopic dermatitis. There certainly are standardized questionnaires that are available but, as far as I know, there is nothing that has really been validated.

*Dr. Björkstén:* Benn et al. [3] in Denmark actually did a big study evaluating a simple questionnaire which was validated by dermatologists. Unfortunately, coming back to Dr. Saavedra, no single question had the specificity and sensitivity that would make it useful. And if I may just continue, there is one word of caution again regarding the family history, and as I said, probably at least half of the population has the genetics for allergic disease and the fact that you don't have it may be the fact that you became tolerant early in life. So the value of a family history is very different in different populations. We cannot use the family history for example in Estonia for the very simple reason that the phenotype is not expressed.

*Dr. Sampson:* I think one of the other problems you run into is that most of these studies have different definitions of positive family history. Some of the questions would ask things such as itchy rash, which may very well not be atopic dermatitis, and have similar vague symptoms for asthma and allergic rhinitis. I think it would be really useful to have a well-validated, standardized questionnaire that we could use but even when we get that, as you point out, the specificity is still unlikely to be very good.

*Dr. von Berg:* The problem with the questionnaires also is that they normally ask for present or past diseases, and actually to diagnose the past disease is very difficult. Another point is that there is atopic and non-atopic asthma or atopic and non-atopic dermatitis, and that these are different phenotypes, which is not considered in these questionnaires.

*Dr. Lake:* A question about tolerance. In studies that go back probably 20 years or more in animal models of immunologically intact rodents, when we attempted to induce tolerance to an intact protein we found that extensively hydrolyzed protein was not capable of inducing tolerance and partially hydrolyzed protein could [4]. Do you have any concerns about altering tolerance development by raising babies on extensively hydrolyzed products from early on?

*Dr. Sampson:* One of the things we have to look at is the age at which we do these studies in rodents; the rodent is highly tolerizable so that giving them almost any protein will generate oral tolerance. What we do in our animal models when we generate cow's milk-allergic mice, i.e., mice that will develop anaphylaxis with ingestion of cow's milk, we give them cow's milk plus cholera toxin which will cause them to develop allergy to that particular protein. If you give it to them in a hydrolyzed formula, they are not going to develop that particular sensitivity. So the question remains is the atopic group or the predisposed group more like the mouse that we give the cholera toxin or is it more like the mouse that has a normal tolerogenic capability. I think the data at this point would suggest that in those high-risk infants, the infants that are likely to develop the sensitization, are probably more like the mouse with cholera toxin; they are not capable of developing that normal tolerance. I think this is analogous to different types of atopic individuals in the sense that some individuals are going to develop transient problems and probably are better off getting the partial hydrolysate that may in fact cause them to tolerize more efficiently whereas the group not destined to have the transient form is going to become reactive regardless.

*Dr. Björkstén:* Perhaps the discussion is becoming slightly confused because I think what you are showing here is less atopic dermatitis. If you don't see an antigen, then you are not sensitized. However I think at this stage there is very little evidence, if any, that the atopic march would be prevented because an early positive skin prick test and early exposure to inhalant antigens is actually associated with a significantly decreased risk for having allergy as at the age of 11. So I am wondering whether the best we can hope from these hypoallergenic formulas is actually that we could prevent atopic dermatitis in infants.

*Dr. Sampson:* I think that with the data that we have right now, all we can say is that we can prevent the development of some atopic dermatitis. We know that many children outgrow their atopic dermatitis and the twopoint prevalence rates come together over the course of time as Dr. Zeiger showed in his study. However, I think the jury is still out on the issue of asthma and allergic rhinitis. One of the problems with the study by Hattevig et al. [5] was that it was done in two different cities and so was not really randomized, which introduces other potential causative effects. One of the things we have to do is to make sure Dr. von Berg keeps going with her study and follows these children for the next 15 years. Perhaps then we will get an answer, but I think right now the answer is not there.

*Dr. Moukarzel:* What is the role of elemental formula, free amino acid formula as prevention? Do you have any comments on non-inducing tolerance in the long term? A free amino acid formula may not induce tolerance as partially hydrolyzed formula.

*Dr. Sampson:* Right now we have no evidence on the use of the amino acid-based formula for prevention. However, if there is concern about the extensively hydrolyzed formulas having insufficient tolerizing effects, then the amino acid formulas would likely be worse. Right now we do not have any data to support the use of amino acid-based formulas for prevention, only for treatment.

*Dr. Sorensen:* You mentioned two interesting aspects of the GINI study and I don't know if you or Dr. von Berg could help us with this. One was that there was a higher attrition rate in the extensively hydrolyzed casein group, another one that only the extensively hydrolyzed casein seemed to be protective against atopic dermatitis in children born to mothers who had active atopic dermatitis. Is that correct?

*Dr. Sampson:* No, it is atopic dermatitis in the parents.

*Dr. Sorensen:* Now I wonder if the attrition rate may have been higher in that group, and that is why it seems to have a better effect.

*Dr. von Berg:* It was slightly higher in the extensively hydrolyzed casein group, but the group was restocked.

*Dr. Seidman:* You began your lecture discussing the fact that the majority of patients who are going to develop atopic disease in fact don't have a positive family history and then very quickly concluded that there is no evidence that any intervention helps, but I wonder if you would comment on the ZUFF study from Switzerland?

*Dr. Sampson:* I am not aware of that.

*Dr. Seidman:* This is a population-based study in two villages, Zug and Frauenfeld, where one city had an intervention and the other didn't. I don't know if there is anybody here who is associated with that study and would like to comment.

*Dr. Exl-Preysch:* We conducted that study. It is a study in a non-selected normal newborn infant population with the aim of finding out if an allergen-reduced nutrition will lead to better health outcome than a regular high allergenic infant nutrition. For very obvious reasons this was not a truly randomized study because feeding recommendations cannot be randomized in normal surroundings. However, it was a prospective study in two cities, 50 km apart, that we compared independently before we started the study. All possible confounding factors were finally included in the evaluation via a logistic regression analysis and worst case evaluation. The nutrition recommendations were the same as in the GINI study only that we had an unselected infant population. There were 566 infants in the regularly fed control group and 564 newborns in the allergen-reduced (NAN HA) prevention group [6–8]. However, it is important to make clear that we didn't only look into allergy, because we were interested in the overall health of the infants. Would they grow healthier on a partially hydrolyzed formula than on a normal formula, would they grow as well? After 2 years we could finally show that the infants in the partially hydrolyzed group (NAN HA) were having less skin problems, only half of the amount of those who got regular infant formula and grew the same.

*Dr. Sampson:* I think you have the same problem as the study by Hattevig et al. [5]; you are doing two different techniques in two different cities. You have different observers in each of the cities and I think there are a lot of potential problems with that.

*Dr. Exl-Preysch:* We knew and discussed the problem of randomization a long time before we started that study. It is just not possible in a normal population to try to randomize feeding recommendations. Finally you will end up in a mess, because people are communicating with each other and will change their views and finally their feeding behavior. That is why we decided with the help of internationally renowned people to choose the 'randomization of two cities' version. To make sure they were comparable, we asked before starting this study an independent institute to make a survey of those two cities that are 50 km apart. We looked into all important parameters in terms of possible confounding factors. Most of them were comparable, those that were not spoke in favor of the control group – ergo against our hypothesis – and secondly in the final analysis that was intention to treat inclusive worst case analysis, we took all of those potentially confounding factors into account. So I don't think that finally this sort of randomization that we did would or could be taken into account for any differences. We analyzed everything that we could, in the end we individually analyzed each doctor's own sort of analysis of the results as confounding factors against the others. Altogether, we had 80 study doctors all coming from that region. They were all trained in several training sectors, and they were again taken into account in the final analysis with the logistic regression. I don't think they will count for any differences between the two cities. So, our final result seems to be very clear: allergen-reduced infant nutrition for all non- or partially breastfed infants seems to be the best state-of-the-art at the moment that we know of.

# References

1 Lack G, Fox D, Northstone K, Golding J: Avon Longitudinal Study of Parents and Children Study Team: Factors associated with the development of peanut allergy in childhood. N Engl J Med 2003;348:977–985.
2 Odelram H, Vanto T, Jacobsen L, Kjellman NI: Whey hydrolysate compared with cow's milk-based formula for weaning at about 6 months of age in high allergy-risk infants: effects on atopic disease and sensitization. Allergy 1996;51:192–195.
3 Benn CS, Benfeldt E, Andersen PK, et al: Atopic dermatitis in young children: diagnostic criteria for use in epidemiological studies based on telephone interviews. Acta Derm Venereol 2003;83:347–350.
4 Strobel S: Development of oral tolerance; in DeWeck AL, Sampson HA (eds): Intestinal Immunology and Food Allergy. Nestlé Nutr Workshop Series Pediatr Program. New York, Raven Press/Vevey, Nestec, 1995, vol 34.
5 Hattevig G, Kjellman B, Sigurs N, et al: Effect of maternal avoidance of eggs, cow's milk and fish during lactation upon allergic manifestations in infants. Clin Exp Allergy 1989;19:27–32.
6 Exl BM, Deland U, Secretin MC, et al: Improved general health status in an unselected infant population following an allergen reduced dietary intervention programme. The ZUFF-study-programme. Part I: Study design and 6-month nutritional behaviour. Eur J Nutr 2000;39: 89–102.
7 Exl BM, Deland U, Secretin MC, et al: Improved general health status in an unselected infant population following an allergen-reduced dietary intervention programme: the ZUFF-STUDY-PROGRAMME. Part II: infant growth and health status to age 6 months. ZUg-FrauenFeld. Eur J Nutr. 2000;39:145–156.
8 Exl BM, Deland U Secretin MC, et al: Improved general health status in and unselected infant population following an allergen reduced dietary intervention programme: the ZUFF study programme. Part IV: infant growth and health status to age 2 years (abstract). J Pediatr Gastroenterol Nutr 2000;31:100.

Lucas A, Sampson HA (eds): Primary Prevention by Nutrition Intervention in Infancy and Childhood.
Nestlé Nutr Workshop Ser Pediatr Program, vol 57, pp 125–134,
Nestec Ltd., Vevey/S. Karger AG, Basel, © 2006.

# Introduction of Solid Foods

*Andrea von Berg*

Research Institute for the Prevention of Allergies and Respiratory Diseases,
Marien-Hospital-Wesel, Wesel, Germany

## Introduction

Feeding guidelines for the prevention of allergic diseases follow the view that allergen avoidance leads to a reduction in allergy, which is understood as being mediated by sensitization. The role of early feeding in the development of allergic disorders has been studied widely. Most of these studies have concentrated on the role of breastfeeding and, in the case of children at a high risk of allergies, on the role of hypoallergenic formulas as substitutes for or supplemental to breastfeeding. Less attention has been paid to the role of solid food introduction into the baby's diet and the conditions under which this has been done. Nevertheless, all guidelines include some recommendations on the introduction of solid food.

According to the joint guidelines of the European Society for Paediatric Allergology and Clinical Immunology (ESPACI), Committee on Hypoallergenic Formulas, and the European Society for Paediatric Gastroenterology, Hepatology and Nutrition (ESPGHAN), Committee on Nutrition [1], as well as the German guidelines [2], breastfeeding for the first 4–6 months of life is recommended, with the introduction of solid foods thereafter. The feeding guidelines of the Committee on Nutrition of the American Academy of Pediatrics in general recommend delaying the introduction of solid foods until 6 months of age, but are more stringent with recommendations for certain foods: cow's milk products should be avoided until 1 year, eggs until 2 years and fish even until 3 years [3]. The guidelines of the WHO recommend the introduction of solids after 6 months of exclusive breastfeeding for all children [4].

The most recent recommendations from an expert group set up by the Section of Pediatrics, European Academy of Allergology and Clinical Immunology, are slightly different, stating that all children should avoid solid foods preferably until 6 months but at least 4 months of age, and that infants

Berg

at a high risk of allergic diseases can be nourished like non-high-risk infants after the age of 4 months [5].

## Evidence for Delaying Solid Food Introduction

The scientific evidence supporting the recommendations to delay solid food introduction until 4–6 months or even longer are scarce. Only a few studies have investigated the effect of early solid food introduction on the development of allergic diseases and their results are inconsistent. The current recommendations are mainly based on 2 older studies.

In 1991, in a prospective, non-randomized trial in children at risk of atopy, eczema and with a history of food allergy, Kajosaari [6], found that allergy was reduced in children in whom solid foods were introduced after 6 months of exclusive breastfeeding compared with children fed solids after 3 months. The effect was seen at 1 year, but had disappeared by the time the children were 5 years old [6]. The second study by Fergusson et al. [7, 8] from 1990, conducted in a large nonselected birth cohort of 1,265 children from New Zealand, has shown that feeding 4 or more diverse solid foods in the first 4 months is associated with a significantly increased risk of eczema (odds ratio (OR) 2.9) in children 2–4 years of age compared to children who had no solids before 4 months of life, and this effect lasted up to age 10 years [7, 8]. From these two studies it seems obvious that the timing and diversity of solid food introduction into the baby's diet are two crucial factors for the later development of allergic diseases.

## Recent Studies

However, more recent studies on solid food introduction have looked in more detail into the conditions under which the decision to introduce solid foods into the baby's diet has been taken, their results adding to the current conflicting data.

In a prospective, observational study following 671 infants from birth to 24 months of age, Forsyth et al. [9] assessed the relationship between the early introduction of solid food and infant weight, gastrointestinal illness and allergic diseases during the first 2 years of life. At 2 years, data from 455 (67.8%) children were available. The timing of solid food introduction was divided into 3 intervals: <8, 8–12, and >12 weeks. 65/671 (9.7%) children were introduced solids at age <8 weeks, and 332/671 (49.5%) between weeks 8 and 12. Infants who received solids early (at <8 weeks and 8–12 weeks) were significantly heavier than those who were fed solids after 12 weeks (p < 0.01) up to 26 weeks of life, thereafter no weight difference between the groups remained. Also, those infants who received solids early were heavier at

126

their first solid feeding than infants of similar age who had not yet received solids [9].

Apart from a birth weight of ≥4,000 g (n = 66, p = >0.05), the characteristics of children who were fed solid foods early were: male sex (p < 0.005), lower social class, and bottle-fed.

Children with the early introduction of solids had a significant but less than twofold increased risk of respiratory illnesses at 14–26 weeks of age and persistent cough at 14–26 and 27–39 weeks. These associations persisted even after adjustment for factors that are known to be related to respiratory symptoms in early childhood, such as parental smoking and poor social conditions. However, the follow-up was too short to answer whether these respiratory conditions were the expression of an atopic condition or were due to viral-induced respiratory disorders. The prevalence of eczema in this study was highest in children who had solids introduced at age 8–12 weeks rather than at an earlier (<8 weeks) or later age (>12 weeks). A possible explanation is offered from animal models showing that hypersensitivity reactions caused by a large antigen load are less strong than those caused by small antigen load [10]. As intestinal permeability decreases gradually from birth during the following weeks, it is possible that less antigen crosses the intestinal epithelium between weeks 8 and 12 than in the first 8 weeks.

In preterm infants solid feeding practices in addition to milk feeding patterns and their association with the development of atopic diseases have recently been studied by Morgan et al. [11]. In their prospective study on 257/329 preterm infants they found a rather high prevalence (35.8%) of eczema, and the introduction of 4 or more solid foods before 17 weeks of age was a risk factor for eczema (OR 3.49) at 1 year of age, independent of the family history of atopy. Prematurity in general may be a risk factor for the development of allergic diseases because of the immature immune system. On the other hand, increasing prematurity is known to be associated with a decreasing risk of atopy [12], which could be due to the higher risk of infections in the very preterm children, and to the later introduction of solids than in healthier, less premature infants. However, the results were not adjusted for the different stages of prematurity, and this could well have biased the results [13].

Solid feeding practices were also studied in the German Infant Nutritional Intervention (GINI) study, which is a prospective, randomized birth-cohort study that was conducted to assess the preventive effect of three different hydrolyzed infant formulas in comparison with a standard cow's milk formula in a double-blind fashion in 2,252 high-risk infants recruited between 1995 and 1998 in two regions of Germany, Munich (n = 1,165) and Wesel (n = 1,087) [14].

Parents received detailed verbal and written recommendations on infant nutrition. Mothers were asked to delay the introduction of solid foods until after the intervention period of 4, better 6, months during which they were advised to use the randomized study formula as the only milk supplement to breastfeeding. Furthermore, it was recommended that potentially allergenic foods such as cow's milk and diary products, eggs, fish, tomatoes, nuts, soy products and citrus fruits should be avoided during the first year.

For the first 24 weeks parents recorded the infant's nutrition in a weekly diary. They were asked to note the type of milk (breast milk, formula) and the time of weaning, as well as the time of the first introduction and the kind of solid food into the baby's diet [14].

One GINI sub-study looked at the influence of solid food introduction on specific sensitization at 12 months of age in a subgroup of 170 children from the GINI cohort [15]. Specific IgE to the following food allergens was determined: apple, banana, pear, peanut, hazelnut, carrot, potato, soy, wheat, cow milk, diary products and egg.

According to the parentally recorded questionnaires, children were divided into 2 groups: group BF which was exclusively breastfed during the first 4 months of life, and group SF which received the study formula.

Solid foods in addition to formula or breastfeeding were given in 37/170 (21.8%) before the end of the 16th week, while 30/170 (17.6%) had their first solids between weeks 17 and 20, and 46/170 (21.7%) in weeks 21–24. 53/170 (31.2%) were fed exactly according to the recommendations and received their first solid feeding after the end of 6 months.

Vegetables/juices and cereals were the most common first solids in the first 16 weeks (12.4 and 10.6%, respectively). The most common vegetable was carrots, with 62% of the children consuming them in the first 24 weeks.

By the age of 24 weeks, only 7% of the children had had dairy products, and only 0.7% had had soy. None of the children were reported to have received egg, fish or nuts during the first 24 weeks.

When children received solids early, that is in the first 16 weeks or in weeks 17–20, sensitization at 12 months to at least one of the 13 allergens tested was low at 5.4 and 6.7%, respectively. In contrast, specific IgE ≥0.35 kU/l to at least one allergen was 17.4% in the children who first had solids in weeks 21–24, and 18.9% when solids were introduced after 24 weeks. Although there was a tendency towards more frequent sensitization with the later introduction of solid foods, this was not significant (p = 0.154).

Data on egg sensitization were available from 111 children. Although 74 children had not received any egg within the first year, 8.1% of them were sensitized to egg at 12 months. Of the other 37 children who had egg in the first year, only 1 child (2.7%) had specific IgE to egg.

Variability of food in the first 24 weeks was divided into 3 categories: 1 = none (n = 53, 31.9%); 2 = 1–2 food groups (n = 66, 39.8%), and 3 = >2 food groups (n = 47, 28.3%). There was an inverse association between the number of foods and sensitization: 20.8% (category 1); 12.1% (category 2), and 8.5% (category 3) [15].

Apart from comparing the 1-year incidence of atopic dermatitis (AD) in children exclusively breastfed during the first 16 weeks of life (BF group) with that of children who were fed with a standard cow's milk formula exclusively or supplemental to breast milk (CMF group), the aim of another GINI sub-study was to examine whether the co-intervention advice of early solid food avoidance has an additional effect on the incidence of atopic eczema [16]. The crude OR of AD for exclusive breastfeeding was 0.60 (95% CI 0.40; 0.91). However mothers in the BF group differ from mothers in the CMF group with regard to several aspects: higher atopic risk level (p = 0.036), higher level of education (p = 0.001), fewer pets in the homes of mothers in the BF group (p = 0.001), and more BF group mothers living in the city of Munich than in the more rural area of Wesel (p = 0.001). After adjustment for the atopic risk factors and confounders, the OR for AD decreased to 0.47 (95% CI 0.30; 0.74).

These differences between the BM and CMF groups have considerably translated into the mothers' feeding behavior with regard to the infants' age at first introduction of solid foods and solid food diversity in the first months of life. Solid foods were classified according to the types of food (dairy products eggs, cereals, legume, vegetable, fruit, nuts, meat, fish and others), the diversity of the children's diet was constructed by summing up the number of different types of solid food that the child had been fed during the first 24 weeks [16]. While only 5.4% of the breastfeeding mothers had introduced solids to the infants' diet in the first 16 weeks after birth, 30.9% of mothers from the CMF group had done so. No solids had been given at the age of 24 weeks in 49% of the breastfed children compared to 19% of the bottle-fed children. The main factor for delaying solid food introduction beyond the first 6 months of life was the presence of AD in one of the child's family members.

The results showed an increasing trend in the AD incidence with the later introduction of solid foods and a decreasing trend with food diversity, but no significant effect modification of solid food was found ($\chi^2$ test, p = 0.89 for the number of food groups).

However, the duration of breastfeeding, age at introduction of solid food and the diversity of solid food are not independent factors because extended breastfeeding is associated with delayed solid food introduction and a reduced diversity of solid food in the diet. On the other hand an extended duration of breastfeeding and consequently delaying the introduction of solid food are associated with parental atopic risk status and educational level.

This study does not confirm the results of the study by Fergusson et al. [7, 8] which showed that a reduced diversity of solid foods in the first 4 months of life, but not breastfeeding itself, had a preventive effect on the incidence of AD. Several reasons for this have been discussed. The main difference was that mothers in the GINI study were provided with detailed recommendations to breastfeed and avoid solid foods for at least 4 months, while parents in the prospective observational development study in New Zealand did not get any nutritional advice. This resulted in a much lower percentage of children who received solid foods in the first 4 months of life (GINI 5.4% in the breast milk group, 30.9% in the CMF group, compared to 38.3 and 80.1%, respectively, in the New Zealand study). Another important difference is that in the GINI study all children came from atopic families, while the population in the New Zealand study was nonselected.

The increased public awareness in the last 1–2 decades regarding the association between the development of allergic diseases in the child and the family history, on the one hand, and the possibility for allergy prevention by certain dietary interventions, on the other hand, has led to behavioral changes [16, 17]. Parents in the GINI study, who were recruited for the study 15 years later than the parents in the New Zealand study, may have been much more prepared to breastfeed longer and to introduce solid foods later because they were atopic themselves. Therefore, one explanation for the results of the GINI study may be reverse causality, that is cause and effect are reversed.

Reverse causality is also considered as one reason for the results in a population-based prospective birth cohort study by Zutavern et al. [17]. They followed 642 children prospectively from birth to 5 years of age and looked into the association between the development of preschool wheezing, transient wheezing, atopy or eczema and solid foods. They could not find a protective effect of late solid food introduction, but instead a statistically increased risk of eczema in relation to the late introduction of egg (adjusted OR 1.6, 95% CI 1.1–2.4) and milk (adjusted OR 1.7, 95% CI 1.1–2.5). The risk of preschool wheezing was also, though not significantly, increased when egg was introduced late (adjusted OR 1.5, 95% CI 0.92–2.4).

From more recent studies [9, 11, 15–17] it seems that evidence for the preventive effect of the late introduction of solid foods and low diversity as recommended in feeding guidelines is rather weak when confounding factors like reverse causality are considered. This is not surprising since the dose of allergen is only one factor in the complex mechanism for the development of allergic disorders and the induction of oral tolerance which protects the individual from food hypersensitivity. In a recent review by Chehade and Mayer [18] factors involved in oral tolerance were discussed, some of which are related to the antigen and antigen handling, and some to the host, where the genetic background, age and intestinal microflora are important players in the complex scenario of allergy development or tolerance.

## Conclusion

Although all feeding guidelines for the prevention of allergic diseases recommend the late introduction of solid foods to the infant's diet, the scientific evidence for this is scarce and mainly based on two studies. More recent studies on the association between solid food introduction and the development of allergic diseases have looked in more detail into the conditions under which solids were introduced. The increasing public awareness of an association between genetic background and the development of childhood allergic diseases, and the possibilities for nutritional preventive interventions has led to changes in feeding behaviors which may explain the conflicting data of older and more recent studies. When the reverse of cause and effect (reverse causality) is considered, early solid food introduction seems to be less harmful than previously thought.

## References

1 Host A, Koletzko B, Dreborg S, et al: Dietary products used in infants for treatment and prevention of food allergy. Joint statement of the European Society for Paediatric Allergology and Clinical Immunology (ESPACI) Committee on Hypoallergenic Formulas and the European Society for Paediatric Gastroenterology, Hepatology and Nutrition (ESPGHAN) Committee on Nutrition. Arch Dis Child 1999;81:80–84.
2 Bauer CP, von Berg A, Niggemann B, Rebien W: Primäre alimentäre Atopieprävention. Allergologie 2004;13:120–125.
3 American Academy of Pediatrics. Committee on Nutrition. Hypoallergenic infant formulas. Pediatrics 2000;106(2 Pt 1):346–349.
4 WHO: 54th World Health Assembly. WHA54.2. Agenda item 13.1: Infant and young child nutrition. Geneva, WHO, 2004.
5 Muraro A, Dreborg S, Halken S, et al: Dietary prevention of allergic diseases in infants and small children. Part III: Critical review of published peer-reviewed observational and interventional studies and final recommendations. Pediatr Allergy Immunol 2004;15:291–307.
6 Kajosaari M: Atopy prophylaxis in high-risk infants: prospective 5-year follow-up of children with six months exclusive breast feeding and solid food elimination. Adv Exp Med Biol 1991; 310:453–458.
7 Fergusson DM, Horwood LJ, Beautrais AL, et al: Eczema and infant diet. Clin Allergy 1981;11: 325–331.
8 Fergusson DM, Horwood LJ, Shannon FT: Early solid feeding and recurrent childhood eczema: a 10-year longitudinal study. Pediatrics 1990;86:541–546.
9 Forsyth JS, Ogston SA, Clark A, et al: Relation between early introduction of solid food to infants and their weight and illnesses during the first two years of life. BMJ 1993;306:1572–1576.
10 Jarrett E: Perinatal influence on IgE responses. Lancet 1984;ii:797–799.
11 Morgan J, Williams P, Norris F, et al: Eczema und early solid feeding in preterm infants. Arch Dis Child 2004;89:309–314.
12 Siltanen M, Kajosaari M, Pohjavuori M, Savilahti E: Prematurity at birth reduces the long-term risk of atopy. J Allergy Clin Immunol 2001;107:229–234.
13 Khakoo GA, Lack G: Introduction of solids to the infant diet. Arch Dis Child 2004;89:295.
14 von Berg A, Koletzko S, Grübl A, et al: The effect of hydrolyzed cow's milk formula for allergy prevention in the first year of life: The German Infant Nutritional Intervention Study, a randomized double-blind trial. J Allergy Clin Immunol 2003;111:533–540.
15 Bartels PR, Zusammenhang zwischen Zeitpunkt und Art der Beikosternährung im ersten Lebensjahr und einer möglichen Sensibilisierung gegen Nahrungsmittelallergene sowie der Inzidenz von Atopischer Dermatitis im Alter von einem Jahr; Diss, Technischen Universität München, 2003.
16 Schoetzau A, Filipiak-Pittroff B, Franke K, et al: Effect of exclusive breast-feeding and early solid food avoidance on the incidence of atopic dermatitis in high-risk infants at 1 year of age. Pediatr Allergy Immunol 2002;13:234–242.
17 Zutavern A, von Mutius E, Harris J, et al: The introductions of solids in relation to asthma und eczema. Arch Dis Child 2004;89:303–308.
18 Chehade M, Mayer L: Oral tolerance and its relation to food hypersensitivities. J Allergy Clin Immunol 2005;115:3–12.

## Discussion

*Dr. Zeiger:* With respect to your last report, what are your recommendations with regard to the more recent data that are available?

*Dr. von Berg:* First of all it is almost impossible to do randomized controlled studies in the area of solid food introduction. But on the basis of what we see here in the latest studies, I think that there is evidence that allows us to be a little less rigid with our recommendations. For example I think the American recommendations on solid food introduction are far too strict. I would say that the introduction of solid foods should be postponed to after the 4th month, but I would not say that the children should not have eggs until 2 years and milk until 1 year of age, I think that is too much.

*Dr. Klish:* The natural way to feed infants is not only to breastfeed but to share solid foods. In most ancient cultures, not only did infants receive antigens of a broad variety through breast milk but mothers tended to share whatever they were eating with their infants by pre-masticating the food and spitting it into the mouths of their babies. So from a teleological point of view it makes sense that exposure to antigens early is good for infants. However, in saying that, one of the recent issues has to do with weight gain of infants who have solid foods introduced to them early and what role this plays in the obesity epidemic. I wonder if you have any comments on either of these points?

*Dr. von Berg:* Yes, as we heard yesterday, I think nobody argues against recommendations to breastfeed for 4–6 months, and what we saw here in this study is that breastfeeding mothers don't give solids early. The normal way of feeding babies is breastfeeding, they don't need to get solid foods in the first 4 or 6 months, and probably by that we reduce the risk of early weight gain.

*Dr. Björkstén:* My comment is actually similar to that of Dr. Klish. There is traditionally no such thing as exclusive breastfeeding. In every culture there has always been early introduction of solids. Exclusive breastfeeding with no solids is a novel situation. Suppose that the introduction of solid foods affects the gut microbiota, you mentioned apples, carrots, potatoes, fibers which all would affect the gut microbiota but are poorly antigenic. There is a difference in time between the New Zealand study and the GINI study and things have changed. The New Zealand diet in the 1980s and late 1970s when this study population was collected was different from a modern diet, and there have been changes in the gut microbiota. I think that your own data fit more nicely into an ecological effect and it has nothing to do with the immunology that we have been searching for years. Is this very provocative to you?

*Dr. von Berg:* No, it is not provocative at all. In all nutritional intervention studies, for example the studies by Halken et al. [1] and Kalliomaki et al. [2], there was hardly any difference in sensitization regardless of what the children were fed. But what was interesting I think, if we look at exposure and sensitization here, the highest sensitization was to egg, and this is probably not because these children got so much egg, but because they are very susceptible for producing IgE antibodies.

*Dr. Björkstén:* Many years ago some studies showed that it is an excellent predictor for allergic disease as the children were followed up to age 15, but it is not the atopic march on which we based many of our studies. It only indicates that you have the propensity for IgE antibody formation as egg is a more common antigen to be exposed to.

*Dr. von Berg:* Yes, and perhaps a very aggressive antigen. One question is if, by manipulations with hydrolysates, for example, we could avoid sensitization to hen's egg, whether we could then avoid asthma, because we know from these epidemiological studies that the early sensitization to hen's egg is almost a predictor for later asthma. I just wanted to add one thing. In the GINI study at 1 year we looked at those children who had hen's egg-associated atopic dermatitis, and saw that the only hydrolysate that actually reduced this atopic dermatitis was the extensively hydrolyzed casein formula. In following these children we will see whether the extensively hydrolyzed casein formula does something on the development from hen's egg-associated atopic dermatitis to asthma.

*Dr. Björkstén:* That is based on the assumption that hen's egg exposure is subsequently a risk factor for respiratory allergies. I think there is absolutely no evidence for that. What it shows is that the person who is prone to make IgE antibodies relieves his propensity to egg and milk, because we know this natural story from the inhalant allergens and we know that the person who develops asthma is often sensitized at an early age, but there is absolutely no evidence that the avoidance of these antigens early in life actually prevents the sensitization. Indeed it is the other way around, it seems to be promoting tolerance, the early exposure, so what I think is that, yes, if you avoid development of IgE antibodies to egg you have a marker but it is a marker for the constitution rather than having anything to do with risk factor.

*Dr. von Berg:* At least this analysis nicely shows that early introduction of vegetables is not a risk factor of sensitization.

*Dr. Hanson:* With due respect to my colleagues I would like to protest against the claim that the procedures from traditional societies are to be accepted as useful and positive, because we are now in the age of evidence-based medicine and I have rather extensive experience of procedures, of handling newborns in rural Pakistan, where we could define a number of these practices as being very dangerous. This includes giving a plant extract that was kept between the delivery of each child and was heavily contaminated, and was given the first day. Furthermore, the start of breastfeeding was delayed for 1–3 days by giving this and other infected material and so on. So I would like to remain with our modern medicine.

*Dr. Sampson:* I just want to ask you, how good an indicator is sensitization? In other words, we know from the food allergy data, for example, that of all the positive skin tests we see, the minority really reflect clinical disease, and I would suspect if we were to do the same thing with aero allergens we would see the same thing. So by simply looking at sensitization, is it even a useful marker?

*Dr. von Berg:* Sensitization in general is not enough. Probably, as you did in food allergy, we should look at the degree of sensitization. We defined sensitization as positive when it was just measurable, and this is probably not enough. But the results were not much different when we took CAP class 2, this is 0.7 kU/l, but what we have not done up to now is to correlate the CAP class with the severity and the course of disease. I think actually sensitization might be a marker or predictor for whether atopic dermatitis is transient or persistent. We have many children with atopic dermatitis in the study who are not sensitized, and these are probably the ones who have transient atopic dermatitis, and we are going to look at that.

*Dr. Lake:* As pediatricians we are asked to delay the introduction of shellfish and peanut until after 15–18 months, even in the absence of a family history of food allergy. Do you have any data, now out 3 years, to support this recommendation?

*Dr. von Berg:* No, not yet.

*Dr. Björkstén:* I would again reiterate this sort of sensitization. I think that we really have to look at the data that there is no causal relationship. One of the things we are learning from the traditional societies, in this case Estonia again, is that over 60% of an unselected cohort of healthy newborn babies have circulating IgE antibodies to foods, which means that we have done something wrong in the laboratory although it is the same people and we actually retested it. In Estonia there is no relationship to disease and it tells us that IgE development is an immunological phenomenon which is part of the development of immune responses and tolerance. So by avoiding egg sensitization, not even today is it reasonable to suspect that it would prevent respiratory allergies or that it obviously can play a role in food allergy in infants.

*Dr. von Berg:* Actually we looked at 'sensitization' at CAP class 0.5 and found a lot of so-called sensitization which had no implication at all, so this is what you found as well?

Berg

*Dr. Björkstén:* No, I am not talking about the borderline, that was one of the Hattevig studies. No, these were actually clearly positive CAP 1 and CAP 2, but we didn't see all 4 classes, but the 1 and 2 are there and they are not related to disease in Estonia, while in Sweden it is beautifully related.

*Dr. Wang:* We see a lot of patients with atopic dermatitis and they are breastfeeding. Do you think the food allergen goes through the breast milk and the infants get these allergens? Did you have this kind of situation in your studies? If so it might have affected your results. On the other hand, we should make sure the mothers aren't giving solid food especially hen's egg and cow's milk.

*Dr. von Berg:* We saw in the GINI study that there were some children who actually developed atopic dermatitis while they were being exclusively breastfed. But whether that comes through the mother or whether that comes, as discussed before, through some dermal sensitization, for example, is not known. In such cases when the child develops atopic dermatitis we tell the mother to stop breastfeeding for a while, but that she should extract the milk by breast pump. If the child got better then of course she should stop breastfeeding altogether, otherwise she could go back. We had many cases where it was not the breast milk to which the child reacted although the atopic dermatitis started while it was being breastfed.

*Dr. Sorensen:* Do you think that eventually there will be different recommendations regarding the introduction of solid foods depending on breastfeeding versus formula feeding or even different types of formula, and that the single recommendation that we presently have from the various regulatory organisms is no longer justified?

*Dr. von Berg:* No, I would say breastfeeding of course for 4–6 months and no different recommendations for breastfed or formula-fed children with regard to solid food introduction. From our studies we don't have any evidence that solid food introduction other than egg has any effect on outcome. Therefore I would at least say that we should not be that rigid anymore.

*Dr. Tjesic-Drinkovic:* The recommendation for exclusive breastfeeding for 4–6 months gives us a rather long 2-month period to start with solids. According to your data and other knowledge, i.e., on inducing tolerance, would you be in favor of earlier introduction of solid foods, say closer to 4 months than 6 months?

*Dr. von Berg:* If a child is hungry he has to have something and that is more often after 4 than after 6 months, and from our data that doesn't make a difference. As you see from our data it depends probably on what you give. If you give carrots and potatoes you should not have any problems.

*Dr. Klish:* It is my impression that the rigidity of the recommendations from the American Academy of Pediatrics has come primarily from the Breast Feeding Task Force of the academy, and they feel that the early introduction of solids (4 months of age) somehow interferes with the continuation of breastfeeding itself. That is why these recommendations have become more rigid. Would you care to comment on that relationship?

*Dr. von Berg:* I can't talk for the Americans here but it sounds logical that if you have a strong breastfeeding task force within the academy they will try to influence the recommendations in order to improve breastfeeding.

## References

1   Halken S, Hansen KS, Jacobsen HP, et al: Comparison of a partially hydrolyzed infant formula with two extensively hydrolyzed formulas for allergy prevention: a prospective, randomized study. Pediatr Allergy Immunol 2000;11:149–161.
2   Kalliomaki M, Salminen S, Poussa T, et al: Probiotics and prevention of atopic disease: 4-year follow-up of a randomised placebo-controlled trial. Lancet 2003;361:1869–1871.

Lucas A, Sampson HA (eds): Primary Prevention by Nutrition Intervention in Infancy and Childhood.
Nestlé Nutr Workshop Ser Pediatr Program, vol 57, pp 135–151,
Nestec Ltd., Vevey/S. Karger AG, Basel, © 2006.

# Osteoporosis: Is Primary Prevention Possible?

*Mary S. Fewtrell*

MRC Childhood Nutrition Research Centre, Institute of Child Health, London, UK

Osteoporosis is a major and increasing cause of morbidity and mortality in developed countries, and set to become so worldwide in the next few decades. Health-care costs are high, principally due to associated hip fractures which often result in loss of independence. An individual's risk of developing osteoporosis is determined by the peak bone mass reached at skeletal maturity, and the rate of bone loss later in adult life. Historically, strategies to prevent osteoporosis concentrated on reducing bone loss, particularly after the menopause in women. However, over the past decade there has been a greater focus on maximizing peak bone mass as an alternative or additional potential strategy. Although peak bone mass is to a great extent (70–80%) genetically determined, it is clear that events during fetal life, infancy and childhood are also important. This chapter will discuss the evidence that osteoporosis may be a disease that is amenable to primary prevention during early life, and the potential role of nutritional interventions.

It is important to appreciate that a number of factors have been shown to result in increased bone mass in the short-term, during the period of intervention. This may in itself have immediate outcome benefits for the individual, for example reducing short-term fracture risk. However, to represent a potential preventative strategy against osteoporosis, any such effect must be shown to persist after the intervention has stopped, resulting in higher peak bone mass and/or favorable effects on bone structure or bone turnover. This has received much less attention, and is the principle focus here.

## Studies in Animal Models

The concept that early life events might program later bone health and risk of osteoporosis in humans is supported to some extent by animal data. For example, malnutrition during the growth period has been shown to result in a slowing and eventually cessation of bone growth in a number of species. Bone histology typically shows an almost complete cessation of osteoblastic activity and the growth plate effectively becomes dormant, but these abnormalities are largely reversible after nutritional rehabilitation [1]. Most such studies did not involve malnutrition during prenatal or very early postnatal life. Consequently, they were potentially beyond the critical period during which permanent programming effects on the skeleton might occur. However, more recent animal experiments have demonstrated permanent effects of manipulating maternal nutrition during either pregnancy or lactation on offspring bone size and histology, including alterations in growth plate morphology [2, 3].

## Studies in Humans

The remainder of this chapter reviews the relevant epidemiological and experimental data for long-term effects of early life events on bone health in humans, in whom investigations are necessarily more difficult and limited. Conceptually, when considering such data it is helpful to distinguish between effects on (i) skeletal (frame) size; (ii) mineral mass, and (iii) bone structure and strength. In practice, most studies include anthropometric measurements (for example, height) which are related to skeletal size, and a measure of bone mass, generally obtained using dual-energy X-ray absorptiometry (DXA). DXA provides a two-dimensional measurement of bone area (BA) and bone mineral content (BMC); BMC is then divided by BA to provide bone mineral density (BMD), but this is not a true 'density'. Both BMC and, to a lesser extent, BMD remain influenced by body size. It is therefore important when interpreting the results of studies using DXA to attempt to disentangle effects on body (and hence skeletal) size and those on mineral mass per se. A further limitation is that DXA measures bone mass, but does not provide information on bone structure or strength which might be at least as important (if not more so) in terms of outcome. This issue is attracting increasing attention but has only really been addressed in more recent studies examining the long-term effects of exercise on the skeleton.

## In Utero Effects on Offspring Bone Mass

Neonatal bone mass is clearly influenced by genetic factors, but also by factors associated with the intrauterine environment. Most studies have been observational, although a randomized trial of maternal calcium supplementation during the second and third trimesters reported higher size-adjusted neonatal bone mass in the offspring of supplemented mothers who were themselves in the lowest quintile for baseline calcium intake [4]. Studies of vitamin D supplementation during pregnancy collectively suggest that the effects are minimal in mothers with adequate vitamin D status, but that in mothers with poor vitamin D status, supplementation may result in improved fetal growth and mineral accretion, and, possibly, improved postnatal weight and length gain [5].

Data from the Southampton Women's study, in which detailed dietary intake data were collected during pregnancy from 145 women, and the infant's bone mass was measured by DXA shortly after birth, suggest that parental birth weight, paternal height and maternal smoking have effects predominantly on skeletal size, whereas maternal skin-fold thickness, and exercise during late pregnancy may influence bone mass independent of size [6]. In a 9-year follow-up of 211 children from the same cohort, whole body BMC was positively associated with both maternal 25-OH vitamin D status during the last trimester and with umbilical venous calcium concentrations [7]. It has been proposed that maternal calcium stress may result in increased fetal and placental parathyroid hormone (PTH) and PTH-related protein (PTH-rP) leading to higher fetal trabecular bone formation (which, due to its greater surface area, provides a better calcium reservoir), and a decrease in cortical bone. After birth, trabecular bone is rapidly remodeled but the effects on the cortical 'envelope' may be more permanent, representing a potential mechanism for permanent effects on skeletal size [8].

## Fetal, Infant and Childhood Growth and Later Bone Mass

### Size in Early Life

Data from a number of studies have shown positive associations between birth weight, birth length and/or weight at 1 year of age, and bone mass during later childhood [9], early adult life [10], and at 60–75 years of age [11]. In each case, associations were strongest for BMC and weakest for size-corrected bone mass, suggesting a predominant association between early size and later bone size rather than bone density per se. In one cohort there was evidence for an environment-gene interaction between vitamin D receptor (VDR) genotype and birth weight, suggesting that environmental factors may modify genetic influences on bone size [12].

### Childhood Growth

One study in children born at term [9] and two studies in populations born preterm [13, 14] reported higher bone mass (after adjusting for current size) in individuals with either the greatest absolute length or weight gain, or with upward centile crossing during infancy and childhood. Consistent with these findings, data from a cohort of around 7,000 Finnish men and women born between 1924 and 1933 [15] showed that the risk of hip fracture was significantly higher in those with a low rate of childhood growth between 7 and 15 years. This study is important since childhood growth was found to predict the clinically meaningful endpoint – osteoporotic fracture. All these studies emphasize that linear growth may be more influential than weight gain – an important observation since this represents a potential mechanism for maximizing bone mass, especially in populations who experience stunting of growth.

## Nutrition and Bone Mass in Term Infants

Few studies have evaluated the long-term effects of infant diet on bone health in term infants. Jones et al. [16] reported that infants who were breast-fed had higher size-adjusted lumbar spine, hip and whole body BMD than formula-fed infants at 8 years of age. The effect remained after adjusting for confounding factors, and was most significant for infants breastfed for at least 3 months, although a greater duration of breastfeeding was not associated with further benefits for childhood bone mass. The frequency of night feeds during the first month of life (arguably a more reliable indicator of the 'amount' of breastfeeding than the number of day feeds) was significantly and positively related to later BMD, providing some evidence of a dose-response effect. Moreover, a mother's intention to breastfeed at delivery (as opposed to her actual breastfeeding behavior) showed no relationship with later BMD. Collectively, these data suggest that the observations reflect a genuine biological effect of breast milk on later bone mass rather than confounding.

Two studies in term infants have demonstrated short-term effects of manipulating calcium intake, via changes to the fat blend used in infant formulas, on bone mass. Infants randomized to receive a formula containing a modified fat blend designed to improve calcium absorption had significantly higher size-adjusted whole body BMC than those who received a standard formula [17]; their BMC was also more similar to that of a group of breastfed term infants. Long-term follow-up of this cohort is underway to determine whether these early effects have persisted. Using an alternative strategy to improve calcium absorption, Koo et al. [18] reported higher bone mass in infants receiving a low palmitate versus a standard infant formula; long-term effects have not yet been evaluated.

## Prospective Studies in Preterm Infants

Preterm infants are an interesting group in which to examine the influence of early factors on later bone health. They are born at a time of normally rapid mineral accretion and bone growth, and are thus at risk of mineral deficiency, as well as more general nutrient deficiencies, during the neonatal period.

They frequently have under-mineralized bones and may develop metabolic bone disease of prematurity. A large number of studies have examined the consequences of early diet on short-term bone health but data on longer-term bone outcomes are generally lacking. Backstrom et al. [19] studied a small group of infants randomized to vitamin D (500 or 1,000 IU/day) and either unsupplemented or mineral-supplemented breast milk. Bone mass measured at age 9–11 years was not influenced by early diet or by the dose of vitamin D. However, the duration of breastfeeding was positively associated with size-adjusted lumbar spine bone mass in mineral-supplemented subjects.

Bone mass was measured by DXA at 10–12 years in 230 children from our large prospective randomized trial of diet during the neonatal period. Subjects with evidence of metabolic bone disease during the neonatal period were significantly shorter at aged 10–12 years [20], suggesting a long-term effect of suboptimal early nutrition on skeletal growth. Compared to children born at term, the preterm group had reduced bone mass in association with their smaller body size, but there was no specific effect of early diet on bone mass. However, children randomized to receive the lowest nutrient diets during infancy had significantly higher plasma osteocalcin, suggestive of increased bone formation rates [21]. Follow-up of this cohort in early adult life is nearing completion and will provide the first experimental data in humans on the effects of early nutrition on peak bone mass and turnover.

### Childhood Lifestyle Factors and Bone Health

Although much of the research into the early origins of bone health has concentrated on events during fetal life or infancy, lifestyle factors later in childhood and adolescence have also received attention as potentially modifiable determinants of later bone health. Adolescence is potentially a particularly important period, since bone mass increases by 25–30% – equivalent to the amount of bone lost after the menopause. The two most studied lifestyle factors are calcium intake and exercise. However, whilst both interventions are generally associated with increased bone mass during the period of intervention, there is less evidence on the persistence of such effects.

*Childhood Diet*
Calcium
Epidemiological studies have shown associations between milk or calcium intake during childhood and both adult bone mass and fracture risk. Such associations are generally stronger at lower levels of calcium intakes. The results from cohort studies relating calcium intake recorded during adolescence and bone mass measured during the third decade are less consistent.

Several prospective randomized trials of calcium supplementation have now been conducted in children. Studies using calcium salts are generally consistent in showing an increase in bone mass (rather than bone size) during the supplementation period. This is accompanied by biochemical evidence of decreased bone formation and reflects reduced bone remodeling. However, in all but one study, the effect reversed on stopping the calcium supplements [22, 23]. The exception, a study in Gambian children with very low baseline calcium intakes, reported a persistent increase in bone mass at the radius 24 months after stopping the supplements [24].

The study with the longest duration of calcium supplementation was conducted in girls starting at pubertal stage 2 and lasting up to 7 years [25]. The results suggested a beneficial effect of calcium supplementation during the period of maximum bone growth, and in subjects with the greatest requirements (those with larger skeletons, and with a low habitual calcium intake). However, once bone growth had largely ceased and consolidation was occurring, the beneficial effects were lost. Presumably, calcium requirements were lower during this period and were met in most girls by their habitual calcium intake.

In contrast to studies using calcium salts, two trials using either milk [26] or milk-based food supplements [27] as the calcium source have shown different effects, with increases in bone mass lasting up to 3 years after the intervention was stopped. Both studies were in girls, and the increased bone mass was associated either with increased height and bone size or with higher plasma IGF-1 concentrations. In one study, the beneficial effect of the intervention was greatest in subjects with the lowest habitual calcium intakes and was most apparent in the appendicular skeleton. It has been postulated that these observations reflect an anabolic effect of milk protein, possibly milk basic protein which is known to enhance bone strength by stimulating bone formation and collagen synthesis [28]. However, another randomized trial (this time in prepubertal boys and girls with high baseline calcium intakes) using a high calcium dairy drink found no effect on body size or bone mass either during an 18-month intervention or at the 12-month follow-up [29].

Vitamin D

Vitamin D in its active form plays a vital role in maintaining bone health, and deficiency states in children are associated with rickets which may have obvious permanent effects on bone structure. However, less is known about the effects of more subtle variations in vitamin D status, or vitamin D intake. In a non-randomized study, infants supplemented with vitamin D during the first year of life had significantly higher BMD at the radius and hip (but not spine) at 7–9 years than unsupplemented infants [30]. Supplemented infants received 400 IU/day of cholecalciferol, and both groups had similar breast-feeding durations. Vitamin D-supplemented subjects were also heavier and taller at the time of the bone measurements, suggesting the findings may reflect the effects of vitamin D predominantly on bone size rather than mineralization.

A study in Finnish girls reported a positive association between baseline concentrations of 25-OH vitamin D and gains in BMD over the subsequent 3 years. The association was present for girls in mid-puberty at enrolment but not for prepubertal subjects, and was also greater at the lumbar spine than the femoral neck [31].

Other Nutrients

Although there are theoretical reasons why other elements of the diet such as vitamin K, zinc, protein, sodium or fruit and vegetables might influence later bone health, no studies have yet been conducted on specific nutrients. Parsons et al. [32] studied Dutch children who had received a macrobiotic diet during infancy and early childhood. These children had very low dietary calcium intakes, marked vitamin D deficiency and demonstrated stunted growth between birth and 8 years of age. Despite subsequent catch-up in weight and height, significant deficits in bone mass were seen at all skeletal sites at 9–15 years. Although it is not possible to identify a specific etiological factor, these findings add to the evidence for long-term bone effects of early malnutrition and stunting.

*Childhood Activity*

Weight-bearing physical activity has attracted increasing interest as a potentially modifiable determinant of peak bone mass. Several studies have reported higher bone mass in elite pediatric gymnasts and athletes compared to matched controls, and a number of randomized intervention studies in children and adolescents have demonstrated increased bone mass in loaded bones during the period of increased activity. The interventions used vary in intensity and ease of application, but include programs designed to be implemented as part of the routine school day (for example, jumping activities for 10 min 3 times/week). Collectively, the results of these studies suggest that effects are site-specific, greatest for cortical bone, and that interventions may be most effective during puberty when bone growth is most rapid. Although the majority of studies have used DXA to measure bone mass, some studies using peripheral quantitative computed tomography (pQCT) have also reported higher cortical cross-sectional area, cortical thickness and increased parameters of bending strength, suggesting that weight-bearing exercise may have benefits for bone structure as well as bone mass.

Despite the generally positive results of short-term interventions, data demonstrating that the beneficial effects of exercise persist and are reflected in higher peak bone mass, improved bone strength or reduced fracture risk are more limited. Follow-up of ballet dancers, gymnasts and other athletes into adult life suggests that they do have higher bone mass than matched controls but such studies are limited by potential biases related to the self-selected nature of the athletes. A 6-year longitudinal study in normally active adolescents reported that those in the highest quartile for activity had significantly greater gains in bone mass than those in the lowest quartile; the differences persisted for at least 1 year after peak bone mineral velocity was reached, but the cohort was not followed until they attained peak bone mass [33]. Lloyd et al. [34] reported that exercise (but not calcium intake) during adolescence positively influenced bone mass and bone-bending strength in the femur in a cohort of 80 young women followed prospectively for 10 years.

Follow-up of individuals who have participated in intervention trials is as yet limited. Fuchs and Snow [35] reported that the gains in hip BMC and BA (but not lumbar spine BMC and BA) seen during a randomized trial of high-impact training in prepubertal children were maintained for at least 7 months after the intervention ceased. The effect of the intervention appeared to operate by increasing bone size, rather than by increasing bone density per se. These results are consistent with those reported in a 12-month follow-up of 3- to 5-year-old children [36] who participated in a randomized trial of activity intervention. The intervention was associated with increased leg BMC and greater tibial periosteal circumference. At follow-up, although there were no persisting changes in leg BMC, the difference in periosteal circumference persisted.

*Interactions Between Activity and Calcium Intake*

In some studies, the effect of weight-bearing exercise was seen only in subjects with the highest calcium intakes. For example, Iuliano-Burns et al. [37] found a positive interaction between calcium supplementation and physical activity on femur bone mass in girls aged 7–11 years, whilst in 3- to 5-year-olds the effect of an activity intervention on leg BMC was seen only in those who were also supplemented with calcium [36]. Interestingly, 12 months after the intervention period, there was no persisting effect of calcium supplementation although the effect of activity was still apparent.

**Conclusions**

Available data are consistent with a predominant association between growth during fetal life, infancy and childhood on later skeletal size. The data suggest that optimizing growth, particularly linear growth, during infancy and childhood is likely to increase peak bone mass, which in turn might reduce the risk of osteoporotic fracture. Proposed mechanisms for these effects include programming of PTH/PTH-rP in utero leading to permanent effects on the size of the cortical envelope [8] and alterations in the set points of the GH-IGF-1 or hypothalamic-pituitary-adrenal axes [38]. Polymorphisms of the VDR are also associated with height and bone size [39] and may interact with environmental factors.

In contrast to the effects of early growth, there is some evidence that infant nutrition may influence bone mineralization and turnover more

***Table 1.*** An 'evidence-based' approach to optimizing later bone health

| In utero | Infancy | Childhood |
|---|---|---|
| Adequate maternal vitamin D status | Breastfeeding | Weight-bearing exercise |
| Adequate maternal calcium intake | Adequate calcium/ phosphorus intake (especially for preterm infants) | Adequate calcium intake (particularly during pubertal growth spurt) |
| | Adequate vitamin D intake | Milk/milk-based products |
| | Maximize linear (bone) growth | $\longrightarrow$ |
| | | $\longrightarrow$ |

directly. For example, breastfeeding may have benefits for later bone mass that are independent of effects on bone size, while suboptimal nutrition in preterm infants influences later bone turnover. This is a difficult area to investigate in children, generally relying on proxy measures of mineral mass (such as size-adjusted bone mass) and biochemical markers of bone turnover, with their limitations.

There are reasonably compelling data that weight-bearing exercise during childhood and adolescence may result in lasting benefits for bone health. Effects are usually region-specific and result predominantly from local responses to stress induced by loading. These studies emphasize the need to obtain measures of bone structure and parameters of bone strength, and not simply measure bone mass. In contrast, the evidence for a lasting effect of calcium supplementation on bone health is less convincing. The use of calcium salts results in a temporary reduction in bone remodeling but probably not in long-term benefit unless supplementation is maintained throughout the growth period. However, supplementation using calcium derived from milk products may have a more lasting but anabolic effect on bones. Furthermore, interactions between VDR genotype and calcium absorption have been demonstrated [40]. VDR genotype could therefore potentially modify the response of individuals to calcium supplementation. Suggested measures for maximizing peak bone mass and optimizing bone health based on current evidence are presented in table 1.

It is relevant to consider the likely practical relevance of the effect sizes observed in intervention studies. The effects of weight-bearing exercise interventions on BMD are in the order of 3–5% (depending on the loading applied), whilst reported effect sizes in follow-up milk supplementation trials vary from 1 to 5%. Whilst there are difficulties and uncertainties inherent in extrapolating bone mass data from children to adults, it has been calculated that a 2–3% increase in peak bone mass could reduce later fracture risk by 10–20%.

Fewtrell

**Table 2.** Suggested areas for future research

| | |
|---|---|
| 1 | Long-term follow-up of existing intervention trials (nutrition, exercise) to determine which interventions affect adult outcome, identify sensitive periods and site specificity of interventions |
| 2 | Use of additional techniques for assessing bone structure and strength (e.g. peripheral quantitative computed tomography, pQCT) as well as bone mass |
| 3 | Identification of environment–gene interactions which might allow targeting of interventions for vulnerable groups |
| 4 | Investigation of potential mechanisms – e.g. effects on hormonal axes, bone structure |

In conclusion, whilst further research is clearly required (table 2), there is evidence that osteoporosis may be at least partly preventable by interventions during early life designed to optimize linear growth, nutrition and weight-bearing activity. Furthermore, available data suggest that the effect sizes observed with such interventions are of a magnitude which could be potentially significant in public health terms in reducing the burden of osteoporosis.

## References

1 Pratt CWM, McCance RA: Severe undernutrition in growing and adult animals. 6. Changes in the long bones during the rehabilitation of cockerels. Br J Nutr 1961;15:121–129.
2 Gudehithlu KP, Ramakrishnan CV: Effect of undernutrition on the chemical composition and the activity of alkaline phosphatase in soluble and particulate fractions of the newborn rat calvarium and femur. II: Effect of preweaning undernutrition in the suckling rat. Calcif Tissue Int 1990;46:378–383.
3 Mehta G, Roach HI, Langley-Evans S, et al: Intrauterine exposure to a maternal low protein diet reduces adult bone mass and alters growth plate morphology in rats. Calcif Tissue Int 2002;71:493–498.
4 Koo WWK, Walters JC, Esterlitz J, et al: Maternal calcium supplementation and fetal bone mineralization. Obstet Gynecol 1999;94:577–582.
5 Pawley N, Bishop NJ: Prenatal and infant predictors of bone health: the influence of vitamin D. Am J Clin Nutr 2004;80(suppl):1748S–1751S.
6 Godfrey K, Walker-Bone K, Robinson S, et al: Neonatal bone mass: influence of parental birthweight, maternal smoking, body composition and activity during pregnancy. J Bone Miner Res 2001;16:1694–1703.
7 Javaid MK, Taylor P, Shore SR, et al: Umbilical vein calcium concentration and maternal vitamin D to predict the bone mass of children at age 9 years. Osteoporosis Int 2003;14(suppl 1): S13.
8 Tobias JH, Cooper C: PTH/PTHrP activity and the programming of skeletal development in utero. J Bone Mineral Res 2004;19:177–182.
9 Jones G, Dwyer T: Birth weight, birth length and bone density in prepubertal children: evidence for an association that may be mediated by genetic factors. Calcif Tissue Int 2000; 67:304–308.
10 Cooper C, Cawley MID, Bhalla A, et al: Childhood growth, physical activity and peak bone mass in women. J Bone Miner Res 1995;10:940–947.
11 Cooper C, Fall C, Egger P, et al: Growth in infancy and bone mass in later life. Ann Rheum Dis 1997;56:17–21.

12 Dennison EM, Arden NK, Keen RW, et al: Birthweight, vitamin D receptor genotype and the programming of osteoporosis. Paediatr Perinat Epidemiol 2001;15:211–219.

13 Fewtrell MS, Prentice A, Cole TJ, Lucas A: Effects of growth during infancy and childhood on bone mineralisation and turnover in preterm children aged 8–12 years. Acta Paediatr 2000; 89:148–153.

14 Weiler HA, Yuen CK, Seshia MM: Growth and bone mineralization of young adults weighing less than 1500g at birth. Early Hum Dev 2002;67:101–112.

15 Cooper C, Erikkson JG, Forsen T, et al: Maternal height, childhood growth and risk of hip fracture in later life: a longitudinal study. Osteoporos Int 2001;12:623–629.

16 Jones G, Riley M, Dwyer T: Breastfeeding in early life and bone mass in prepubertal children: a longitudinal study. Osteoporos Int 2000;11:146–152.

17 Kennedy K, Fewtrell MS, Morley R, et al: Double-blind randomised trial of a synthetic triacylglycerol in formula-fed infants: effects on stool biochemistry, stool characteristics and bone mass. Am J Clin Nutr 1999;70:920–927.

18 Koo WW, Hammami M, Margeson DP, et al: Reduced bone mineralization in infants fed palm olein-containing formula: a randomized, double-blinded, prospective trial. Pediatrics 2003; 111:1017–1023.

19 Backstrom MC, Maki R, Kuusela A-L, et al: The long-term effect of early mineral, vitamin D and breast milk intake on bone mineral status in 9- to 11-year old children born prematurely. J Paediatr Gastroenterol Nutr 1999;29:575–582.

20 Fewtrell MS, Cole TJ, Bishop NJ, Lucas A: Neonatal factors predicting childhood height in preterm infants: evidence for a persisting effect of early metabolic bone disease? J Pediatr 2000;137:668–673.

21 Fewtrell MS, Prentice A, Jones SC, et al: Bone mineralisation and turnover in preterm infants at 8–12 years of age: the effects of early diet. J Bone Miner Res 1999;14:810–820.

22 Slemenda C, Peacock M, Hui S, et al: Reduced rates of skeletal remodelling are associated with increased bone mineral density in teenage girls. J Bone Mineral Res 1997;12:676–682.

23 Lee WTK, Leung SSF, Leung DMY, Cheng JCY: A follow-up study on the effects of calcium-supplement withdrawal and puberty on bone acquisition of children. Am J Clin Nutr 1996;64: 71–77.

24 Dibba B, Prentice A, Ceesay M, et al: Bone mineral content and plasma osteocalcin concentrations of Gambian children 12 and 24 mo after the withdrawal of a calcium supplement. Am J Clin Nutr 2002;76:681–686.

25 Matkovic V, Goel PK, Badenhop-Stevens NE, et al: Calcium supplementation and bone mineral density in females from childhood to young adulthood: a randomized controlled trial. Am J Clin Nutr 2005;81:175–188.

26 Barker ME, Lambert H, Cadogan J, et al: Milk supplementation and bone growth in adolescent girls: is the effect ephemeral? Bone 1998;23:S606.

27 Bonjour JP, Chevalley T, Ammann P, et al: Gain in bone mineral mass in prepubertal girls 3.5 years after discontinuation of calcium supplementation: a follow-up study. Lancet 2001;358: 1208–1212.

28 Toba Y, Takada Y, Yamamura J, et al: Milk basic protein: a novel protective function of milk against osteoporosis. Bone 2000;27:403–408.

29 Gibbons MJ, Gilchrist NL, Frampton C, et al: The effects of a high calcium dairy food on bone health in pre-pubertal children in New Zealand. Asia Pac J Clin Nutr 2004;13:341–347.

30 Zamora SA, Rizzoli R, Belli DC, et al: Vitamin D supplementation during infancy is associated with higher bone mineral mass in prepubertal girls. J Clin Endocrinol Metab 1999;84: 4541–4544.

31 Lehtonen-Veromaa MKM, Mottonen TT, Nuotio IO, et al: Vitamin D and attainment of peak bone mass among peripubertal Finnish girls: a 3-y prospective study. Am J Clin Nutr 2002;76: 1446–1453.

32 Parsons TJ, van Dusseldorp M, van der Vliet M, et al: Reduced bone mass in Dutch adolescents fed a macrobiotic diet in early life. J Bone Miner Res 1997;12:1486–1494.

33 Bailey DA, McKay HA, Mirwald RL, et al: A six-year longitudinal study of the relationship of physical activity to bone mineral accrual in growing children: the University of Saskatchewan Bone Mineral Accrual Study. J Bone Miner Res 1999;14:1672–1679.

34 Lloyd T, Petit MA, Lin H-M, Beck TJ: Lifestyle factors and the development of bone mass and bone strength in young women. J Pediatr 2004;144:776–782.

Fewtrell

35  Fuchs RK, Snow CM: Gains in hip bone mass from high-impact training are maintained: a randomized controlled trial in children. J Pediatr 2002;141:357–362.
36  Binkley T, Specker B: Increased periosteal circumference remains present 12 months after an exercise intervention in preschool children. Bone 2004;35:1383–1388.
37  Iuliano-Burns S, Saxon L, Naughton G, et al: Regional specificity of exercise and calcium during skeletal growth in girls: a randomized controlled trial. J Bone Miner Res 2003;18: 156–162.
38  Fall C, Hindmarsh P, Dennison E, et al: Programming of growth hormone secretion and bone mineral density in elderly men: an hypothesis. J Clin Endocrinol Metab 1998;83:135–139.
39  Lorenzton M, Lorenzton R, Nordstrom P: Vitamin D receptor gene polymorphism is associated with birth height, growth to adolescence and adult stature in healthy Caucasian men: a cross-sectional study. J Clin Endocrinol Metab 2000;85:1666–1671.
40  Ames SK, Ellis KJ, Gunn SK, et al: Vitamin D receptor gene Fok1 polymorphism predicts calcium absorption and bone mineral density in children. J Bone Miner Res 1999;14:740–746.

## Discussion (Also refer to the Presentation "Nutrition and Cancer Prevention: Targets, Strategies, and the Importance of Early Life Interventions" by S.D. Hursting et al)

*Dr. Laron:* I have 3 questions for Dr. Fewtrell. One, which norms do you propose for BMD for young children, and which norms for DXA? The second question is with regard to volumetric DXA; you mentioned it but didn't discuss it further. We know that short children may have a below normal DXA which normalizes when bone volume is calculated, so that somebody who may seemingly need treatment may actually not need it. What is your opinion? The last question is what do you think about the new approach of passive exercise in small babies which Eliakim and Nemet [1] recently described and which improves bone density as measured by the ultrasonography method?

*Dr. Fewtrell:* With regard to the norms for DXA BMD, there are now pediatric reference data incorporated into most machines, and databases are being improved and updated. For example, there is the new large Hologic pediatric database from the US that is just becoming available. I think the problem of size issues with DXA is very important, and applies both to research and clinical settings, although in different ways. Essentially, many patients have stunted growth and appear to have low areal bone density, although this may simply reflect their small size rather than indicating that they have undermineralized bones. A number of approaches have been suggested to adjust for the effect of size, including the use of so-called 'volumetric' bone density such as BMAD, or adjusting for weight and height. In fact we have recently done some work showing that different size correction approaches actually produce similar results in terms of categorizing groups of patients as having normal or abnormal bone mineralization [2], so it probably doesn't matter which correction you use as long as size is considered. But I think there is actually another issue here because once you have done your size correction and come to the conclusion that a child is small and has an appropriate amount of mineral for their size, that still doesn't tell you whether they are at increased risk. That is where techniques that measure other parameters of bone geometry or strength might be important. We need to know more about the distribution of the bone mineral, and the shape and geometry of the bones because these factors may determine things like fracture risk.

*Dr. Laron:* I asked this question because of IGF1 and growth hormone. In patients who have growth hormone or IGF1 deficiency, when a simple DXA is used they are found to be osteoporotic [3] but if the volumetric BMD is calculated they become normal [4], and the same might be true for the children who are short by other causes.

146

*Dr. Fewtrell:* That is true, I think we should not be using the term 'osteoporosis' in children based on DXA measurements with the criteria established for adults. I know that in the US this has resulted in problems where children who are small and consequently have a low areal BMD Z score have been erroneously diagnosed as having osteoporosis. This is why it is so important to apply some form of size correction. In the UK we are currently compiling our own reference database from which we will be able to get a size-adjusted BMD Z score and not just the areal BMD Z score, to get around this problem.

*Dr. Laron:* What was the respective machine?

*Dr. Fewtrell:* Our reference data come from different GE Lunar machines that have been cross-calibrated. Cross-calibration could also be performed with other machine makes as well.

With regard to your earlier question about the use of passive exercise in preterm infants, I am not aware of the ultrasound study you mentioned, but I know Moyer-Mileur et al. [5] have done some work previously suggesting that passive exercise in preterm infants improves their bone mass in the short-term, and that makes sense. Whether the effect persists in the long-term is another matter – this has not been investigated.

*Dr. Roma:* Since most hypoallergenic diets and formulas, elemental and semi-elemental, are lactose-free, is there any influence on calcium absorption? Do you recommend calcium and vitamin D when children are on steroids for a long time?

*Dr. Fewtrell:* There is certainly some evidence that children who are on a milk-free diet have a greater risk of fracture during childhood, but I don't know specifically about hypoallergenic diets. With regards to calcium and vitamin D when children are on steroids, we know there is an increased risk of low bone mass and fractures associated with steroid treatment, but whether that is reduced or prevented by giving additional calcium or vitamin D is not clear, although it is presumably important to make sure they have at least an adequate intake. I know in practice that most patients in our own hospital who have a low bone mass are put on calcium and vitamin D supplements, although the hard evidence that this has benefits is perhaps not there.

*Dr. Abrams:* I have a brief comment about lactose-free formulas and calcium absorption. We looked at that and did not find a very large effect. Most of the non-whole milk-based formulas do have additional calcium in them, so we don't think that this probably has a big effect on the overall calcium absorption. The total amount was greater than what would be achieved from breast milk, so I don't think that is a big issue.

*Dr. Lucas:* Dr. Hursting that was really a wonderful presentation, I really enjoyed it. When you restrict animals or humans for that matter with food, they are less obese, live longer and get less cancer. But specifically how do we understand what elements you are actually reducing in the diet that have cancer protection, because theoretically you could just be reducing the carcinogens in the diet by reducing food intake?

*Dr. Hursting:* In the animal model system we used purified diets, so I think the carcinogen exposure was reduced. We would measure that in our diets, and they were getting equal, basically no amounts of carcinogen. We have done some studies in terms of the type of calories, where one sees the most effect, and so you can restrict carbohydrate calories, fat calories, protein calories, and the bottom line is that the effect is obesity prevention. Now the sharpest effect is with carbohydrate calorie restriction, and we think that is because the sharpest effect is seen with an IGF drop, and some of the other factors that we are looking at are seen primarily with carbohydrate restriction. But it has been done with a total diet or with fat restriction, protein restriction, and protection from cancer is seen. So it appears that the obesity prevention component is the critical step to this. One should think about the exercise that when we have done the head studies with that we don't see the degree of protection, even though we can achieve a body weight to a similar degree we don't see the de degree of protection

Fewtrell

that we do with that carbohydrate calorie restriction. We don't see the drop in IGF1. So we are trying to move a little beyond but we do think that that is a part of the story.

*Dr. Lucas:* But that would be the link between nutritional protection from both cancer and cardiovascular disease.

*Dr. Hursting:* Yes, that is right. The downside is that when we do DXA on our mice and try to look at any effects of our energy restriction approaches, the only one that we come up with is that their bones are less dense. We found that if we do a combination of calorie restriction with the running wheel for example we can reverse that. Obviously that is the recommendation for humans. Part of the answer to this obesity issue is watching caloric intake and increasing physical activity, and that combination, at least based on our mouse data, is sufficient to raise any IGF drop related to a decrease in bone.

*Dr. Hamburger:* At the bottom of your list of inflammatory responses that lead to cancer you had asthma, and I recall that throughout 30 years, in 1970s, 1980s and 1990s, allergy and elevated IgE was said to cause cancer, then it was said to protect against cancer, asthma was associated with cancer, asthma was associated with less cancer, and finally after 30 years of studies it was decided that there was no relationship between allergy, asthma and cancer. Would you comment on that?

*Dr. Hursting:* That is the most mixed story of those conditions that I talked about. There are some recent data suggesting that perhaps there is a bit of risk for lung cancer. But you are right, historically that has been a more mixed bag. In other allergic situations, generally like an acute allergic response, it does not appear to be like these chronic long-term inflammatory conditions.

*Dr. Pereira-da-Silva:* Two questions for Dr. Fewtrell. It is well known that premature babies are prone to osteopenia. Two weeks after delivery of the preterm baby the mother's milk may have insufficient calcium and phosphorus to fulfill the needs and demands of the growing premature baby. During the stay in the intensive care unit, it is easy to provide fortifiers to human milk but after discharge this is a problem in exclusively breastfed babies [6]. Would you suggest continuing supplementing these babies with calcium and phosphorus? At present we use hypophosphatemia to monitor early osteopenia, but recent studies suggest that this is a poor marker for bone mineral content in premature babies compared to DXA measurements [7]. Which biochemical marker would you suggest for early detection of osteopenia?

*Dr. Fewtrell:* I think there is potentially a problem of inadequate nutrient intake in preterm infants who go home exclusively breastfeeding – not just for calcium and phosphorus but for other nutrients as well. While these infants are in hospital, human milk is supplemented with phosphorus or with a multi-nutrient breast milk fortifier, but typically when the infant is discharged these supplements are stopped. This is certainly the case in the UK. The only potential source of additional minerals and other nutrients for these infants during this period is top-ups with infant formula – and it makes sense if a nutrient-rich post-discharge formula is used for this purpose. Whether a low mineral and nutrient intake during the post-discharge period in breastfed infants actually makes any difference to their longer-term bone health is not known. The evidence is that preterm infants who are breastfed do have lower bone mass during the neonatal period than those who receive formula, but that they eventually catch up in terms of their size and bone mass. What was your other question?

*Dr. Pereira-da-Silva:* Which biochemical marker would you suggest for the early diagnosis of osteopenia?

*Dr. Fewtrell:* I am not actually a neonatologist but I don't think there is any available marker for osteopenia that performs better than monitoring the degree of hypophosphatemia together with alkaline phosphatase. We and others are looking at quantitative ultrasound as a potential monitoring tool, bit I don't think it looks particularly promising at the moment.

*Dr. Chad:* I would like Dr. Hursting to comment on the studies involving modulation by dietary manipulation of fatty acids n-3 and n-6 in cancer prevention. And the other comment would be the relationship between celiac disease and lymphoma later in life.

*Dr. Hursting:* I don't know the latter data so I can't comment on that. The n-3s are back, and I think primarily because of this inflammatory issue and the identification of this prostaglandin and the COX-2-related pathway, it is a great target for cancer prevention. Actually the n-3s were coming back even before that but it has accelerated the research on that pathway through fatty acid manipulation, e.g. the fish oils. It is definitely an important area and quite effective. It has expanded not only into the prostaglandin and cancer story but is a modulator of angiogenesis and other targets along the pathway. We are going to see a lot of work on that in the next few years.

*Dr. Greef:* Obviously from what you have said and I accept that there is a lack of evidence, should we now be recommending that our patients consume an ideal diet, which nobody does, and supplement with natural vitamins, possibly with the antioxidant mix, phytochemical mix, n-3 mix? Do you think we should recommend this? I often think we hide behind something for which there is no evidence-based medicine to support it. It is a sort of deck and dive issue, but at the rock face we have got to make decisions.

*Dr. Hursting:* I am not a big fan of supplementing mega doses, but I am a fan of a multivitamin approach. Particularly if we can work it and keep the caloric intake at a reasonable level, I think it is reasonable to recommend a multivitamin approach.

*Dr. Hanson:* I would assume that the inflammation also contains neutrophils and I would suggest that that could have two effects, one proinflammatory and one anti-inflammatory. The reason is that we have shown recently that lactoferrin which is often present in such cells interferes with the NF-κB pathway and prevents production of the proinflammatory cytokines IL-1, IL-6, TNF-α. We also see that lactoferrin gets into cell lines like melanoma cells and kills the malignant cells, so perhaps the neutrophils could also be helpful.

*Dr. Hursting:* We think of the inflammation, at least from the cancer side, as being a bad thing, but you are right, those inflammatory cells have to be present to fight infection and other things. I am intrigued by the fact that there are so many macrophages and other inflammations related to immune cells in adipose tissue. This is a fairly recent sort of finding and it has opened the eyes of a lot of us to start to look for those. Also the calorie restriction, for example, does seem to be knocking not only the COX-2 path down but IL-6, and we are trying to get in quickly and look whether we are in some way preventing such an influx of those macrophages in the adipose tissue for example. I think this is an important piece of it in the whole immune story and how it relates to inflammation. We are going to see a lot of good work on that, and it will become a topic in the cancer field.

*Dr. Saavedra:* Would you care to speculate on the potential effect of changes in bone mineral content or density in the first 2 years of life and later on? You showed some good relationships within what would be accomplished or prevented by improving bone density in adolescence, for example, and maybe even later. There has been a trend towards increasing calcium levels, because those are the few things we can manipulate, both in complementary foods as well as in breast milk substitutes. With some formulas the bone mineral content is even higher than breast milk controls. Do you see their benefits and how much are we influencing potential bone health in later in life?

*Dr. Fewtrell:* The short answer is that I don't think we know, because we don't have long-term data from populations in whom the short-term effects of early calcium intake on bone mass have been monitored. The data from the calcium supplementation trials which tend to be later in childhood or adolescence are not consistent, and it seems to me that the response probably depends on other factors such as genes and other elements of the diet. That is something that has perhaps been neglected. We have all tended to focus on calcium which I suppose is an obvious thing, but calcium requirements are likely to vary depending on what else you are eating. This may partly explain the low rates of osteoporosis seen in some populations with very low habitual calcium intakes but who also have low intakes of animal protein and salt. Overall, I'm not at all convinced that simply increasing calcium intake in healthy term infants is likely to have a long-term benefit. Obviously preterm infants have a mineral deficit so the situation is different.

*Dr. Abrams:* I would just like to make a comment that in infancy and early childhood we are trying to make sure that the children don't have fractures, and rickets is associated with very low vitamin D and extremely low calcium intakes as occur in parts of Africa. So there is minimal intake of calcium and vitamin D needed in early childhood to prevent fractures, but we have no reason to think that it has a long-term effect with the high levels of calcium that catch-up growth isn't entirely possible, and the data from breastfeeding would even suggest that perhaps some lower intakes are beneficial but a little balance must be found to make sure that rickets doesn't occur.

*Dr. Schofer:* I was a little surprised about your remarks on vitamin D and calcium supplementation that there are no efficacy data in children. Is that true also for chronic inflammatory conditions like chronic inflammatory bowel disease or hematic diseases, where it is a common practice to substitute these patients with vitamin D and calcium?

*Dr. Fewtrell:* I assume you are referring to my comments about the efficacy of calcium and vitamin D during my presentation. What I was saying was that there simply aren't a lot of randomized trials looking at the effects of vitamin D intake in childhood on later bone health, although obviously we need adequate intake to prevent rickets. With regard to the other part of your question about calcium and vitamin D supplements in various chronic diseases, I don't think this has been looked at systematically in randomized trials, although it is certainly common practice and is unlikely to do any harm. I am aware of a randomized trial of calcium and vitamin D supplementation in patients with cystic fibrosis that is being conducted by an Italian group at the moment, but I am not aware of trials in other chronic conditions.

*Dr. Schofer:* I have one more question for Dr. Hursting. Are there any data that you are aware of linking *Helicobacter* infections in children with lymphoma? We are very often in the situation that we find *Helicobacter* and then we need to think about whether eradication therapy should be used or not.

*Dr. Hursting:* I am not aware of anything with lymphoma; I mean childhood cancers specifically, although there are certainly animal data as well as human data on various *Helicobacter* species in adult cancer development. It appears again to be related to a chronic inflammation that perhaps requires 10 or more years to manifest, to cause trouble, but clearly in the animal systems there are a number of *Helicobacter* species that are linked over time and increased tumor development, and also some human data go on with it.

*Dr. Arvanitakis:* Considering the fact that peak bone mass is almost complete at 25 years of age, how effective do you think we shall be in treating the adult with cystic fibrosis and osteoporosis? Is there any evidence in the literature regarding the relationship between beef meat and the human colon cancer?

*Dr. Fewtrell:* It is increasingly recognized that young adults with cystic fibrosis have a low bone mass and are at an increased risk of fractures. The evidence is that most patients with cystic fibrosis probably don't attain a normal peak bone mass. They seem to have relatively normal bone mass until puberty but do not show the expected rapid gain in bone mass during puberty. The etiology is likely to be multifactorial, involving nutritional factors, chronic inflammation, delayed puberty and drug treatment. The recent consensus statement published by Aris et al. [8] suggests that all cystic fibrosis patients should have calcium, vitamin D and probably vitamin K supplements, and they should be treated with bisphosphates if they also have low bone mass, bone pain or fractures.

*Dr. Hursting:* Regarding the beef question, there are mixed data on beef consumption that have sharpened in the last few years and that sharpening has to do with two components: cured meats, cured beef and other meat products are clearly linked to colon cancer risk. The second is charred meat that is also clearly emerging as a risk factor, not a very strong one but a consistent one. So beef in general doesn't seem to be, but cured and charred meat are probably the two conditions you want to avoid.

## References

1 Eliakim A, Nemet D: Osteopenia of prematurity – the role of exercise in prevention and treatment. Pediatr Endocr Rev 2005;2:675–682.
2 Fewtrell MS, Gordon I, Biassoni L, Cole TJ: Dual X-ray absorptiometry (DXA) of the lumbar spine in a clinical paediatric setting: does the method of size-adjustment matter? Bone 2005;37:413–419.
3 Laron Z, Klinger B: IGF-I treatment of adult patients with Laron syndrome: preliminary results. Clin Endocrinol (Oxf) 1994;41:631–638.
4 Benbassat CA, Eshed V, Kamjin M, Laron Z: Are adult patients with Laron syndrome osteopenic? A comparison between dual-energy X-ray absorptiometry and volumetric bone densities. J Clin Endocrinol Metab 2003;88:4586–4589.
5 Moyer-Mileur LJ, Brunstetter V, McNaught TP, et al: Daily physical activity program increases bone mineralization and growth in preterm very low birth weight infants. Pediatrics 2000;106:1088–1092.
6 Griffin IJ: Postdischarge nutrition for high risk neonates. Clin Perinatol 2002;29:327–344.
7 Faerk J, Peitersen B, Petersen S, Michaelsen KF: Bone mineralisation in premature infants cannot be predicted from serum alkaline phosphatase or serum phosphate. Arch Dis Child Fetal Neonatal Ed 2002;87:F133–F136.
8 Aris RM, Merkel PA, Bachrach LK, et al: Consensus Conference Report: guide to bone health and disease in cystic fibrosis. J Clin Endocrinol Metab 2005;90:1888–1896.

Lucas A, Sampson HA (eds): Primary Prevention by Nutrition Intervention in Infancy and Childhood.
Nestlé Nutr Workshop Ser Pediatr Program, vol 57, pp 153–202,
Nestec Ltd., Vevey/S. Karger AG, Basel, © 2006.

# Nutrition and Cancer Prevention: Targets, Strategies, and the Importance of Early Life Interventions

*Stephen D. Hursting*[a,b], *Marie M. Cantwell*[a,b],
*Leah B. Sansbury*[a,b], *Michele R. Forman*[a]

[a]Laboratory of Biosystems and Cancer, Center for Cancer Research, and
[b]Cancer Prevention Fellowship Program, Division of Cancer Prevention,
National Cancer Institute, Bethesda, Md., USA

## Introduction

More than one million Americans will be diagnosed with cancer in 2005. This is especially tragic given that many cancers are preventable. Doll and Peto [1] estimated in 1981 that 30% of cancers were due to tobacco use while 35% could be attributed to poor dietary practices, and there is mounting evidence that diet-related conditions, such as obesity, can also greatly influence cancer risk [2]. Some significant progress in tobacco control in the United States has been made since the 1964 Surgeon General's Report on Smoking and Health identified cigarette smoking as the cause of lung cancer [3]. Smoking cessation at the individual level, as well as several effective community-based interventions, including regulations to restrict smoking in public places and tobacco product advertising to adolescents and children, have led to declines in tobacco use and lung cancer rates [4]. However, the development and application of diet-related strategies for cancer prevention remain an ongoing challenge to the medical, scientific and public health communities.

Adding to this challenge is the recent recognition of the role of perinatal and childhood nutritional exposures in cancer development across the life course. The established role of perinatal nutrition in neurological development and the relation of maternal and perinatal nutritional status to birth weight and subsequent risk of hypertension, diabetes and cardiovascular disease identify pregnancy and early childhood as critical windows for nutritional interventions to prevent these diseases. The influence of early life dietary exposures on carcinogenesis has been less studied, but evidence

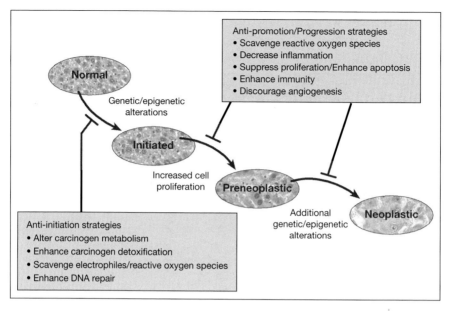

**Fig. 1.** Multi-step carcinogenesis pathway. A schematic presentation of the multi-stage process of carcinogenesis as well as stage-specific prevention strategies. The initiation stage is characterized by the conversion of a normal cell to an initiated cell in response to genetic or epigenetic changes in the cell's DNA. The conversion of an initiated cell to a preneoplastic population of cells and ultimately to a tumor is determined by additional genetic/epigenetic changes that effect the balance between growth and death in these cells. Strategies to intervene in these processes, using nutritional or other preventive strategies to decrease rates of mutation and epigenetic change and maintain the growth/death balance in cancer cells, are listed.

from human and animal studies suggest that nutrition during early time points along the life course can also have a major impact on cancer risk later in life.

It is beyond the scope of this paper to comprehensively review the field of diet and carcinogenesis. Rather, the objective of this review is to use our current knowledge about carcinogenesis to suggest opportunities for nutritional interventions, including during infancy and childhood. In the following sections, each of the potential targets for the nutritional modulation of cancer depicted in figure 1 will be examined, and examples of how these carcinogenesis-associated processes can be modulated will be presented. In addition, a brief discussion is included of the literature on early life exposures and the risk of breast cancer, the best studied cancer to date regarding nutritional effects across the life course. The information sources for this review include the MEDLINE (from January 1, 1993 through January 1, 2004) and CANCERLIT (from January 1, 1983 through January 1, 2004) databases, which were searched with the key words 'carcinogenesis'; 'nutrition and neoplasms'; and 'diet and neoplasms'. For the early life nutritional exposure and breast cancer section, subject search terms included breast cancer risk or incidence and the following: 'in utero', fetal, preeclampsia, birth weight, birth length, preterm, breast or infant feeding, infancy, childhood, puberty, adolescence, (catch-up) growth, age at menarche, maternal and paternal age, birth order or parity, intergenerational, and programming. Reviews, editorials and primary journal articles identified by this search, along with chapters from textbooks on cancer etiology and prevention available at the National Institutes of Health Medical Library, were used to summarize our current knowledge of carcinogenesis and the effects of nutritional factors on that process.

## Multistage Carcinogenesis: Pathways and Targets for Nutritional Intervention

Humans are exposed to a wide variety of endogenous and exogenous carcinogenic insults, including chemicals, radiation, physical agents, bacteria and viruses. Recent progress in the study of the multi-step process of carcinogenesis, particularly on the mechanisms of chemically and virally induced cancer, has revealed several points along the carcinogenesis pathway that may be amenable to cancer prevention strategies [5]. The classic view of experimental carcinogenesis, in which tumor initiation is followed by tumor promotion and progression in a sequential fashion, has undergone significant revision as our understanding of cancer-related genes and the biosystem has evolved [6–8]. However, the concepts and underlying processes of initiation, promotion, and progression remain theoretically important. Tumor initiation begins in cells with DNA alterations resulting from inherent genetic mutations or, more commonly, from spontaneous or carcinogen-induced genetic or epigenetic changes. Alterations in specific genes modify the responsiveness of the initiated cell to its microenvironment, eventually providing a growth advantage relative to normal cells [6]. The tumor promotion stage is characterized by clonal expansion of initiated cells due to alterations in the expression of genes whose products are associated with hyperproliferation, apoptosis, tissue remodeling and inflammation [7]. During the tumor progression stage, preneoplastic cells develop into invasive tumors through further clonal expansion, usually associated with alterations in gene expression and additional genetic damage due to progressive genomic instability [9].

As depicted in figure 1, possible ways of interfering with tumor initiation events include: (1) modifying carcinogen activation by inhibiting the enzymes responsible for that activation or by directly scavenging DNA-reactive electrophiles and free radicals; (2) enhancing carcinogen detoxification by altering the activity of detoxifying enzymes, and (3) modulating certain DNA repair processes. Possible ways of blocking the processes involved in the promotion and progression stages of carcinogenesis include: (1) scavenging reactive oxygen species (ROS); (2) altering the expression of genes involved in cell signaling, particularly those regulating cell proliferation, apoptosis, and differentiation; (3) decreasing inflammation; (4) enhancing immune function, or (5) suppressing angiogenesis.

In 1976, Sporn [10] defined the term chemoprevention as the use of natural or synthetic agents to reverse or suppress multistage carcinogenesis. There are numerous examples in the literature demonstrating that bioactive food components or chemopreventive nutrients can influence one or more of these targets and interfere with the carcinogenesis process, and specific examples will be discussed later in this review. We now appreciate that the nature of initiation, promotion and progression events is complex. For instance, we know from the work of Fearon and Vogelstein [11] and Spitz and Bondy [12] that multiple mutational and epigenetic events are involved in the formation of cancers. Furthermore, humans are generally exposed to mixtures of agents that can simultaneously act at different stages of the carcinogenesis process. Thus, rather than three discrete stages occurring in a predictable order, human carcinogenesis is best characterized as an accumulation of alterations in genes regulating cellular growth, death, and malignant properties. These alternations occur through a series of clonal selections influenced by endogenous and exogenous factors. Concomitant epigenetic instabilities often develop in a cancer and may significantly contribute to tumorigenesis [13]. Nonetheless, the processes involved in cancer initiation, promotion and progression described above remain important and relevant targets for cancer prevention. Nutritional interventions that increase or decrease rates of mutation, rates of epigenetic change, or the balance between growth and death in cancer cells can significantly influence the ultimate development of cancer.

## Targets for Anti-Initiation Strategies

### Carcinogen Activation
Most chemicals are not carcinogenic, but a wide variety of chemicals and chemical classes can cause cancer in animals and humans. Most chemical carcinogens are genotoxic, causing DNA damage by reacting with DNA bases. The carcinogens form covalent adducts with DNA in the nucleus and mitochondria. Endogenous carcinogens, which are often ROS generated as part of normal oxidative metabolism or as a result of xenobiotic metabolism, as well as ultraviolet radiation and gamma radiation, can also cause extensive DNA damage. For instance, proto-oncogenes and tumor suppressor genes are normal cellular genes that can be mutated to cause uncontrolled cell growth or other characteristics that increase the probability of neoplastic transformation [11–16].

Metabolic activation of procarcinogens (i.e., carcinogens requiring enzymatic conversion to DNA-reactive intermediates) is generally catalyzed by cytochrome P450 enzymes through oxidation. More than 100 distinct mammalian P450 enzymes have been identified [17]. In addition, there are other enzyme systems involved in carcinogen activation, such as peroxidases (including the cyclooxygenases, which will be discussed in more detail below) and certain transferases such as N-acetyltransferase and sulfotransferase [18, 19]. Each of these enzymes provides a potential target for modulating carcinogen activation.

One common feature of the metabolic activation of all procarcinogens is that their ultimate DNA-reactive carcinogenic species are electrophilic [20]. In addition, many direct-acting carcinogens damage DNA through electrophilic intermediates [21]. Thus the electrophilicity of the ultimate carcinogenic species serves as a shared intervention target for most chemical carcinogens. The electrophilic metabolites may themselves be ROS and interact as such with DNA [22]. Oxygen free radicals may also be involved in a step required for activation of a procarcinogen, and thus the reactions involved in metabolic activation of carcinogens may release ROS which can in turn attack DNA [22]. Thus, directly scavenging DNA-reactive intermediates with antioxidants or other agents that can scavenge electophiles constitutes a plausible strategy for modulating this early stage of carcinogenesis.

*Carcinogen Detoxification*

In addition to the carcinogen-activating enzymes, a series of enzymes (the so-called phase-II enzymes) detoxify activated carcinogens, thus preventing their binding to DNA. The induction of the glutathione S-transferases (GSTs) is an important response for the detoxification of xenobiotics [23]. This class of enzymes couples a number of diverse substrates to glutathione to excrete them from the body. GSTs are segregated into three classes based on their sequence homology and specificity for substrates [24]. Other detoxification enzymes include uridine diphosphate-glucuronosyl transferase, quinone reductase, and the epoxide hydrolases [25, 26]. The efficiency with which these and other enzymes detoxify carcinogens is a critical factor in determining the carcinogenicity of a particular xenobiotic.

*DNA Repair Processes*

The generation of DNA-reactive intermediates by most chemical carcinogens leads to the production of DNA adducts or other types of damage. As reviewed by Mitchell et al. [27], normal mammalian cells can efficiently remove DNA damage induced by carcinogens. Cells use different strategies to repair DNA damage, depending on the structure of the damage and its location in the genome. For example, small lesions, such as alkylated DNA bases, can be repaired by a mechanism termed base excision repair [28]. This process involves removal of the damaged base followed by a 'small cut and patch' repair involving removal of a few nucleotides. When methylation occurs at either the $O^6$ or $O^4$ positions of guanine or thymine, the modified bases can be repaired by the direct transfer of the methyl group to a methyl transferase [29]. Bulky carcinogen-induced DNA adducts and ultraviolet light photodimers can be repaired through a 'large cut and patch' mechanism involving approximately 27–29 nucleotides that include the damaged bases; this is termed nucleotide excision repair [30]. The integrity of the genetic information is threatened not only by various environmental exposures but also by errors produced during normal DNA replication, for example, non-Watson-Crick base-pairing and slippage during DNA replication. Cells have also developed a mismatch repair mechanism to correct the errors resulting from mis-replication [31].

## Nutritional Modulation of Tumor Initiation Processes: Examples

*Inhibiting Carcinogen Activation*

Fruits, vegetables, herbs and other foodstuffs, as well as non-edible plants, contain numerous bioactive food components known to affect the metabolic activation of chemical carcinogens. Examples of food sources containing agents that decrease carcinogen activation are the cruciferous vegetables, such as cauliflower, broccoli and cabbage. The crucifers are sources of isothiocyanates, which are known to interfere with the metabolism of nitrosamines and other carcinogens. For example, studies by Chung et al. [32], Hecht [33], and Stoner and Mukhtar [34] have shown conclusively that the metabolism and carcinogenicity of the tobacco carcinogen 4-(methylnitrosamino)-1-(3-pyridyl)-1-butanone are decreased by the administration of phenylisothiocyanate. Extensive structure-activity studies by these investigators have also shown that the carbon chain length of the isothiocyanate moiety correlates with tumor prevention activity, with a longer chain isothiocyanate apparently more suitable for insertion into the cell due to increased lipophilicity [35, 36]. Also, diallyl sulfide, a common volatile in garlic, has been shown to be a potent inhibitor of cytochrome P450 2E1 [37, 38]. This cytochrome P450 metabolizes ethanol, acetone, and several known chemical carcinogens, including several nitrosamines that target the nasal tissues, oral cavity, liver and esophagus, as well as dimethylhydrazine and its metabolites, which induce colon tumors in rodents [39].

Members of several other classes of plant compounds have demonstrated anti-initiation activity, including the flavonoids, isoflavonoids, and coumarins. For example, earlier studies suggested that coumarins, which are widely distributed in nature and are found in all parts of plants [40], could modulate drug-metabolizing enzymes and cytochrome P450s [41]. Cai et al. [42]

showed that several naturally occurring coumarins can block skin tumor initiation by polycyclic aromatic hydrocarbons such as benzo[a]pyrene and 7,12-dimethylbenz[a]anthracene by inhibiting cytochrome P450s involved in the metabolic activation of the carcinogens.

As reviewed by MacLeod and Slaga [20], several compounds have been proposed as scavengers for the ultimate electrophilic metabolites of carcinogens such as benzo[a]pyrene diol epoxide (BPDE), a metabolite of benzo[a]pyrene. Earlier studies showed that several sulfhydryl compounds, including cysteine and 2-mercaptoethanol, were effective as nucleophilic traps for BPDE [43]. In addition, riboflavin has been shown to promote the detoxification of BPDE by enhancing hydrolysis [44]. Also, a group of plant phenols, notably ellagic acid, has been identified which reacts facilely with BPDE and thereby blocks the mutagenicity of BPDE in in vitro systems [45]. Ellagic acid has been shown to be an anticarcinogen in vivo, having protective activity against topically applied BPDE in the mouse skin model [46]. In addition, a major polyphenolic antioxidant found in green tea, epigallocatechin-3-gallate (EGCG), has been shown to have strong anticarcinogenic effects in several models, including the mouse skin, lung, fore stomach, esophagus, duodenum, pancreas, liver, breast, and colon models [47]. EGCG reportedly can trap the activated metabolites of several procarcinogens [34].

*Enhancing Carcinogen Detoxification*

As mentioned above, the process by which potentially dangerous xenobiotics are conjugated to an endogenous cellular nucleophile and then excreted from the body is also an important target for the prevention of tumor initiation. Detoxification of chemical carcinogens by enzymes such as GSTs and uridine diphosphate-glucuronyl transferase is enhanced by several constituents of garlic and onions, cruciferous vegetables, and certain spices. For example, in animals phase-II enzymes are induced by oral exposure to diallyl sulfide and s-allyl-cysteine which are found in garlic; both compounds enhance GST levels in liver and colon [48]. As previously discussed, these organosulfur compounds are also known to inhibit the activity of several cytochrome P450s [37]. Thus, the tumor-inhibiting effects of diallyl sulfide and related compounds may be due to the dual effect of decreased carcinogen activation and enhanced carcinogen detoxification [49]. The isothiocyanates also play a dual role: they suppress carcinogen activation as well as enhance carcinogen detoxification by increasing GST activity [33]. The antischistosomal drug oltipraz [50] and the antioxidative agent N-acetylcysteine [32] are also highly effective inducers of GSTs and are potent inhibitors of induced colon, lung, and bladder carcinogenesis. The phytoalexin resveratrol, found in grapes and other food products and an inhibitor of the two-stage mouse skin carcinogenesis model, also has been shown to induce phase-II enzymes such as quinone reductase [51].

*Enhancing DNA Repair*

Although the gene products and general mechanisms of DNA repair in prokaryotes are fairly well characterized, mammalian repair systems have only recently been elucidated, and little is known about the influence of dietary factors on these processes. In animal studies, calorie restriction [52, 53], EGCG [54], and selenium [55] enhance unscheduled DNA synthesis and other measures of repair capacity. Calorie restriction in mice has also been shown to increase apoptotic cell death in heavily damaged cells, thereby accelerating the elimination of cells with irreparable DNA damage [56].

## Targets for Anti-Promotion and Anti-Progression Strategies

*Epigenetic Changes in Cell Signaling*

The tumor promotion phase of multistage carcinogenesis involves the clonal expansion of initiated cells. Tumor-promoting agents are not mutagenic like carcinogens but rather alter the expression of genes whose products are associated with hyperproliferation, apoptosis, tissue remodeling, and inflammation. At some point, the developing tumor constitutively expresses these genes and thus becomes tumor promoter independent. The identification of the mechanisms by which tumor promoters alter gene expression has been a major goal during the past decade, particularly because determining the critical events will reveal targets for the development of new prevention strategies. It has also become clear in the past few years that apoptosis and mitogenesis are equally important in cell number homeostasis, and that the growth advantage manifested by initiated cells during promotion is usually the net effect of increased proliferation and decreased apoptosis. Thus, in addition to cell proliferation, apoptosis has emerged as a critical target for cancer prevention [57].

As described earlier (fig. 1), the mouse skin model of multistage carcinogenesis is an excellent system for studying the molecular alterations associated with the various stages of tumor development and so will be the primary focus of the following discussion on mechanisms involved in tumor promotion. Among the most potent mouse skin tumor promoters are the phorbol esters; tumor promoter 12-*O*-tetradecanoylphorbol-13-acetate (TPA) has been the prototype for many years [7]. However, a wide variety of compounds are tumor promoters and bring about both biologic and molecular changes similar to those elicited by TPA [58]. Changes in gene expression as a consequence of external tumor promoter stimuli usually activate (but sometimes inactivate) specific signal transduction pathways. The nature of the initial interaction of tumor promoters with the cell depends on the type of promoter used. For example, TPA interacts with specific receptors that are isoforms of protein kinase C (PKC) [59]. The identification of PKC as the major target for phorbol esters and other promoters such as mezerein, indole alkaloids, and polyacetates suggests that activation of PKC is a critical event in carcinogenesis. By activating PKC, phorbol esters and related tumor promoters appear to bypass the normal cellular mechanisms for regulating cell proliferation. Several oncogenes (particularly ras), hormones, growth factors, and cytokines are also known to activate this signaling pathway. Other promoters such as okadaic acid are potent inhibitors of phosphatases and increase the level of phosphorylated proteins, which often has an activating effect similar to the activation of kinases [60]. However, regardless of the disparity in the tumor promoters' initial signaling events, the key biologic and molecular changes they elicit, such as increased DNA synthesis, induction of ornithine decarboxylase, induction of growth factors and cytokines, and increased production of eicosanoids, are all similar. This overall alteration in signal transduction and gene expression contributes significantly to the selection and growth of the initiated cell population.

As discussed by Fischer and DiGiovanni [60], not all tumor promoters work through receptor-mediated mechanisms. Organic peroxides such as benzoyl peroxide and hydroperoxides are examples. Unlike the phorbol esters, the peroxides require metabolic activation. The molecular targets of benzoyl peroxide have not been elucidated, although it has been shown to produce macromolecular damage, particularly covalent adducts with proteins [22]. Altering signaling by non-receptor-mediated mechanisms would require considerably higher doses of promoter than required by receptor-dependent modulators, e.g., a 20-mg dose of benzoyl peroxide is needed for tumor promotion, whereas only microgram amounts of TPA are required [60].

Despite its importance, activation of PKC alone does not appear to be sufficient for mediating phorbol ester-induced hyperproliferation in vivo, in part because a major consequence of PKC activation in keratinocytes is the induction of terminal differentiation. The regulation of keratinocyte proliferation and differentiation is a complex process and probably involves interaction of different cell types in the epidermis and dermis as well as multiple signaling pathways within the keratinocytes themselves. Several receptor tyrosine kinases and their ligands appear to be linked to keratinocyte proliferation. The four main receptors are the epidermal growth factor receptor (EGFR), insulin-like growth factor-1 (IGF-1) receptor, basic fibroblast growth factor receptor, and hepatocyte growth factor receptor [60]. All four of these receptors are expressed on the surfaces of keratinocytes; however, with the exception of transforming growth factor-$\alpha$ (TGF-$\alpha$), which is the ligand for EGFR, the ligands for the receptors are produced by dermal fibroblasts or inflammatory cells and act in a paracrine manner.

Several lines of evidence suggest that tumor promoters generally increase the expression of a number of growth factors and cytokines. TPA induces TGF-$\alpha$, TGF-$\beta$, tumor necrosis factor-$\alpha$, granulocyte-macrophage stimulating factor, and interleukins (IL)-1 and 6 [61]. The profile of growth factor induction is different for promoters with different initial mechanisms of action, although most seem to induce TGF-$\alpha$ mRNA expression. TPA treatment also increases expression of EGFR, possibly as a consequence of activating c-Ha-ras. Alternatively, high TGF-α levels may lead to autoinduction of EGFR [60]. Regardless of how it occurs, elevated levels of EGFR and its principal ligand, TGF-α, are strongly correlated with the development of neoplasias.

### Inflammation

In addition to inducing changes in gene expression by activating specific signaling pathways, tumor promoters can elicit the production of protein factors such as IL-1 and several non-protein factors through intracellular activation mechanisms [60]. Of critical importance to the promotion process is the release of arachidonic acid and its metabolism to eicosanoids [62]. Eicosanoids, which include the prostaglandins and hydroperoxy forms of arachidonic acid, are involved in such processes as inflammation, the immune response, tissue repair, and cell proliferation.

Prostaglandin synthesis is regulated by cyclooxygenase (COX) gene expression. Two separate gene products, COX-1 and 2, have similar COX and peroxidase activities, although they are differentially regulated [62, 63]. While a variety of factors, including serum, growth factors, and phorbol esters, can upregulate the mRNA levels of both COXs, the COX-2 gene generally responds in a much more dramatic fashion and thus has been referred to as a phorbol ester-inducible immediate early gene product [64].

In the mouse two-stage skin carcinogenesis model, tumor promotion is a distinct, rate-limiting step that determines the formation of premalignant tumors. As discussed above, the role of tumor promoters in human cancer is more complex because human exposure tends to involve sporadic low doses of complex mixtures of carcinogens, co-carcinogens, and tumor-promoting agents. Nonetheless, studies of rodent tumor models of liver, bladder, colon and mammary cancer and analyses of human tumor formation suggest that processes analogous to tumor promotion by TPA on the mouse skin, including COX-2 overexpression, prostaglandin release and other aspects of inflammation, are a common feature of carcinogenesis [6]. Thus, epigenetic changes in cell signaling such as altered growth factor production and receptor expression, and elevated synthesis of inflammatory and mitogenic factors such as cytokines and eicosanoids, are key targets for inhibiting tumor promotion.

### Tumor Progression

As noted earlier, tumor progression involves the accumulation of additional genetic and/or epigenetic alterations in an initiated cell clone, and generally gives a growth advantage to the progressing clone. In progression a focal lesion consisting of a population of initiated and promoted cells ultimately becomes an invasive malignant tumor mass. One frequently observed genetic alteration that appears to contribute to malignant progression is mutation in the p53 tumor-suppressor gene [65]. The p53 gene product is a transcription factor that regulates the expression of a number of DNA-damage and cell cycle-regulatory genes, and genes regulating apoptosis. By enhancing transcription of these critical genes, p53 regulates the cellular response to DNA damage [66]. p53 also plays a role in maintaining genomic stability [67]. Genomic instability, a hallmark of spontaneous malignant progression, is characterized by sequential chromosomal aberrations such as duplications, deletions, and loss of heterozygosity, which lead to rapid accumulation of unfavorable genetic alterations and eventually to malignant cell growth. Cell numbers, normally maintained by a balance of genes regulating cell proliferation and apoptosis, are altered. DNA hypomethylation, frequently observed in malignant tumors, may also contribute to malignant progression [68]. Thus, p53, other cell cycle and apoptosis regulators, and other genes regulating genomic instability and DNA methylation are critical targets for cancer prevention at later stages (i.e. progression) of carcinogenesis.

## Nutritional Modulation of Tumor Promotion and Progression: Examples

### Scavenging ROS

ROS play an important role in a variety of normal processes within the body, including the immune response against pathogens, intracellular signaling, and vascular permeability. However, the accumulation of ROS as byproducts of normal energy metabolism and in response to inflammatory conditions or ROS-generating environmental exposures (i.e. to particulates in tobacco smoke), has been associated with the pathogenesis of cancer in rodents and humans [22, 69]. Experimental studies have shown that ROS can act as both initiators and promoters of tumors by damaging critical cellular macromolecules such as DNA, proteins, and lipids and by acting as cell-signaling molecules, as nitric oxide does [22, 69]. Antioxidants, including ascorbic acid, α-tocopherol, selenium, and several polyphenolic compounds found in green tea, spices, fruits, and vegetables have been shown to effectively inhibit TPA promotion in mouse skin [19]. Calorie restriction, which is one of the best documented and most effective experimental manipulations for decreasing rodent tumor development [70], including TPA-induced skin carcinogenesis [71], may exert its antitumor effects largely by decreasing ROS production and enhancing antioxidant defenses. Calorie restriction decreases the rate of accumulation of oxidized DNA and protein that accompanies aging in rodents [72]. In addition, a number of intracellular antioxidant defense systems, including superoxide dismutase, catalase, and glutathione peroxidase, are reportedly enhanced by calorie restriction [73]. Thus, evidence is mounting that calorie restriction may decrease oxidative stress by decreasing oxidant production and enhancing antioxidant capacity, although the exact mechanisms involved have yet to be fully established. On the other hand, obesity increases the risk of many types of cancer [2], probably at least in part by increasing ROS production and inflammation.

### Altering the Expression of Genes Regulating Cell Proliferation, Apoptosis, and Differentiation

Many studies using the two-stage carcinogenesis model in mouse skin have identified dietary components that act through diverse mechanisms to alter tumor promotion and progression. A number of retinoids, particularly all-*trans* retinoic acid, are specific inhibitors of TPA-induced tumor promotion in the mouse skin [74, 75]. Although the retinoids' mechanism of action is not fully understood, data indicate that they affect epithelial differentiation and also reduce elevated polyamine levels by inhibiting the induction of epidermal ornithine decarboxylase [76]. Several reports indicate that polyamines are involved in regulating cellular differentiation and growth [76, 77]. Retinoids bring about many of their effects by interacting with nuclear receptors. These nuclear receptors are *trans*-activating factors that can regulate the expression of specific genes involved in differentiation, proliferation, and apoptosis [78, 79]. The synthetic retinoid fenretinide, which has shown promising chemo-preventive activity against several cancers, appears to exert its antitumor effects primarily by inducing apoptosis in damaged cells [80]. As mentioned earlier, it has become clear in the past few years that apoptosis and mitogenesis are equally important in maintaining cell number homeostasis; thus, in addition to cell proliferation, apoptosis has emerged as a critical target for prevention.

Perhaps the clearest example of dietary modulation of skin carcinogenesis through alteration of the PKC pathway comes from the laboratory of Birt et al. [71] showing that calorie restriction, which inhibits skin tumor promotion by TPA, inhibits PKC activity and decreases the concentrations of different PKC isoforms (particularly PKCα and PKCζ). Birt et al. [81] have also shown that feeding diets high in corn oil increases PKC activity in epidermal cells, apparently by influencing intracellular lipid metabolism rather than altering the distribution of PKC isoforms.

### Decreasing Inflammation

A number of prostaglandin synthesis inhibitors are effective in counteract-ing skin tumor promotion and carcinogenesis. Compounds such as anti-inflammatory steroids (i.e. glucocorticoids) are potent inhibitors of mouse skin tumor promotion by phorbol esters [61]. These compounds are effective phospholipase A2 inhibitors, which may explain their ability to decrease the amount of arachidonic acid available for metabolism to important proinflam-matory end-products. Inhibitors of the COX pathway, such as indomethacin and flurbiprofen, have been best studied as colon cancer chemopreventives [82] and also inhibit skin tumor promotion in most mouse strains [83]. The COX pathway is a major prevention target, primarily because these enzymes (particularly COX-2) play a role in inflammation as well as in apoptosis and cellular adhesion in some cells [84]. Recent findings have raised questions about the possible increased risk of myocardial infarction with the class of agents termed selective COX-2 inhibitors, such as rofecoxib [85]. However, several safe, effective, and inexpensive agents that can perturb the COX pathway, such as the nonsteroidal anti-inflammatory drugs, are readily available. In addition, numerous dietary factors, such as several organosulfur compounds in garlic and onions, and resveratrol in grapes, can also safely target the COX pathway [86, 87].

## Early Life Nutritional Exposures and Childhood Cancer Risk

The impact of early life nutritional exposures on childhood cancer has not been well studied. The primary focus of research on the relationship between childhood diet and childhood cancer risk has focused on N-nitroso compound exposure in cured meats and brain cancers. No clear picture of a link between early-life consumption of these meats, such as hot dogs, and brain cancer development has emerged [88, 89]. The leading cause of cancer morbidity under age 5 is childhood leukemia, and four studies have now been published assessing the link between early life exposures and leukemia risk [90–93]. Two of these [90, 91] focused on consumption of N-nitroso compounds, again without conclusive findings that cured meat intake is an important risk factor. A recent report [92] suggests that consumption of fruits or fruit juices that contain vitamin C and potassium (particularly oranges and bananas) may reduce the risk of childhood leukemias, but these findings need to be confirmed. Breast cancer in adulthood is the best studied cancer regarding early life nutritional exposures as a risk factor [94], and this will be the focus of the remainder of the review.

## Early Life Nutritional Exposures and Adult Breast Cancer Risk

In this section, we describe: (1) animal experimental studies of dietary modulations in pregnancy and cancer risk; (2) certain concepts and underlying processes of human pregnancy, highlighting growth factors, hormones, and hypoxic states in pregnancy, and (3) explore hormonal and nutritional exposures during pregnancy, infancy and childhood to determine the extent of their association with breast cancer risk.

### Animal Experimental Studies
Adult female offspring of alcohol-exposed dams in pregnancy developed significantly more 7,12-dimethylbenz[a]anthracene-induced mammary tumors, compared to adult offspring of non-exposed dams in pregnancy [95]. In addition, compared to the mammary gland structure in the offspring of non-exposed

dams, the mammary epithelial tree of the alcohol-exposed offspring was denser and contained more structures, illustrated by elevated levels of estrogen receptor-α, that are susceptible to DNA damage and other initiation events that begin the breast carcinogenesis process.

Maternal diet during pregnancy affects estrogen levels and leads to reproductive system tumors in the offspring. Specifically, pregnant rats fed a high-fat diet have higher estradiol levels than controls. Female offspring of mice fed a high-fat diet during pregnancy developed more reproductive system tumors and metastases than offspring of pregnant mice fed a low-fat diet [96]. But in a subsequent study, female mice who were exposed in utero to low-fat diets and then nursed from dams who were fed high-fat diets during their pregnancy had a higher frequency of mammary tumors than mice exposed in utero to high-fat diets but nursed from dams who were fed low-fat diets in pregnancy [97]. Thus diet during the early postnatal life of rodents appears to have its greatest effect when the hypothalamus matures in females. Indeed, this model may be appropriate for women who were very preterm births and as newborns had immature hypothalamic-pituitary feedback systems.

Nutritional perturbation of epigenetic gene regulation is a likely link between early nutrition and later metabolism and risk of cancer in Agouti mice [98]. Specifically, dietary methyl supplementation of $a/a$ dams with extra folic acid, vitamin $B_{12}$, choline, and betaine altered the phenotype (fur color) of their $A^{vy}/a$ offspring via increased $C_pG$ methylation at the $A^{vy}$ locus [99]. Thus, maternal supplementation in pregnancy permanently affected the offspring's DNA methylation at epigenetically susceptible loci. Further studies in the role of epigenetic mechanisms in pregnancy and cancer risk are needed to address the implications for mothers and children.

### Human Pregnancy

Pregnancy is a set of dynamic interactions between the mother, placenta, and the fetus. Endogenous hormonal and metabolic exposures in utero are modulated by maternal energy expenditure, her diet, pre-pregnancy body mass, weight gain and physical activity in pregnancy, and by fetal growth and development.

During the first trimester of a normal, healthy pregnancy, the placenta is undergoing angiogenesis under hypoxic conditions [100]. Vasculogenesis, whereby blood vessels arise from blood islands and angiogenesis from existing vessels, is initiated around 3 weeks of gestation [101]. Blood islands arising from the mesoderm are induced by fibroblast growth factor-2 (FGF-2) to form hemangioblasts, precursors for vessels and blood cell formation. Hemangioblasts in the center of the blood islands form hematopoietic stem cells, the precursors of all blood vessels.

Growth factors such as the placental growth factors, vascular endothelial growth factors, and others well-known in carcinogenesis are upregulated by the placenta as are leptin and other hormones required for growth [102]. The trophoblasts differentiate into the layers associated with the maternal contact, the syncytiotrophoblasts, and the layers proximal to the fetus, choriotrophoblasts. By 5–7 weeks of gestation, hypoxia-inducing factor-1 (HIF-1) and TGF-β are also upregulated, leading to an increase in oxygen tension by 9 weeks of gestation. By 11–14 weeks of gestation, the Von Hippel-Lindau tumor-suppressor gene has downregulated certain growth factors and HIF-1α and 1β with the advent of low-resistance channels that have developed across the placenta to increase the flow of nutrients and hormones from the mother to the fetus and the outflow of waste from the fetus. Maternal hormonal trajectories reveal patterns of decreasing levels of IGF-binding protein-1 (IGFBP-1), and increasing levels of IGF-1 and 2, progesterone, estrogens, and insulin; while glucose is the fuel that drives the fetal engine [103, 104]. This is the dynamic state of a well-tuned clavier, in which angiogenesis is arrested once the placenta has penetrated the spiral arteries and is capable of sustaining the fetus until birth, and hyperinsulinemia is a characteristic maternal state.

During the remaining two trimesters, the fetus will be exposed to many other factors which may influence the risk of cancer for which gestational age at birth is a marker. Compared to the preterm (<38 weeks gestation), the full-term newborn has undergone the androgen surge late in the third trimester, while the post-term (≥42 weeks gestation) newborn will have higher exposures to estrogens and insulin beyond the levels of the full-term neonate. These elevated hormonal exposures have been hypothesized to lead to large-for-gestational age (LGA) or high birth weight (>4,000 g) neonates and in turn risk of breast cancer [105]. Yet the high birth weight is a heterogeneous group, including offspring of gestational diabetics, an intergenerational component, as well as gender- and ethnic-group specificity. More males than females are higher birth weight, which is reflected in the gender-specific distribution of childhood acute lymphoblastic leukemia [106]. More Hispanic and non-Hispanic whites have LGA than African-Americans, an ethnic group specificity reflected in childhood acute lymphoblastic leukemia. In an analysis of the 1958 British Birth Cohort, Hennessey and Alberman [107] identified the following determinants of birth weight-for-gestational age: maternal birth weight, height, smoking, age at menarche, and weight gain in pregnancy plus gender of the offspring.

### The Fetal Period: Birth Weight

#### Rationale
A woman's life-time hormonal exposure from endogenous metabolism and exogenous preparations is associated with breast cancer risk [108, 109]. Hormonal exposure begins in utero when estrogen levels are as high as in puberty [105]. One indicator of intrauterine hormonal exposure is birth weight, which varies directly with: levels of maternal estrogen in pregnancy

[110–112]; peak placental growth hormone at 37 weeks gestation [113], and umbilical-cord blood IGF-1 [114–117] and leptin levels [118]. IGF-1 promotes postnatal somatic growth [119] and is a potent mitogen and anti-apoptotic agent in vivo [120], and stimulates aromatization of estrone to the more biologically active estradiol in breast cancer cells in vitro [121]. Adult IGF-1 levels are positively associated with breast cancer risk in premenopausal women [122]. Leptin increases breast cancer cell growth in vitro [123]. Body mass index (BMI) varies directly with serum leptin concentrations and is positively associated with a risk of postmenopausal breast cancer [124].

Birth weight reflects intrauterine nutritional exposures, and correlates directly with maternal weight gain in pregnancy [125, 126], parental birth weight [127], and maternal pre-pregnancy BMI [128, 129]. An estimated 40% of the variance in birth weight can be explained by genetic contributions [130, 131] or by a form of transgenerational epigenetic inheritance [132]. The proportion of macrosomic ($\geq$4,000 g) newborns peaked in the United States in the 1980s at 11% and declined to 9.2% in 2002; this percentage varies by ethnic group [133]. African-American and non-Hispanic white women from families where previous generations delivered neonates of low or high birth weight have a twofold increased risk of delivering a low or high birth weight neonate, respectively [134, 135].

*Birth Weight-Breast Cancer Association*

Table 1a shows the risk estimates from four cohort studies [135–139] and 12 case-control studies [140–151], three of which were nested within cohort studies [140, 142, 143]. Compared to normal birth weight neonates (2.5–2.99 kg), the high birth weight ($\geq$4,000 g) experienced a 20% to fivefold increased risk of premenopausal breast cancer, except for a study in young women where a U-shaped relation of birth weight and breast cancer was observed [150]. In studies analyzing pre- and postmenopausal women in the same model, four of ten reported a significantly increased risk in the category with the highest birth weight [139, 146, 148] or reduced risk in those weighing <4,000 g at birth compared to those weighing $\geq$4,000 g [142]. Research on birth weight and postmenopausal breast cancer is also inconsistent. Therefore, the literature is most suggestive of an association of high birth weight neonates and risk of premenopausal breast cancer after adjustment for adult risk factors (in the comments to table 1a). Of note, the research has largely been conducted in non-Hispanic white women. Two studies in Asians [144, 151] report no association between birth weight and breast cancer. Asians have a more peaked birth weight distribution and a smaller proportion of low and high birth weight neonates than Caucasians [152] to detect an association in the extremes of the distribution.

Three linked birth-cancer registry studies examine the relation of birth length and breast cancer risk [136, 140, 148] (table 1b). All three studies demonstrate a positive trend of higher breast cancer risk in premenopausal or

*Table 1a.* Adjusted relative risk of breast cancer by study design, birth year, ethnic group, menopausal status and birth weight

| Reference | Birth year | Ethnic group | Cases[a] | Birth weight, kg | | | | | p trend | Comments |
|---|---|---|---|---|---|---|---|---|---|---|
| | | | | <2.5 | 2.5–2.9 | 3.0–3.4 | 3.5–3.9 | ≥4.0 | | |
| **Cohort studies** | | | | | | | | | | |
| McCormack et al. [136], 2003 | 1915–1929 | NHW | 63[1] | | 1.0 (ref) | 1.6 | 2.4* | 3.5* | 0.01 | B-ca registry, proxy indicators of adult risk |
| | | NHW | 296[2] | | 1.0 (ref) | 0.8 | 1.0 | 0.9 | NS | |
| dos Santos Silva et al. [137], 2004 | 1946 | NHW | 21[0] | | 1.0 (ref) | 1.4 | 2.2 | 5.0* | 0.03 | Adjusted for childhood and adult risk factors |
| | | NHW | 59[3] | | 1.0 (ref) | 1.0 | 1.4 | 1.6 | NS | |
| | | | | <2.0 | 2.0–2.9 | >3.0 | | | | |
| Kaijser et al. [138], 2003 | 1925–1949 | NHW | 19[1] | 1.5 | 0.7 | 2.5 | | | | Std incidence ratio reported; B-ca registry, sampled neonates <35 weeks gestation or 2,000 g and >35 weeks gestation, no adjustment for adult risk factors; standardized incidence ratios shown |
| | | NHW | 39[3] | 1.1 | 0.7 | 2.6* | | | | |
| | | | | 2.5[c] | 3.0 | 3.4 | 3.6 | 4.0 | | |
| Ahlgren et al. [139], 2004 | 1930–1975 | NHW | 2,74[3] | 1.0 (ref) | 1.0 | 1.1 | 1.1 | 1.2* | _[d] | Adjusted for childhood and adult risk factors |

**Table 1a.** (continued)

| Reference | Birth year | Ethnic group | Cases[a] | Birth weight, kg | | | | | | p trend | Comments |
|---|---|---|---|---|---|---|---|---|---|---|---|
| | | | | <2.5 | 2.5–2.9 | 3.0–3.4 | 3.5–3.9 | ≥4.0 | >4.5 | | |
| **Case-control studies** | | | | | | | | | | | |
| Ekbom et al. [140][e], 1997 | 1874–1961 | NHW | 1,068[30.8] | 1.0 (ref) | 1.0 | 1.0 | 1.0 | | | NS | B-ca registry, no adult risk factors; nested within cohort |
| Titus-Ernstoff et al. [141], 2002 | 1911–1945 | NHW | 1,716[2] | 1.1 | 0.9 | 1.0 (ref) | 1.1 | 0.9 | 1.2 | NS | Self-reported data after diagnosis; nested within a cohort |
| Michels et al. [142], 1996 | 1921–1965 | NHW | 550[3] | 0.6 | 0.7* | 0.7* | 0.9 | 1.0 (ref) | | <0.01 | Self-reported after diagnosis; adjusted for adult risk factors; nested within cohort |
| Lahmann et al. [143], 2004 | 1924–1950 | NHW | 88[2] | | 1.0 (ref) | 1.9 | 2.3 | 2.7 | | –[d] | Birth records; adjusted for adult risk factors; nested within cohort |
| Sanderson et al. [144], 2002 | 1932–1973 | Asian | 288[3] | 0.9 | 1.0 (ref) | 1.1 | 0.8 | 0.7 | | NS | Maternal recall after diagnosis; adjusted for adult risk factors |
| Sanderson et al. [146], 1996 | 1944–1969 / 1924–1940 | NHW | 746[3] / 401[3] | 1.3 / 0.9 | 1.0 (ref) / 1.0 (ref) | 1.3* / 1.1 | 1.2 / 0.8 | 1.7* / 0.6 | | 0.06 / 0.06 | Self-reported after diagnosis; no adjustment for adult risk factors |
| Sanderson et al. [145], 1998 | 1945–1947 | NHW | 510[1] | 1.2 | 1.0 (ref) | 1.0 | 1.0 | 1.3 | | NS | Maternal recall after diagnosis; adjusted for adult risk factors |

| Reference | Birth years | Group | No. cases[a] | Exposure category (birth weight) and OR | | | | | p | Comments |
|---|---|---|---|---|---|---|---|---|---|---|
| Mellemkjaer et al. [147], 2003 | 1935–1966 | NHW | 881[1] | 1.6 | 0.8 | | 1.0 | 1.3 | | B-ca registry, no adult risk factors |
| Vatten et al. [148], 2002 | 1910–1970 | NHW | 373[3] | <3.1: 1.0 (ref) | 3.1–3.4: 1.1 | 3.5–3.7: 1.2 | >3.7: 1.4* | | 0.02 | B-ca registry, adjusted for adult risk factors |
| Hodgson et al. [149], 2004 | 1949–1978 | AA | 83[3] | 1.1 | 1.0 (ref) | 0.4 | | | NS | Birth hospital record data |
| | | NHW | 108[3] | 0.9 | 1.0 (ref) | 0.9 | | | NS | |
| Innes et al. [150], 2000 | 1958–1981 | AA, NHW | 484[1] | <1.5: 3.0* | 1.5–2.4: 1.5* | 2.5–3.4: 1.0 (ref) | 3.5–4.4: 1.1 | ≥4.5: 3.1* | | B-ca registry, no adjustment for adult risk factors |
| Le Marchand et al. [151], 1988 | 1946 on | Asian, NHW | 71[1] | 1.16–2.94: 1.0 (ref) | 2.95–3.34: 0.7 | 3.341–4.45: 0.8 | | | NS | B-ca registry, no adjustment for adult risk factors |

NHW = Non-Hispanic white; AA = African American; B-ca registry = birth-cancer registry; NS = non-significant.
*95% Confidence interval excludes one.
[a]Menopausal status: [0]premenopausal; [1]premenopausal based on age <50 years; [2]postmenopausal based on age >50 years; [3]both.
[b]Includes case from De Stavola (2000).
[c]Median of each quintile.
[d]Ahlgren et al. [139] OR per kg increase 1.1 (95% CI 1.01–1.20); Lahmann et al. [143] OR per 100 g increase 1.1 (95% CI 1.00–1.12).
[e]Includes cases from Ekbom (1992).

*Table 1b.* Adjusted relative risk of breast cancer by study design, birth year, ethnic group, menopausal status and birth length

| Reference | Birth year | Ethnic group | Cases[a] | Birth length, cm | | | | | p trend | Comments |
|---|---|---|---|---|---|---|---|---|---|---|
| **Cohort study** | | | | | | | | | | |
| McCormack et al. [136], 2003 | 1915–1929 | NHW | 65[1] | <49.0 | 49.5–50.0 | 50.5–51.0 | 51.5–52.0 | <52.5 | | B-ca registry, proxy indicators for adult risk |
| | | | | 1.0 (ref) | 2.1 | 2.9* | 3.5* | 3.4* | 0.001 | |
| | | NHW | 294[2] | 1.0 (ref) | 1.0 | 1.1 | 0.8 | 1.3 | NS | |
| **Case-control studies** | | | | | | | | | | |
| Vatten et al. [148], 2002 | 1910–1970 | NHW | 373[3] | <50.0 | 50.0 | 51.0 | >51.5 | | | B-ca registry, adjusted for adult risk factors |
| | | | | 1.0 (ref) | 1.2 | 1.5* | 1.3 | | 0.02 | |
| Ekbom et al. [140][a], 1997 | 1874–1961 | NHW | 1,068[3] | Quartile 1 | Quartile 2 | Quartile 3 | Quartile 4 | | | B-ca registry, no adult risk factors; nested within a cohort |
| | | | | 1.0 (ref) | 1.1 | 1.2 | 1.1 | | NS | |

NHW = Non-Hispanic white; B-ca registry = birth-cancer registry; NS = non-significant.
*95% Confidence interval includes one.
[a]Menopausal status: [1]premenopausal based on age <50 years; [2]postmenopausal based on age >50 years; [3]both.

172

pre- and postmenopausal patients who were 51 cm or more in length at birth. Two report significant trends after adjustment for gestational age and adult risk factors. The risk is larger than the risk for birth weight alone, indicating that growth factors specific to linear bone growth may play an important role in breast cancer etiology [136, 148].

### The Fetal Period: Preterm Births

#### Rationale

Women who deliver preterm have higher estradiol levels than those who deliver full-term [114]. Preterm neonates (<37 weeks gestation) have higher levels of gonadotrophins than full-term neonates in early infancy. Gonadotrophins stimulate the ovary to produce excessive amounts of estradiol, which are associated with an increased risk of ovarian cysts in adolescence. And since estrogens may have a direct mutagenic potential [153], exposure to higher levels of estrogens in early postnatal life may lead to an increased risk of breast cancer.

#### Preterm Birth-Breast Cancer Association

Based on linked birth-cancer registry data, there appears to be a significant trend of increasing risk (or SIR) of breast cancer with decreasing gestation age of the neonate [138, 154, 155] and a significantly higher risk of breast cancer in newborns of gestation ages <33 or 30–38 weeks [136, 140]. In contrast, no association is observed in the case-control studies [142, 145] (table 2). Several caveats should be noted: (1) the cutoff for preterm births and therefore the referent group varies by study; (2) research is based on small numbers, and (3) women who deliver early may incorrectly recall gestational age of the index child because they never reached the landmark 'due date' [156]. Misclassification of preterm births based on maternal-reported gestational age might attenuate the relation of preterm births to breast cancer. Of note, in birth cohorts before the 1980s, neonatal intensive care units were not in existence to support survival of the preterm; therefore survivors might be LGA (>90th percentile of birth weight for newborns delivered each week of gestation) babies who had a high growth rate in utero (during a short pregnancy). Factors that stimulated intrauterine growth and a higher rate of mitotic division in the LGA neonate might have eventually led to an increased risk of breast cancer [109].

### The Fetal Period: Maternal Age and Preeclampsia

#### Rationale

Maternal age-specific hormone levels in pregnancy have not been examined extensively. Pregnancy estriol levels do not vary by maternal age in one

**Table 2.** Adjusted relative risk (RR) of breast cancer by study design, birth year, ethnic group and preterm birth

| Reference | Birth year | Ethnic group | Cases[a] | Gestational age, weeks | RR | Comments |
|---|---|---|---|---|---|---|
| **Birth cancer registry studies** | | | | | | |
| Ekbom et al. [140] | 1874–1961 | NHW | 10[3] | <33 | 4.0* | Referent: >33 weeks |
| Le Marchand et al. [151] | 1946 on | Asian, NHW | 9[0] | <36 | 1.2 | Referent: 36–40 weeks |
| Vatten et al. [148] | 1910–1970 | NHW NHW | 77[3] 291[3] | <32 32–36 | 1.2 1.1 | Referent: >40 weeks; p for trend = 0.02 |
| McCormack et al. [136] | 1915–1929 | NHW | 63[1] | 30–38 | 2.1* | Referent: >41 weeks; p for trend = 0.03 |
| | | | | | Std incidence ratio | |
| Kaijser et al. [138] | 1925–1949 | NHW | 19[1] | ≤32 33–34 | 1.4 0.9 | Referent: birth weight <2,000 g and gestation >35 weeks |
| | | NHW | 39[3] | ≤32 33–34 | 1.1 0.9 | |
| Ekbom et al. [155] | 1925–1934 | NHW | 12[3] | <31 31–32 33–34 ≥35 | 6.7* 2.3 0.7 0.2 | Referent: birth weight <2,000 g and gestation >35 weeks |
| **Case-control studies** | | | | | RR | |
| Michels et al. [142] | 1921–1965 | NHW | 8[3] | Preterm | 1.0 | Referent: not preterm |
| Sanderson et al. [145] | 1945–1947 | NHW | 18[1] | <37 | 0.9 | Referent: 37–42 weeks; crude OR provided |

NHW = Non-Hispanic white.
*95% Confidence interval excludes one.
[a]Menopausal status: [0]premenopausal; [1]premenopausal based on age <50 years; [2]postmenopausal based on age >50 years; [3]both.

study [111], but total estrogen (TE) and estradiol ($E_2$) levels are highest in women aged 20–24 years, lowest in teenagers and intermediate in women aged 25+ years in another study [157]. Maternal age co-varies with parity, which exhibits a consistent hormonal pattern across three studies. Specifically, TE and $E_2$ levels (at 16 and 27 weeks gestation in one study or at 26 and 31 weeks gestation in another study) are higher among women in their first than those in their second full-term pregnancy and higher in the same woman in her first than in her second pregnancy [112, 158]. Maternal age is associated with a risk of poor pregnancy outcomes. Compared to women aged 20–24 years, women aged 35+ are at increased risk of delivering a newborn with birth defects, a marker of chromosomal aberrations and in turn cancer risk [159]. Compared to primiparous women aged 20–24 years, primiparous women aged 30+ are at increased risk of delivering low birth weight neonates [160]. Compared to women aged 20–24 years, teenagers have fewer pregnancies and higher rates of small-for-gestational age (SGA; <10th percentile of birth weight for newborns delivered each week of gestation) and preterm births, thus, women aged 20–24 years are considered the referent group in maternal and child health research. In sum, if maternal age at the birth of the index case is related to breast cancer risk in the offspring, then the association may be via parity (and hormone levels), birth weight and/or adverse pregnancy outcomes.

*Maternal Age-Breast Cancer Association*
Because the maternal age-breast cancer association has breast cancer rates of offspring of teenage mothers as the referent group, the relative risks (RRs) are re-calculated using cancer rates of daughters of women aged 20–24 years as the referent group (for the reasons mentioned above; table 3). Data are presented from 10 case-control studies [141, 146, 147, 150, 151, 161–165], one of which is a birth-cancer registry study, and two cohort studies [166, 167]. The RR of breast cancer increases with increasing maternal age to 35–39 years in five studies and is slightly higher in the offspring of teenagers in four. The RR for the maternal age-breast cancer association remains the same after stratification by reproductive risk factors in the patient [163, 164, 166], while a J-shaped relation was observed after adjustment for her birth weight [150]. Thus maternal age is probably not a marker for hormonal exposures in utero, because the RR of breast cancer in the offspring of the 20- to 24-year-olds, who have reportedly the highest hormone levels in pregnancy, are not higher than those in the offspring of other mothers.

*Rationale for Preeclampsia*
Preeclampsia, a condition characterized by pregnancy-induced hypertension, edema, and proteinuria, is diagnosed in 2–10% of pregnant women. Preeclampsia, known as the 'disease of theories', may be more than one disease of heterogeneous origin with early and late onset patients who vary by severity of disease [168–170] and who deliver neonates at risk of being SGA or LGA [171, 172]. Increased cardiac output of late onset preeclamptics may enhance uteroplacental profusion, which increases the risk of delivering LGA neonates, while severe, early onset patients may experience reduced uteroplacental profusion, which increases the risk of delivering a SGA [171]. The levels of dehydroepiandosterone sulfate (DHEAS) in the cord blood of

***Table 3.*** Revised relative risk (RR) of breast cancer by maternal age at birth of the index case, stratified by study design, year of study, ethnic group and number of cases

| Reference | Birth year | Ethnic group | Cases[a] | Maternal age by year[b] | | | | | | Comments |
|---|---|---|---|---|---|---|---|---|---|---|
| | | | | <20 | 20–24 | 25–29 | 30–34 | 35–39 | 40+ | |
| **Cohort studies** | | | | | | | | | | |
| Colditz et al. [166] | 1921–1946 | NHW | 1,799[3] | 1.0 | 1.0 (ref) | 1.1 | 1.1 | 1.1 | 1.0 | p for trend: NS |
| Zhang et al. [167] | 1886–1919 | NHW | 149[3] | | <25: 1.0 (ref) | 25–29: 1.2 | 30–35: 1.3 | >35: 1.1 | | |
| **Case-control studies** | | | | <20 | 20–24 | 25–29 | 30–34 | 35–39 | 40+ | |
| Rothman et al. [161] | NR | AA, NHW, Asian | 4,339[3] | 0.9 | 1.0 (ref) | 1.2 | 1.1 | 1.2 | 1.1 | |
| Thompson and Janerich [162] | 1926–1962 | AA, NHW | 2,492[3] – parous | 1.1 | 1.0 (ref) | 1.2 | 1.2 | 1.5* | 1.3 | |
| | | AA, NHW | 499[3] – nulliparous | 1.3 | 1.0 (ref) | 1.1 | 1.2 | 1.6 | 0.7 | |
| Janerich et al. [163] | 1875–1947 | NHW | 2,414[3] | 1.0 | 1.0 (ref) | 1.1 | 1.1 | 1.0 | 1.0 | |
| Newcomb et al. [164] | 1913 on | NHW | 1,253[3] | 1.2 | 1.0 (ref) | 1.2 | 1.1 | 1.4 | 1.1 | Subject report after diagnosis; p for trend: NS |
| Sanderson et al. [146] | 1944–1969 | NHW | 746[3] | | 1.0 (ref) | 1.0 | 1.2 | 1.0 | | |
| Mellemkjaer et al. [147] | 1935–1966 | AA, NHW | 881[1] | | 1.0 (ref) | 1.1 | 1.1 | | | B-ca registry; p for trend: NS |
| Titus-Ernstoff et al. [141] | 1911–1945 | NHW | 1,555[2] | 1.0 | 1.0 (ref) | 1.0 | 1.2 | 1.2 | 1.3 | p for trend = 0.04 |

| Study | Years | Population | N | | | | | | p for trend |
|---|---|---|---|---|---|---|---|---|---|
| Innes et al. [185] | 1958–1981 | AA, NHW | 484[1] | 1.2 | 1.0 (ref) | 1.4* | 1.5* | 2.0* | p for trend = 0.01 |
| Weiss et al. [165] | 1948 on | AA, NHW | 2,106[3] | 1.0 | 1.0 (ref) | 1.0 | 1.0 | 1.0 | p for trend: NS |
| | | | | | 15–22 | 23–26 | 27–30 | 31–46 | |
| Le Marchand et al. [151] | 1946 on | Asian, NHW | 153[1] | 1.2 | 1.0 (ref) | 1.2 | 1.7 | | |

NHW = Non-Hispanic white; AA = African American; NR = not reported; NS = non-significant.
*95% Confidence interval excludes one.
aMenopausal status: 0premenopausal; 1premenopausal based on age <50 years; 2postmenopausal based on age >50 years; 3both.
bWhen a column is left blank the reader assumes that the OR includes all age categories older or younger.

neonates are highest in severe hypertensives in pregnancy, intermediate in the moderate hypertensives, and lowest in mild hypertensives who have comparable levels to the neonates of normotensive women [173, 174]. Within strata of birth weight-for-gestational age, cord blood levels of IGF-1 are lower, but levels of IGFBP-1 and leptin are higher in the offspring of severe preeclamptics than normotensive controls [175, 176]. Estrogen and androgen concentrations do not differ in the cord blood of preeclamptic compared to normotensive offspring in another study [177].

*Preeclampsia Exposure in Utero and Breast Cancer Risk*

In several studies, the daughters of preeclamptics have a 10–60% lower risk of breast cancer than the daughters of normotensives [140, 145, 150] (table 4). Although so far breast cancer risk in the offspring of preeclamptics has been discussed, preeclampsia also influences the risk of breast cancer in the mothers. Compared to normotensive pregnant women, preeclamptics have higher levels of progesterone, androgen precursors of estrogen (e.g. DHEAS), cortisol, insulin, and human chorionic and other gonadotropins in pregnancy, but lower levels of estrogen and of IGF-1 [173, 174, 178, 179]. Twenty-two women with prior preeclampsia and a similar number of normotensive control women, matched on age and BMI, were studied on average 17 years postpartum [180]. Compared to the normotensives, women with a history of preeclampsia had elevated levels of free testosterone, free androgen, and free testosterone to estradiol ratios in serum.

*Preeclampsia-Maternal Breast Cancer Association*

Women who report a diagnosis of preeclampsia (eclampsia, toxemia, or pregnancy-induced hypertension) have a 10–70% lower risk of breast cancer [181–185], except in one cohort study [186] that describes a 40% higher risk in prior preeclamptics (table 4). All but the cohort study of Middle Eastern women in Jerusalem, Israel, by Paltiel et al. [186] were conducted in European/non-Hispanic white populations. RRs vary by criteria for diagnosis and by parity, as illustrated by the RR of 0.3 in nulliparous preeclamptic women [181]; the RR of 0.7 in all women diagnosed with pregnancy-induced hypertension in contrast with a RR of 1.1 in nulliparous women in the same study [182]. Thus the criteria for diagnosis of preeclampsia may alter the magnitude of breast cancer risk; while the as yet unknown underlying disease etiology may be protective or conducive to breast cancer. Potential mechanisms underlying the lower risk of breast cancer in preeclamptics include: the index pregnancy may lower estrogen and/or IGF-1 levels postpartum and in turn lower breast cancer risk; or complex mechanisms related to programming from life-long androgenic exposures and genetic variants associated with preeclampsia may influence breast cancer risk.

**Table 4.** Adjusted relative risk (RR) of breast cancer in the mother or daughter by maternal preeclampsia (yes vs. no), birth year and ethnic group

| Reference | Birth year | Ethnic group | Number of cases[a]/Total number of cases[b] | Diagnosis criteria | RR | Comments |
|---|---|---|---|---|---|---|
| **Daughter's risk** | | | | | | |
| Ekbom et al. [140] | 1874–1961 | NHW | 14/1,068[3] | Toxemia | 0.4* | B-ca registry; no adult risk factors |
| Sanderson et al. [145] | 1944–1947 | NHW | 20/509[3] | Preeclampsia or eclampsia | 0.8 | Maternal recall, adjusted for adult risk factors |
| Innes et al. [150] | 1957–1981 | AA, NHW | 6/462[1] | Toxemia | 0.9 | B-ca registry; no adult risk factors |
| **Maternal risk** | | | | | | |
| Polednak and Janerich [181] | 1926 on | NHW | 2/314[1] | Toxemia | 0.3* | Case-control; hospital record data |
| Thompson et al. [182] | 1926–1962 | AA, NHW | 139/3,897[3] | Hypertension | 0.7* | Diagnosed with hypertension before the end of the most recent term pregnancy; case recall |
| Troisi et al. [183] | 1946–1972 | AA, NHW | 97/1,236[3] | Toxemia | 0.8 | Case-control; case recall |
| Vatten et al. [184] | NR | NHW | 280/5,474[3] | Preeclampsia or hypertension | 0.8* | B-ca registry; analysis restricted to primiparous women |
| Innes and Byers [185] | NR | AA, NHW, Hispanic | 95/2,404[3] | Preeclampsia | 0.9 | B-ca registry, case-control; analysis restricted to primiparous women |

179

**Table 4.** (continued)

| Reference | Birth year | Ethnic group | Number of cases[a]/Total number of cases[b] | Diagnosis criteria | RR | | | Comments |
|---|---|---|---|---|---|---|---|---|
| | | | | | | Delivery | | |
| | | | | | | preterm | term | |
| | | | | Normotensive | RR | 1.0 | 1.0 NS | |
| | | | | Preeclampsia or hypertension | | 0.9 | 0.8* | |
| | | | | | RR | | | |
| Paltiel et al. [186] | NR | Includes Israel, WA and NA | 40/91[3] | Preeclampsia | 1.4* | | | Cohort of births 1964–1976; linked to cancer registry |

NHW = Non-Hispanic white; AA = African American; WA = West Africa; NA = North Africa; NR = not reported ; NS = non-significant. *95% Confidence interval excludes one.
[a]Number of breast cancer cases diagnosed with toxemia, preeclampsia or hypertension in pregnancy.
[b]Menopausal status: [0]premenopausal; [1]premenopausal based on age <50 years; [2]postmenopausal based on age >50 years; [3]both.

*Infancy: Breast and Bottle Feeding*

*Rationale*

Human breast milk and infant formula from cow's milk or soy are the major sources of nutrition in infancy. Breast milk composition reflects maternal diet, nutritional status, hormone levels, and environmental exposures. Hormones such as IGF-1 in breast milk vary in concentration by age of the infant as well as by phase of the menstrual cycle in the mother [187]. The major hypothesis relating breast milk intake to breast cancer risk arises from the animal work done by Bittner [188] in the 1930s wherein a factor (later identified as a retrovirus) present in mouse milk was essential for the development of breast cancer [189]. The evidence that a similar virus appeared in human breast milk has not been consistently documented [189–192]. Breastfeeding has undergone a dramatic secular trend in the United States, from a low frequency of breastfeeding in 29% of infants aged 1 week old in 1955 [193] to a high proportion of breastfeeding in 67.5% of infants aged 1 week in 1998 [194, 195]. Birth weight of the neonate, ethnic group, and socioeconomic status influence the proportion of infants who are breastfed and the duration of breastfeeding [196]. Since the 1960s, approximately 10% of infants are exclusively fed by soy formula, and breastfed infants may be supplemented with soy formula [197].

*Breast Feeding-Breast Cancer Association*

Epidemiologic research, primarily designed as case-control studies, has demonstrated a modest, but not significant, lower risk of premenopausal breast cancer in those who reported having been breastfed [145, 165, 198–201] with two exceptions [202, 203] (table 5). Of the three studies in postmenopausal breast cancer, the RRs vary above [202, 203] and below the null value [198], but none are significant. Having been breastfed is not associated with risk of breast cancer in women whose mothers later developed breast cancer [198]. In two studies, the duration of breastfeeding is not associated with breast cancer risk [145, 203].

Breastfeeding has also been shown to influence weight status and has been extensively reviewed by Butte [204]. Breastfeeding was associated with a reduced risk of being overweight as a child in four of the 16 studies discussed. However, several factors make interpretation of these results difficult including small sample sizes, and different definitions of the exclusivity and duration of breastfeeding. The evidence to date suggests that breastfeeding reduces the risk of being overweight as a child to a moderate extent. Gillman et al. [205] for example reported that adolescents (9–14 years) who were breastfed for at least 7 months were 20% less likely to be overweight (OR 0.80; 95% CI 0.67–0.96) than those breastfed for 3 months or less. The duration of breastfeeding was also inversely related to the risk of being overweight at adolescence. Specifically, compared to those who were never breastfed or

181

**Table 5.** Adjusted relative risk (RR) of breast cancer by study design, birth year, ever breastfed (bottle-fed) as well as duration of breastfeeding

| Reference | Birth year | Ethnic group | Breastfeeding, % | | | RR | Comments |
|---|---|---|---|---|---|---|---|
| | | | cases[a] | controls | | | |
| **Cohort studies** | | | | | | | |
| Michels et al. [142] | 1921–1964 | NHW | 36.3[0] | | Ever | 1.0[b] | Referent: never breastfed |
| | | | | | Duration | RR | |
| | | | | | <3 | 0.7[b] | Referent: never breastfed; adjusted for multiple covariates; p for trend: NS |
| | | | | | 4–8 | 1.0[b] | |
| | | | | | >9 | 0.9[b] | |
| | | NHW | 73.5[2] | | Ever | 1.1 | Referent: never breastfed |
| | | | | | Duration | RR | |
| | | | | | <3 | 1.3[b] | Referent: never breastfed; adjusted for multiple covariates; p for trend: NS |
| | | | | | 4–8 | 0.9[b] | |
| | | | | | >9 | 1.3[b] | |
| **Case-control studies** | | | | | | | |
| Brinton et al. [199] | NR | NHW | 73.7[3] | 74.3 | Ever | 0.9[b] | Referent: never breastfed |
| Ekbom et al. [200] | 1874–1954 | NHW | 88.9[3] | 88.1 | Ever | 1.0 | Referent: never breastfed |
| Freudenheim et al. [198] | 1901–1951 | NHW | 48.9[0] | 58.5 | Ever | 0.7 | Referent: never breastfed; adjusted for age and education |
| | | | 80.6[2] | 85.7 | Ever | 0.7 | |
| Weiss et al. [165] | 1936–1972 | NHW | 41.7[1] | 49.5 | Ever | 0.7[b] | Referent: never breastfed |
| Titus-Ernstoff et al. [202] | 1942–1945 | NHW | 42.0[0] | 48.1 | Ever | 0.7 | Referent: never breastfed |
| | | | 55.6[2] | 55.8 | Ever | 1.0 | |
| Sanderson et al. [156] | 1944 on | NHW | 44.5[1] | 44.6 | Ever | 1.0 | Referent: never breastfed |
| | | | | | Duration | RR | |
| | | | | | <3 | 1.0 | Referent: never breastfed |
| | | | | | 3–5.9 | 1.1 | |
| | | | | | >6 | 1.0 | |

NHW = Non-Hispanic white; NS = non-significant.
[a]Menopausal status: [0]premenopausal; [1]premenopausal based on age <50 years; [2]postmenopausal based on age >50 years; [3]both.
[b]Relative risk.

breastfed for <1 month, an 8% reduction in the risk was demonstrated for every increment of 3 months of breastfeeding (adjusted OR 0.92; 95% CI 0.87–98) or breastfed for <1 month. It has been suggested that this may be due to the latent effect of the infant feeding mode and not solely to lower fatness during the first 2 years of life [206]. This is of biological interest as obesity during and after adolescence is highly predictive of adult obesity [207, 208] and increased risk of postmenopausal breast cancer [209].

Several possible mechanisms have been put forward to explain how breastfeeding could be related to lower rates of overweight in children including behavioral and hormonal pathways. Birch and Fisher [210] have shown that children who are breastfed are better able to adjust intake at a meal in response to a high calorie pre-load and concluded that breastfed children may learn to self-regulate caloric intake better than non-breastfed infants. In addition, infant formula feeding compared with breastfeeding evokes a higher and more prolonged insulin response and therefore earlier fat deposition [211]. The effect may also be due to different metabolic programming of breastfed from formula-fed infants due to variations in milk composition, protein intake, fatness and/or rate of weight gain in early life and residual confounding by variables such as child feeding practices and physical activity.

Research has shown that mothers' child feeding practices are directly related to children's energy intake, food preferences, the ability to regulate food intake and body weight [212–214]. In addition to the association between infant feeding and the risk of being overweight in childhood or adolescence, infant feeding may alter dietary intake during childhood. This could be due to demographic and physiologic differences between mothers who breastfeed versus those who bottle-feed. Indeed it may be possible that food preferences subsequent to breastfeeding are affected by the mode of infant feeding. Of note, very little information is currently known regarding differences in the age at introduction of solid foods and the type of solid food given in breastfed versus bottle-fed infants by ethnic group, energy expenditure and other metabolic markers of body size.

*Linear Growth and Body Size from Infancy Through Adolescence*

*Rationale*
Infancy and childhood are periods of rapid growth in weight, height, and brain size. Recent analyses of birth weight, childhood growth, and breast cancer risk have led to the exploration of factors influencing catch-up or -down growth in early childhood. In the Avon Longitudinal Study of Pregnancy and Childhood (ALSPAC), Ong et al. [215] describe how thinner, shorter newborns with tall fathers experience the greatest catch-up in weight compared with those who show no change from birth to 2 years. Moreover, ALSPAC children with early catch-up growth have higher serum IGF-1 levels at 5 years

***Table 6.*** Growth patterns and relative risk (RR) of breast cancer by birth year, ethnic group and menopausal status

| Reference | Birth year | Ethnic group | Cases | Ages at which measurements were taken | RR | Comment |
|---|---|---|---|---|---|---|
| **Cohort studies** | | | | | | |
| De Stavola et al. [223] | 1946 | NHW | 51 | 2–4 | 0.9 | Linear velocity (cm/year), adjusted for age at menarche, age at first birth, parity and social class |
| | | | 53 | 4–7 | 1.3* | |
| | | | 49 | 7–11 | 1.0 | |
| | | | 43 | 11–15 | 1.1 | |
| | | | 37 | 15–adulthood | 0.9 | |
| | | | | 7 years | Hazard ratio | |
| Hilakivi-Clarke et al. [95] | 1924–1933 | NHW | 22 | <114.5 cm | 1.0 (ref) | p for trend in linear growth = 0.01; adjusted for birth weight and birth length |
| | | | 32 | 117.5 | 1.3 | |
| | | | 39 | 120 | 1.7* | |
| | | | 41 | 123 | 1.7* | |
| | | | 43 | >123 | 1.9* | |
| | | | | 15 years | | |
| | | NHW | 23 | <153 | 1.0 (ref) | |
| | | | 34 | 157 | 1.3 | |
| | | | 33 | 160 | 1.3 | |
| | | | 38 | 163 | 1.8* | |
| | | | 49 | >163 | 1.9 | |
| **Case-control studies** | | | | | | |
| Herrinton and Husson [254] | 1934–1963 | NHW, AA | 77 | 12–14 | 1.7* | Tall vs. short height-at-age, controls matched on birth year, age at entry, marital status, alcohol use, race, parity, age at first birth and menopausal status |
| | | NHW, AA | 59 | 15–18 | 2.2* | |
| | | | | | RR | |
| Ahlgren et al. [139] | 1930–1975 | NHW NHW | 3,340 | 7–8 years | 1.1* | Adjusted RR per 5-cm increase; p for trend = 0.01 |
| | | | | 8–14 years | 1.2* | |

NHW =Non-Hispanic white; AA = African American.
*95% Confidence interval excludes one.

than those remaining on trajectory or experiencing catch-down, after adjustment for current size [216]. A similar pattern of higher IGF-1 concentrations appear at 4 and 9 years of age in children who are thinner and smaller newborns, experience catch-up in linear growth, and have tall fathers [217, 218]. Thus, in utero effects may be modulated by childhood growth velocity, by genetic factors, and may correlate with IGF-1 concentrations in childhood.

In addition, adult height is known to be positively associated with breast cancer risk [219, 220]. Furthermore, there was a trend of decreasing risk of breast cancer with increasing age at attainment of height and women had a 30% reduction (OR = 0.7; 95% CI 0.5–1.0) in risk of breast cancer for pre- and postmenopausal women who reached their maximum height at 18 years or older compared with women who reached their maximum height at age 13 or younger [221, 222]. De Stavola et al. [223] suggested that women who grow faster in childhood and reached adult height above the average for their menarche category are at particularly increased risk of breast cancer. For example for each 1-standard deviation increase in height velocity at age 4–7 years, the breast cancer risk increased by 54% (OR 1.54; 95% CI 1.13–2.09).

Alberman et al. [224] stated that factors in early life which contributed to a significant increase in adult height included gender and parental height, birth weight and maternal pre-pregnant weight, while increasing gestational age had a negative effect. In addition, a woman's final adult height can also be influenced by the onset of ovarian function during adolescence. However, other early life exposures which could potentially affect age at final height and adult height, such as infant feeding practices have not been extensively studied. One study by Zadik et al. [225] showed that despite their slower growth rate, breastfed children reach the same final height as bottle-fed children. The American Dietetic Association advocates exclusive breastfeeding for 4–6 months and breastfeeding with weaning foods for at least 12 months [226]. It is therefore of interest to assess the effect of infant feeding (type and duration) on age at final height and actual adult height.

### Diabetes and Breast Cancer Risk

Epidemiologic studies suggest that type-2 diabetes is associated with a 10–20% increased risk of breast cancer [227–230]. Although this association has been observed in both premenopausal and postmenopausal women, most reports only observed a significant increase in risk among postmenopausal women and many did not have the statistical power or data to investigate the association by menopausal status [227–230]. Furthermore, hyperinsulinemia with insulin resistance may promote breast cancer through several mechanisms including: activation of the insulin pathway, activation of the IGF pathway, and impaired regulation of endogenous sex hormones [228]. The proposed carcinogenic effects of insulin in relation to increased breast cancer

**Table 7.** Summary of literature on early life exposures and breast cancer

| Exposure | Number of studies with significant findings*/total number of studies | Range RR |
|---|---|---|
| High birth weight | | |
|   Premenopausal | 3/7 | 3.1–5.0 |
|   Postmenopausal | 0/3 | – |
|   Both | 5/11 | 1.2–2.6 |
| Birth length | 2/4 | 1.5–3.5 |
| Preterm | 3/8 | 2.1–6.7 |
| Preeclampsia | 6/9 | 0.3–1.4 |
| Maternal age | 2/12 | 1.5–2.0 |
| Infant feeding | 0/7 | 0.7–1.3 |
| Linear growth | 4/4 | 1.1[a]–1.9 |

*95% Confidence interval excludes one.
[a]Adjusted RR per 5-cm increase.

risk may result from insulin's ability to directly target breast cells or the related IGF-1 polypeptide [228]. IGF-1 is synthesized in the liver, but is also present in breast cells and functions as an autocrine growth factor [231]. Circulating IGF-1 is bound with high affinity to IGFBP-3 and evidence suggests that IGFBP-3 plays a regulatory role in the proliferation of breast cancer cells as a result of its inhibition of IGF-1, the binding protein for cellular integration [231]. High circulating concentrations of IGF-1 and IGFBP-3 are associated with an increased risk of breast cancer and IGF-1 appears to be an important link between obesity and increased risk of breast cancer [228].

Type-2 diabetes is characterized as a high insulin state caused by insulin resistance in fat and muscle tissues and leads to an increased production of insulin, whereas type-1 diabetes is a state of absolute deficiency of insulin caused by autoimmune destruction of pancreatic β cells. The main risk factors for type-2 diabetes include: older age, obesity, and genetic predisposition. The etiology of type-1 diabetes is much less understood than that of type-2, but evidence suggests that both genetics and environmental exposures early in life, including nutrition, could play a role in the disease process. Early infant feeding patterns, such as reduced duration of exclusive breastfeeding, early age at introduction to dairy products, or early age at introduction to gluten-containing solid foods, have been associated with a risk of type-1 diabetes. Furthermore, it is possible that the aforementioned infant feeding patterns are associated with a risk of type-2 diabetes later in life, or that particular infant feeding patterns could modify exposures later in child- or adulthood that in turn increases one's risk for type-2 diabetes, hyperinsulinemia, and the subsequent risk of breast cancer. To date, most studies investigating the association between early infant feeding patterns and risk of diabetes focused solely on the association between ever-breastfeeding and the duration of overall breastfeeding and the risk of type-1 diabetes. To our knowledge, very few studies have investigated the association between early life feeding patterns other than ever-breastfeeding, or have extensively investigated the association between early infant feeding patterns and the risk of type-2 diabetes in the US.

*Breastfeeding and Risk of Diabetes*

Reported findings on the association between the duration of breastfeeding (total and exclusive breastfeeding), age at introduction of supplementary milk products or solid foods and the risk of type-1 diabetes are mixed. Several older studies have observed an increase in the incidence of type-1 diabetes in individuals who have not been breastfed or who were breastfed for <4 months [232]. Data from more recent studies investigating this hypothesis are mixed. Perez-Bravo et al. [233] observed a statistically significant difference in the reported duration of breastfeeding (5.4 vs. 7.6 months, p < 0.02) among children with type-1 diabetes compared to controls, while Couper et al. [234] did not observe an association between the total duration of breastfeeding and the risk of diabetes-associated autoantibodies. Furthermore, a study of German children with a first-degree family history of type-1 diabetes reported that breastfeeding duration, either exclusive or partial, was not associated with an increased islet autoantibody risk by 8 years of age [235]. Recent data suggest that there may be an association between the duration of exclusive breastfeeding and the risk of diabetes. A study of Finnish children found no difference in the duration of any breastfeeding or in the age at introduction of solid food and the risk of type-1 diabetes; however, they did observe a statistically significant decrease in the risk of type-1 diabetes among children who were exclusively breastfed for at least 2 (OR 0.60, 95% CI 0.41, 0.89) or 3 months (OR 0.63; 95% CI 0.43, 0.95) [236]. Adjustment for mother's age and education, child's birth weight, or birth order did not affect the results [236]. In addition, a recent study of Finnish children with a family history of diabetes reported that those infants who were breastfed exclusively for at least 4 months had a lower risk of seroconversion to all autoantibodies, including IA-2A, ICA, GADA, and insulin (IAA) [237]. There was no association between the duration of any breastfeeding and the presence of diabetes-associated autoantibodies, or any of the antibodies [237]. It is possible that exclusive breastfeeding itself is not associated with an increased risk of type-1 diabetes, and that the observed association between breastfeeding and diabetes may be completely explained by the correlation of duration breastfed and timing of exposure to cow's milk, cereal, or other solid foods. Finally, the association between breastfeeding and diabetes may be biased due to residual confounding by the sociodemographic and other characteristics of the women who chose to exclusively breastfeed for 4 months or longer.

The relationship between early infant diet and the risk of type-2 diabetes has not been well documented compared to the association with risk of type-1 diabetes. Furthermore, the etiology of type-2 diabetes remains unclear, which hampers our ability to target specific exposures and time periods that may play a role in the risk of type-2 diabetes. Three studies to date indicate that there may be a link between early infant feeding and the risk of type-2 diabetes later in life. One investigation of breastfeeding and the incidence of type-2 diabetes among the Pima Indians reported that exclusive breastfeeding for the first 2 months of life was associated with a significantly lower rate of type-2 diabetes [238]. Another study investigated the association between early life exposures and the risk of insulin resistance and type-2 diabetes among middle-aged men living in rural and urban areas near Bangladesh, India [239]. The researchers observed that men living in urban compared to rural areas and those with increased adult weight gain over the 10 years of follow-up compared to those men without adult weight gain were at significant higher risk for insulin resistance and type-2 diabetes [239]. Canadian children who were breastfed for at least 12 months had a lower risk of developing type-2 diabetes compared to children breastfed for less than 12 months (OR = 0.24; 95% CI 0.13, 0.99) [240]. The estimate remained protective, but non-significant (OR = 0.27; 95% CI 0.06, 1.26), after adjustment for maternal smoking, maternal alcohol use, birth weight, maternal BMI, and maternal diet [240]. Finally, a study in Holland observed that men and women aged 48–53 years who were exclusively breastfed had lower fasting insulin and post-challenge glucose levels compared to those who were bottle-fed [241]. It is possible that susceptibility to type-2 diabetes may be a function of the interaction between genetic factors, intrauterine exposures, infant and childhood diet, as well as lifestyle across the lifespan.

*Age at Introduction of Milk Supplementation and Risk of Diabetes*
Ecologic studies provide evidence to support an association between diabetes incidence and cow's milk consumption based upon their observations of a positive correlation between the regional incidence of type-1 diabetes and per capita milk consumption [232, 242]. These observations lead to investigations into the association between cow's milk-based infant formula consumption early in life and later development of insulin-dependent diabetes [232, 242]. Two meta-analyses showed a moderate increase in the risk for type-1 diabetes in children exposed to cow's milk before 3 months of age. The first meta-analysis by Gerstein et al. [243] of 13 studies found a 1.5 times higher risk of developing diabetes for people who were exposed to milk-based products before 4 months of age compared to those exposed at or after 4 months of age. In addition, the second meta-analysis of early infant diet and the risk of type-1 diabetes found a similar relationship between exposure to cow's milk (OR = 1.61; 95% CI 1.31, 1.98) and exposure to breast-milk substitutes (OR = 1.38; 95% CI 1.18, 1.61) before the age of 3 months [244]. In contrast,

no association was observed in prospective studies of diabetes-related autoantibodies and the age when cow's milk or cow's milk-based formulas were introduced. A small study of Australian children with a first-degree family history of type-1 diabetes found no association between age at introduction of cow's milk and the development of islet autoantibody [234]. Another similar study of children with a first-degree family history of type-1 diabetes in Germany also reported no association between early age at milk supplementation and risk of increased islet autoantibodies in the children by 8 years of age [235].

*Intrauterine Exposures, Age at Introduction of Gluten-Containing Foods, and Risk of Diabetes*

Among infants with a first-degree family history of type-1 diabetes, those who received food supplementation with gluten-containing foods before 3 months of age were at an increased risk of islet autoantibodies (HR = 4.0; 95% CI 1.4–11.5) compared to children who were exclusively breastfed until 3 months of age [235]. In addition to these findings, American children with a family history of type-1 diabetes were at an increased risk of islet autoimmunity if they were exposed to cereals at 3 months of age or younger or at 7 months of age or older, compared to those exposed from 4–6 months of age [245].

It is possible that there is a window of exposure to cereals outside which the risk of autoimmunity is increased, however further investigation into the association between timing and type of cereal supplementation and risk of autoimmunity or type-1 diabetes is needed. Additional studies may elucidate whether the observed risk from the aforementioned study is due to exposure to specific antigens or to other components of cereals or possibly the combination of the ingredients (i.e. type of milk or type of cereal).

In addition to the proposed association between early childhood diet and risk of islet autoimmunity and type-1 diabetes, it is possible that intrauterine nutritional or other exposures may play a role in the subsequent risk of diabetes in the offspring. In a study of the association between intrauterine nutritional exposure and the risk of islet autoimmunity in children with a family history of type-1 diabetes, an inverse association was observed between maternal dietary intake of vitamin D during pregnancy and the risk of islet autoimmunity in offspring [246]. Thus the offspring of women who consumed higher levels of vitamin D from food were at a decreased risk of islet autoimmunity compared to the offspring of mothers who reported lower vitamin D intake (HR = 0.49; 95% CI 0.26, 0.94) [20]. A significant association remained, even after adjustment for HLA genotype, family history of type-1 diabetes, presence of gestational diabetes mellitus, and ethnicity (HR = 0.37; 95% CI 0.17, 0.78) [246]. The researchers did not observe any association between maternal fatty acid intake and the risk of islet autoimmunity in the offspring. These results suggest that maternal intake of vitamin D though foods may have a protective effect on the appearance of islet autoimmunity and the risk of type-1 diabetes in their offspring.

### Biological Mechanism of Infant Feeding Patterns and Risk of Diabetes

The biological mechanisms responsible for the association between early infant feeding patterns and the risk of diabetes remain unclear and further research is necessary before any conclusions can be drawn. It is possible that differences in feeding methods may play a role in both intrauterine and post-natal development of metabolic disorders either directly or indirectly through immune responses to maternal nutritional intake, cow's milk proteins, and/or accelerated childhood growth and adiposity. There are several proposed mechanisms by which infant feeding may affect childhood overweight and obesity, including altered plasma insulin and leptin levels [247].

Endocrine responses to dietary intake in infancy may play a direct role in later risk of diabetes through increased weight gain associated with infant feeding patterns. In one study of endocrine responses of breastfed and bottle-fed infants, bottle-fed infants had significantly higher plasma concentrations of insulin after feeding compared to infants who were exclusively breastfed [248]. Infant feeding patterns may also play a role in the infant's response to insulin and in the fat deposition of the infant. Higher insulin levels stimulate greater adipose tissue deposition and have been associated with a subsequent increase in weight gain and obesity [247]. Since insulin enhances cell glucose uptake and inhibits lipolysis, bottle-fed infants may have a different composition of body fat or increased BMI compared to breastfed infants, that in turn may play a role in the later risk of diabetes. Several studies have documented that infant-feeding practices are associated with differences in weight and body mass during infancy, early childhood, and in adolescence. In six studies of individuals between 3 and 26 years, all but one showed a significant association between ever-breastfeeding and reduced risk of child overweight [247]. Significant associations remained after controlling for several covariates including: paternal BMI and education level, maternal smoking, child birth weight, number of siblings, physical activity of the index, and dietary factors [247]. Another mechanism by which infant feeding may play a role in adult risk of increased body mass and diabetes is through the effects of leptin, a key regulator of appetite and body fatness. Early infant diet has been associated with leptin levels in adolescents. Specifically, adolescents who were born prematurely and randomized at birth to receive a high-protein preterm formula had a significantly greater ratio of leptin to fat mass compared to children who received banked donated breast milk [249]. Human milk intake was significantly associated with lower leptin concentrations relative to fat mass in adolescence, independent of potential confounders [249].

As mentioned previously, the association between short-term breastfeeding and the risk of diabetes could be due in part to early age at introduction of cow's milk. Breast milk protects the infant against infections by maternally transmitted immunity and this could also influence the child's resistance to other potential triggers of diabetes-associated autoimmunity, including exposure to autoantibodies in cow's milk [232, 237, 242]. Proteins present in cow's milk have been proposed to activate the immune system in a destructive process in some individuals leading to type-1 diabetes; this process may be mediated by exposure to and/or duration of breastfeeding as well as the age at introduction to cow's milk [237]. Thus short-term exclusive breastfeeding and early introduction of cow's milk could predispose individuals to autoimmunity or diabetes.

Large-scale studies are needed to disentangle the association between intrauterine, infant, childhood, and adult risk factors and the risk of type-2 diabetes and insulin resistance as well as determine the association between exclusive breastfeeding, age at introduction to breast milk substitutes and gluten-containing solid foods, as well as other childhood dietary exposures and risk of breast cancer.

## Conclusions

Carcinogenesis is a multi-step process, and the cellular and molecular pathways associated with each step provide targets for cancer prevention via nutritional interventions throughout the life course. This includes early life nutritional exposures, an area which has been understudied but has tremendous promise for impacting cancer risk. In fact, preventing or reversing the genetic and epigenetic changes associated with initiation and promotion processes early in life can be expected to have far greater preventive activity than late-in-life interventions that primarily act at the progression stage of carcinogenesis, when multiple genetic and epigenetic alterations have accumulated.

In the above case series describing early life nutritional exposures and breast cancer, over 20 studies of birth weight, birth length, and preterm births were examined, but no consistent association between a birth parameter and breast cancer risk appeared. The strongest effects on breast cancer can be seen in birth length, albeit research is limited, and linear growth velocity in childhood and adolescence, for which the most consistent associations appear.

What will we need to identify nutrition interventions in pregnancy and in early life that could reduce adult cancer risk? Future etiologic research needs to focus on measurement of the newborn's length of the trunk and limbs to explore the source of variation in birth length. Care should be taken in linear growth measurements from birth through infancy and childhood, because anthropometrics are riddled with error from inadequate standardization and training of anthropometrists, improper calibration of equipment, and lack of growth reference data. Finally, cord blood analysis of immunologic parameters, such as CD19 and macrophages, and hormone levels of insulin, IGF-1, IGFBP-3, and leptin could be correlated with the birth size (length of limb vs. trunk) of the neonate to identify underlying hormonal-nutritional mechanisms related to those who have longer birth length than the average birth length for gestational age.

Maternal height and pre-pregnancy BMI along with weight gain in pregnancy, dietary intake and physical activity in pregnancy are important elements of the picture puzzle related to the birth size of the offspring and later breast cancer risk. More detailed information about the duration of exclusive and partial breastfeeding, the ages at introduction of breast milk supplements and substitutes as well as solid foods are needed in tandem with the anthropometric data. Access to anthropometric data collected at multiple points in infancy, childhood and adolescence along with parental anthropometry would enhance the opportunity to examine the factors influencing linear growth velocity, body fat distribution, and insulin resistance, all three endpoints of which are currently being investigated in relation to breast cancer research.

Methodological research in physical activity assessment has led to the development of the International Physical Activity Questionnaire, a version of which has been validated for children and one for adults (IPAQ website). This tool in tandem with the use of pedometers, accelerometers or another mode of calibration of actual physical activity will advance our understanding of the interplay of energy balance from diet and physical activity. Along this line, considerable research in energy expenditure (assessed by whole room indirect calorimetry, by $VO_{2max}$ or another vehicle utilized during exertion) in children aged 5–17 years has revealed ethnic group differences in expenditure. In particular, African-American children have a consistently lower average resting, and basal energy expenditure than non-Hispanic white children, after taking into consideration pubertal stage, diet, and age [250]. These findings follow along with the secular trend in obesity [251] and in age at onset of puberty and menarche, where the African-American girls and boys enter puberty earlier than the non-Hispanic whites [252], and the average age at menarche is several months earlier in African-American than non-Hispanic white girls [253]. No data have been reported on energy expenditure in Hispanic children by ethnic subgroup. Moreover, gaps in energy expenditure research during pregnancy and lactation preclude the development of nutritional programs in early life.

Another area for future research examines the effect of weight loss from dieting and/or physical activity on risk factors for breast cancer. Neither animal nor human studies have reportedly examined whether weight loss during different phases of the life course will reduce cancer risk. While dieting in pregnancy and early childhood is not advocated for most individuals, extremely obese children have been placed on weight loss plans and enhanced physical activity. The components of the diet in the weight loss plans have not been elucidated nor have the children been followed after intervention to assess any long-term effects. Key areas for consideration include the identification of biomarkers other than hormones for breast cancer prevention research. Thus the area of energy balance, weight loss and physical activity in relation to cancer prevention will be greatly enhanced by multidisciplinary research combining animal experimentation and human exploration.

## References

1 Doll R, Peto R: The causes of cancer: quantitative estimate of avoidable risks of cancer in the United States today. J Natl Cancer Inst 1981;66:1191–1308.
2 Calle EE, Rodriguez C, Walker-Thurmond K, Thun MJ: Overweight, obesity, and mortality from cancer in a prospectively studied cohort of U.S. adults. N Engl J Med 2003;348: 1625–1638.
3 Report of the Advisory Committee to the Surgeon General of the Public Health Service: 1964 Smoking and Health: US Public Health Service, Office of the Surgeon General. Washington, US GPO, 1964.
4 Weir HK, Thun MJ, Hankey BF, et al: Annual report to the nation on the status of cancer, 1975–2001, featuring the use of surveillance data for cancer prevention and control. J Natl Cancer Inst 2003;95:1276–1299.
5 Hursting SD, Slaga TJ, Fischer SM, et al: Mechanism-based cancer prevention approaches: targets, examples and the use of transgenic mice. J Natl Cancer Inst 1999;91:215–225.
6 Yuspa SH, Shields PG: Etiology of cancer: chemical factors; in Devita VT Jr, Hellman SH, Rosenberg SA (eds): Cancer: Principles and Practices of Oncology, ed 5. Philadelphia, Lippincott-Raven, 1997, pp 185–202.
7 Slaga TJ: Mechanisms involved in two-stage carcinogenesis in mouse skin; in Slaga TJ (ed.): Mechanisms of Tumor Promotion. Boca Raton: CRC Press, 1984, pp 1–93.
8 Yuspa SH, Poirier MC: Chemical carcinogenesis: from animal models to molecular models in one decade. Adv Cancer Res 1988;50:25–70.
9 Pitot HC: Progression: the terminal stage in carcinogenesis. Jpn J Cancer Res 1989;80: 599–607.
10 Sporn MB: Approaches to prevention of epithelial cancer during the preneoplastic period. Cancer Res 1976;36:2699–2702.
11 Fearon ER, Vogelstein B: A genetic model of human colorectal tumorigenesis. Cell 1990;61: 759–767.
12 Spitz MR, Bondy ML: Genetic susceptibility to cancer. Cancer 1993;72:992–995.
13 Sugimura T: Multistep carcinogenesis: a 1992 perspective. Science 1992;258:603–607.
14 Gonzalez F: Genetic polymorphism and cancer susceptibility. 14th Sapporo Cancer Seminar. Cancer Res 1995;55:710–775.
15 Drinkwater NR, Bennett LM: Genetic control of carcinogenesis in experimental animals. Prog Exp Tumor Res 1991;33:1–20.
16 Stanley LA: Molecular aspects of chemical carcinogenesis: the roles of oncogenes and tumor suppressor genes. Toxicology 1995;96:173–194.
17 Nebert DW, Nelson DR, Coon MR, et al: The P450 superfamily: update on new sequences, gene mapping and recommended nomenclature. DNA Cell Biol 1991;10:1–14.
18 Guengerich FP: Metabolic activation of carcinogens. Pharmacol Ther 1992;54:17–61.
19 Eiling TE, Thompson DC, Foureman GL: Prostaglandin H synthase and xenobiotic oxidation. Annu Rev Pharmacol Toxicol 1990;30:1–45.
20 MacLeod MC, Slaga TJ: Multiple strategies for the inhibition of cancer induction. Cancer Bull 1995;47:492–498.
21 Miller EC, Miller JA: Searches for ultimate chemical carcinogens and their reactions with cellular macromolecules. Cancer 1981;47:2327–2345.

22 Perchellet J-P, Perchellet EM, Gali HU, Gao XM: Oxidant stress and multistage carcinogenesis; in Mukhtar H (ed): Skin Cancer: Mechanisms and Human Relevance. Boca Raton, CRC Press, 1995, pp 145–180.
23 Mantle TJ, Pickett CB, Hayes JD (eds): Glutathione S-Transferases and Carcinogenesis. Philadelphia, Taylor and Francis, 1987, pp 1–121.
24 Ketterer B: Protective role of glutathione and glutathione transferases in mutagenesis and carcinogenesis. Mutat Res 1988;202:343–361.
25 Oesch F, Doehmer J, Friedberg T, et al: Control of ultimate mutagenic species by diverse enzymes. Prog Clin Biol Res 1990;340B:49–65.
26 James MO, Schell JD, Boyle SM, et al: Southern flounder hepatic and intestinal metabolism and DNA binding of benzo[a]pyrene (BAP) metabolites following dietary administration of low doses of BAP, BAP-7,8-dihydrodiol, or a BAP metabolite mixture. Chem Biol Interact 1991;79:305–321.
27 Mitchell DL, Adair GM, MacLeod MC, et al: DNA damage and repair in the initiation phase of carcinogenesis. Cancer Bull 1995;47:449–455.
28 Friedberg EC, Walker GC, Siede W: DNA Repair and Mutagenesis. Washington, American Society of Microbiology Press, 1995, pp 1–79.
29 Sancar A: Mechanisms of DNA repair. Science 1995;266:1954–1956.
30 Sancar A, Tang M-S: Nucleotide excision repair. Photochem Photobiol 1993;57:905–921.
31 Modrich P: Mismatch repair, genetic stability and cancer. Science 1995;266:1959–1960.
32 Chung FL, Kelloff G, Steele V, et al: Chemopreventive efficacy of arylalkyl isothiocyanates and N-acetylcysteine for lung tumorigenesis in Fischer rats. Cancer Res 1996;56:772–778.
33 Hecht SS: Chemoprevention by isothiocyanates. J Cell Biochem Suppl 1995;22:195–209.
34 Stoner GD, Mukhtar H: Polyphenols as cancer chemopreventive agents. J Cell Biochem 1995;22:169–180.
35 Morse MA, Wang CX, Stoner GD, et al: Inhibition of 4-(methylnitrosoamino)-1(3-pyridyl)-1-butanone-induced DNA adduct formation and tumorigenicity in the lung of the F344 rat by dietary phenethyl isothiocyanate. Cancer Res 1989;49:549–553.
36 Morse MA, Elkind KI, Amin SG, et al: Effects of alkyl chain length on the inhibition of NNK-induced lung neoplasia in A/J mice by arylalkyl isothiocyantes. Carcinogenesis 1989;10:1757–1759.
37 Brady JF, Wang MH, Hong JY, et al: Modulation of rat hepatic microsomal monooxygenase enzymes and cytotoxicity by diallyl sulfide. Toxicol Appl Pharmacol 1991;108:342–354.
38 Brady JF, Ishizaki H, Fukuto JH, et al: Inhibition of cytochrome P450IIE1 by diallyl sulfide and its metabolites. Chem Res Toxicol 1991;4:642–647.
39 Chen L, Lee M, Hong JY, et al: Relationship between cytochrome P450 2E1 and acetone catabolism in rats as studied with diallyl sulfide as an inhibitor. Biochem Pharmacol 1994;48:2199–2205.
40 Murray RDH, Mendez J, Brown SA (eds): The Naturally Occurring Coumarins: Occurrence, Chemistry and Biochemistry. New York, Wiley, 1982, pp 97–111.
41 Bickers DR, Mukhtar H, Molica SJ, Pathak MA: The effect of psoralens on hepatic and cutaneous drug metabolizing enzymes and cytochrome P450. J Invest Dermatol 1982;79:201–205.
42 Cai Y, Ivie W, DiGiovanni J: Effect of naturally occurring coumarins on the formation of mouse epidermal DNA adducts and skin tumors induced by benzo[a]pyrene and 7,12-dimethylbenz[a]anthracene. Carcinogenesis 1997;18:1521–1527.
43 Kootstra A, Haas BL, Slaga TJ: Reactions of benzo[a]pyrene diol epoxides with DNA and nucleosomes in aqueous solution. Biochem Biophys Res Commun 1980;94:1432–1438.
44 Wood AW, Sayer JM, Newmark HL: Mechanism of the inhibition of mutagenicity of benzo[a]pyrene 7,8-diol 9,10-epoxide by riboflavin 5′-phosphate. Proc Natl Acad Sci USA 1982;79:5122–5126.
45 Wood AW, Huang M-T, Chang RL, et al. Inhibition of the mutagenicity of bay-region diol epoxides of polycyclic aromatic hydrocarbons by naturally occurring plant phenols: exceptional activity of ellagic acid. Proc Natl Acad Sci USA 1982;79:5513–5517.
46 Lesca P: Protective effects of ellagic acid and other plant phenols on benzo[a]pyrene-induced neoplasia. Carcinogenesis 1983;4:1651–1653.
47 Katiyer SK, Mukhtar H: Tea in chemoprevention of cancer. Epidemiologic and experimental studies. Int J Oncol 1996;8:221–238.

48 Sparnins VL, Barany G, Wattenberg LW: Effects of organosulfur compounds from garlic and onions on benzo[a]pyrene-induced neoplasia and glutathione-S-transferase activity in the mouse. Carcinogenesis 1988;9:131–134.
49 Sumiyoshi H, Wargovich MJ: Chemoprevention of 1,2-dimethylhydrazine-induced colon cancer in mice by naturally occurring organosulfur compounds. Cancer Res 1990;50:5084–5087.
50 Rao CV, Tokomo K, Kelloff G, Reddy BS: Inhibition of dietary oltipraz of experimental intestinal carcinogenesis induced by azoxymethane in male F344 rats. Carcinogenesis 1991;12: 1051–1055.
51 Jang M, Cai L, Udeani GO, et al: Cancer chemopreventive activity of resveratrol, a natural product derived from grapes. Science 1997;275:218–220.
52 Srivastava VK, Busbee DL: Decreased fidelity of DNA polymerases and decreased excision repair in aging mice: effects of caloric restriction. Biochem Biophys Res Commun 1992;182: 712–721.
53 Haley- Zitlin V, Richardson A: Effect of dietary restriction on DNA repair and DNA damage. Mutat Res 1993;295:237–245.
54 Weisburger JH, Rivenson A, Kingston DG, et al: Dietary modulation of the carcinogenicity of the heterocyclic amines. Princess Takamatsu Symp 1995;23:240–250.
55 Birt DF, Julius AD, Runice CE, et al: Enhancement of BOP-induced pancreatic carcinogenesis in selenium-fed Syrian golden hamsters under specific dietary conditions. Nutr Cancer 1988; 11:21–33.
56 James SJ, Muskhelishvili L: Rates of apoptosis and proliferation vary with caloric intake and may influence incidence of spontaneous hepatoma in C57BL6 x C3H F1 mice. Cancer Res 1994;54:5508–5510.
57 Thompson HJ, Strange R, Schedin PJ: Apoptosis in the genesis and prevention of cancer. Cancer Epidemiol Biomarkers Prev 1992;1:597–602.
58 Slaga TJ, Klein-Szanto AJP, Fischer SM, et al: Studies on the mechanism of action of anti-tumor promoting agents: their specificity in two-stage promotion. Proc Natl Acad Sci USA 1980;77:2251–2254.
59 Blumburg PM: Protein kinase C as the receptor for the phorbol ester tumor promoters. Cancer Res 1988;48:1–8.
60 Fischer SM, DiGiovanni J: Mechanisms of tumor promotion: epigenetic changes in cell signaling. Cancer Bull 1995;47:456–463.
61 DiGiovanni J: Multistage carcinogenesis in mouse skin. Pharmacol Ther 1992;54:63–128.
62 Fürstenberger G, Marks F: Prostaglandins, epidermal hyperplasia and skin tumor promotion; in Honn KV, Marnett LJ (eds): Prostaglandins, Leukotrienes and Cancer. Boston, Nijhoff, 1985, pp 22–37.
63 Sigal E: The molecular biology of mammalian arachidonic acid metabolism. Am J Physiol 1991;260:L13–L51.
64 Simonson MS, Wolfe JA, Dunn MJ: Regulation of prostaglandin synthesis by differential expression of the gene encoding prostaglandin endoperoxide synthase. Adv Prostaglandin Thromboxane Leukot Res 1991;21A:69–82.
65 Harris CC: p53: at the crossroads of molecular carcinogenesis and risk assessment. Science 1993;262:1980–1981.
66 Smith ML, Chen I-T, Zhan Q, et al: Involvement of the p53 tumor suppressor in repair of UV-type DNA damage. Oncogene 1995;10:105–109.
67 Livingstone LR, White A, Sprouse J, et al: Altered cell cycle arrest and gene amplification potential accompany loss of wild-type p53. Cell 1992;71:587–597.
68 Guinn BA, Mills KI: p53 mutations, methylation and genomic instability in the progression of chronic myelogenous leukemia. Leuk Lymphoma 1997;26:211–226.
69 Trush MA, Kensler TW: An overview of the relationship between oxidative stress and chemical carcinogenesis. Free Rad Biol Med 1991;10:201–207.
70 Hursting SD, Lavigne JA, Berrigan DA, et al: Calorie restriction, aging and cancer prevention: mechanisms of action and applicability to humans. Annu Rev Med 2003;54:131–152.
71 Birt DF, Kris ES, Luthra R: Modification of murine skin tumor promotion by dietary energy and fat; in Mukhtar H (ed.): Skin Cancer: Mechanisms and Human Relevance. Boca Raton, CRC Press, 1995, pp 371–381.
72 Ames BN, Shigenaga MK, Hagen TM: Oxidants, antioxidants and the degenerative diseases of aging. Proc Natl Acad Sci USA 1993;90:7915–7922.

73  Weindruch R, Walford RL (eds): The Retardation of Aging and Disease by Dietary Restriction. Springfield, Thomas, 1988, pp 1–291.
74  Weeks CE, Slaga TJ, Hennings H, et al: Inhibition of phorbol ester-induced tumor promotion in mice by vitamin A analog and anti-inflammatory steroid. J Natl Cancer Inst 1988;63:401–406.
75  Gensler HI, Sim DA, Bowden GT: Influence of the duration of topical 13-cis retinoic acid treatment on inhibition of mouse skin tumor promotion. Cancer Res 1986;46:2767–2770.
76  Verma AK, Shapas BG, Rice HM, Boutwell RK: Correlation of the inhibition by retinoids of tumor promoter induced mouse epidermal ornithine decarboxylase activity and of skin promotion. Cancer Res 1978;39:419–425.
77  Pegg AE: Polyamine metabolism and its importance in neoplastic growth and as a target for chemotherapy. Cancer Res 1988;48:759–774.
78  Petkovich AM, Brand NJ, Krust A, Chambon P: A human retinoic acid receptor which belongs to the family of nuclear receptors. Nature 1987;330:444–450.
79  Lotan R: Retinoids in cancer chemoprevention. FASEB J 1996;10:1031–1039.
80  Lotan R: Retinoids and apoptosis: implications for cancer chemoprevention and therapy. J Natl Cancer Inst 1995;87:1655–1657.
81  Birt DF, White LT, Choi B, Pelling JC: Dietary fat effects on the initiation and promotion of two-stage skin tumorigenesis in the SENCAR mouse. Cancer Res 1989;49:4170–4174.
82  Sandler RS: Aspirin and other non-steroidal anti-inflammatory agents in the prevention of colorectal cancer. Important Adv Oncol 1996;96:123–137.
83  Tsujii M, DuBois RN: Alterations in cellular adhesion and apoptosis in epithelial cells overexpressing prostaglandin endoperoxide synthase-2. Cell 1995;83:493–501.
84  Slaga TJ, DiGiovanni J: Inhibition of chemical carcinogenesis; in Searle CE (ed.): American Chemical Society Monograph 182. Washington, American Chemical Society, 1984, vol 2, pp 1279–1294.
85  Graham DJ, Campen D, Hui R, et al: Risk of acute myocardial infarction and sudden cardiac death in patients treated with cyclooxygenase 2 selective and non-selective non-steroidal anti-inflammatory drugs: nested case-control study. Lancet 2005;365:475–481.
86  Sale S, Tunstall RG, Ruparelia KC, Potter GA, Steward WP, Gescher AJ: Comparison of the effects of the chemopreventive agent resveratrol and its synthetic analog trans 3,4,5,4′-(tetramethoxystilbene (DMU-212) on adenoma development in the APC (Min+) mouse and cyclooxygenase-2 in human-derived colon cancer cells. Int J Cancer 2005;115:194–201.
87  Sengupta A, Ghosh S, Das S: Modulatory influence of garlic and tomato on cyclooxygenase-2 activity, cell proliferation and apoptosis during azoxymethane induced colon carcinogenesis in rat. Cancer Lett 2004;208:127–136.
88  Preston-Martin S, Yu MC, Benton B, et al: N-Nitroso compounds and childhood brain tumors: a case-control study. Cancer Res 1982;42:5240–5245.
89  Blot WJ, Henderson BE, Boice JD: Childhood cancer in relation to cured meat intake: a review of the epidemiologic evidence. Nutr Cancer 1999;34:111–118.
90  Peters JM, Preston-Martin S, London SJ, et al: Processed meats and risk of childhood leukemia. Cancer Causes Control 1994;5:195–202.
91  Sarasua S, Savitz DA: Cured and broiled meat consumption in relation to childhood cancer. Cancer Causes Control 1994;5:141–148.
92  Kwan ML, Block G, Selvin S, et al: Food consumption by children and the risk of childhood acute leukemia. Am J Epidemiol 2004;160:1098–1107.
93  Ross J, Potter J, Robison L, et al: Maternal exposure to potential inhibitors of DNA topoisomerase II and infant leukemia: a report from the Children's Cancer Group. Cancer Causes Control 1996;7:581–590.
94  Okasha M, McCarron P, Gunnell D, Smith GD: Exposures in childhood, adolescence and early adulthood and breast cancer risk: a systematic review of the literature. Breast Cancer Res Treat 2003;78:223–276.
95  Hilakivi-Clarke L, Forsen T, Eriksson JG, et al: Tallness and overweight during childhood have opposing effects on breast cancer risk. Br J Cancer 2001;85:1680–1684.
96  Hilakivi-Clarke L, Clarke R, Lippman ME: Perinatal factors increase breast cancer risk. Breast Cancer Res Treat 1994;31:273–284.
97  Walker BE, Kurth LA: Effects of fostering on the increased tumor incidence produced by a maternal diet high in fat. Nutr Cancer 1996;26:31–35.

98   Waterland RA, Jirtle RL: Early nutrition, epigenetic changes at transposons and imprinted genes, and enhanced susceptibility to adult chronic disease. Nutrition 2004;20:63–68.

99   Waterland RA, Jirtle RL: Transposable elements: targets for early nutritional effects on epigenetic gene regulation. Molec Cell Biol 2003;23:5293–5300.

100  Regnault TR, Galan HL, Parker TA, Anthony RV: Placental development in normal and compromised pregnancies – a review. Placenta 2002;23(suppl A):S119–S129.

101  Sadler TW: Langman's Medical Embryology, ed 9. Baltimore, Lippincott Williams & Wilkins, 2004.

102  Bajoria R, Sooranna SR, Ward BS, Chatterjee R: Prospective function of placental leptin at maternal-fetal interface. Placenta 2002;23:103–115.

103  Hay WW: Nutrition-gene interaction during intrauterine life and lactation. Nutr Reviews 1999;57:S20–S30.

104  Hoppe C, Molgaard C, Thomsen BL, et al: Protein intake at 9 months of age is associated with body size but not with body fat in 10 year old Danish children. Am J Clin Nutr 2004;79: 494–501.

105  Trichopoulos D: Hypothesis: does breast cancer originate in utero? Lancet 1990;335: 939–940.

106  Linet M, Forman MR, Anderson L, et al: Gene-environment interactions in the etiology of childhood cancer: report of a workgroup. Submitted.

107  Hennessey E, Alberman E: Intergenerational influences affecting birth outcome. Birthweight for gestational age in the children of the 1958 British Birth Cohort. Pediatr Perinatal Epidemol 1998;12:S45–S60.

108  Rossouw JE, Anderson GL, Prentice RL, et al: Writing Group for the Women's Health Initiative Investigators: Risks and benefits of estrogen plus progestin in healthy postmenopausal women: principal results from the women's health initiative randomized controlled trial. JAMA 2002;288:321–333.

109  Bernstein L: Epidemiology of endocrine-related risk factors for breast cancer. J Mammary Gland Biol Neoplasia 2002;7:3–15.

110  Petridou E, Panagiotopoulou K, Katsouyanni K, et al: Tobacco smoking, pregnancy estrogens, and birth weight. Epidemiology 1990;1:247–250.

111  Kaijser M, Granath F, Jacobsen G, et al: Maternal pregnancy estriol levels in relation to anamnestic and fetal anthropometric data. Epidemiology 2000;11:315–319.

112  Wuu J, Hellerstein S, Lipworth L, et al: Correlates of pregnancy oestrogen, progesterone and sex hormone-binding globulin in the USA and China. Eur J Cancer Prev 2002;11:283–293.

113  Chellakooty M, Vangsgaard K, Larsen T, et al: A longitudinal study of intrauterine growth and the placental growth hormone (GH)-insulin-like growth factor I axis in maternal circulation: association between placental GH and fetal growth. J Clin Endocrinol Metab 2004;89: 384–391.

114  Spencer JA, Chang TC, Jones J, et al: Third trimester fetal growth and umbilical venous blood concentrations of IGF-1, IGFBP-1, and growth hormone at term. Arch Dis Child Fetal Neonatal Ed, 1995;73:F87–F90.

115  Wang HS, Lim J, English J, et al: The concentration of insulin-like growth factor-I and insulin-like growth factor-binding protein-1 in human umbilical cord serum at delivery: relation to fetal weight. J Endocrinol 1991;129:459–464.

116  Verhaeghe J, Van Bree R, Van Herck E, et al: C-peptide, insulin-like growth factors I and II, and insulin-like growth factor binding protein-1 in umbilical cord serum: correlations with birth weight. Am J Obstet Gynecol 1993;169:89–97.

117  Bernstein IM, Goran MI, Copeland KC: Maternal insulin sensitivity and cord blood peptides: relationships to neonatal size at birth. Obstet Gynecol 1997;90:780–783.

118  Ochoa R, Zarate A, Hernandez M: Serum leptin and somatotropin components correlate with neonatal birth weight. Gynecol Obstet Invest 2001;52:243–247.

119  Jones JI, Clemmons DR: Insulin-like growth factors and their binding proteins: biological actions. Endocr Rev 1995;16:3–34.

120  Rosen CJ: Serum insulin-like growth factors and insulin-like growth factor-binding proteins: clinical implications. Clin Chem 1999;45:1384–1390.

121  Yu H, Levesque MA, Khosravi MJ, et al: Associations between insulin-like growth factors and their binding proteins and other prognostic indicators in breast cancer. Br J Cancer 1996; 74:1242–1247.

122 Yu H, Rohan T: Role of the insulin-like growth factor family in cancer development and progression. J Natl Cancer Inst 2000;92:1472–1489.
123 Hu X, Juneja SC, Maihle NJ, Cleary MP: Leptin – a growth factor in normal and malignant breast cells and for normal mammary gland development. J Natl Cancer Inst 2002;94: 1704–1711.
124 McConway MG, Johnson D, Kelly A, et al: Differences in circulating concentrations of total, free and bound leptin relate to gender and body composition in adult humans. Ann Clin Biochem 2000;37:717–723.
125 Klebanoff MA, Mills JL, Berendes HW: Mother's birth weight as a predictor of macrosomia. Am J Obstet Gynecol 1985;153:253–257.
126 Johnson JW, Longmate JA, Frentzen B: Excessive maternal weight and pregnancy outcome. Am J Obstet Gynecol 1992;167:353–372.
127 Hennessy E, Alberman E: Intergenerational influences affecting birth outcome. I. Birthweight for gestational age in the children of the 1958 British birth cohort. Paediatr Perinat Epidemiol 1998;12:45–60.
128 Boulet SL, Alexander GR, Salihu HM, Pass M: Macrosomic births in the united states: determinants, outcomes, and proposed grades of risk. Am J Obstet Gynecol 2003;188: 1372–1378.
129 Kramer MS, Morin I, Yang H, et al: Why are babies getting bigger? Temporal trends in fetal growth and its determinants. J Pediatr 2002;141:538–542.
130 Morton NE: The inheritance of human birth weight. Ann Hum Genet 1955;20:125–134.
131 Magnus P: Further evidence for a significant effect of fetal genes on variation in birth weight. Clin Genet 1984;26:289–296.
132 Jablonka E: Epigenetic epidemiology. Int J Epidemiol 2004;33:929–935.
133 Martin JA, Hamilton BE, Sutton PD, et al: Births: final data for 2002. Natl Vital Stat Rep 2003;52:1–113.
134 Coutinho R, David RJ, Collins JW Jr: Relation of parental birth weights to infant birth weight among African Americans and whites in Illinois: a transgenerational study. Am J Epidemiol 1997;146:804–809.
135 Klebanoff MA, Graubard BI, Kessel SS, Berendes HW: Low birth weight across generations. JAMA 1984;252:2423–2427.
136 McCormack VA, dos Santos Silva I, De Stavola BL, et al: Fetal growth and subsequent risk of breast cancer: results from long term follow up of Swedish cohort. BMJ 2003;326:248.
137 dos Santos Silva I, De Stavola BL, Hardy RJ, et al: Is the association of birth weight with premenopausal breast cancer risk mediated through childhood growth? Br J Cancer 2004;91: 519–524.
138 Kaijser M, Akre O, Cnattingius S, Ekbom A: Preterm birth, birth weight, and subsequent risk of female breast cancer. Br J Cancer 2003;89:1664–1666.
139 Ahlgren M, Melbye M, Wohlfahrt J, Sorensen TIA: Growth patterns and the risk of breast cancer in women. N Engl J Med 2004;351:1619–1626.
140 Ekbom A, Hsieh CC, Lipworth L, et al: Intrauterine environment and breast cancer risk in women: a population-based study. J Natl Cancer Inst 1997;89:71–76.
141 Titus-Ernstoff L, Egan KM, Newcomb PA, et al: Early life factors in relation to breast cancer risk in postmenopausal women. Cancer Epidemiol Biomarkers Prev 2002;11:207–210.
142 Michels KB, Trichopoulos D, Robins JM, et al: Birthweight as a risk factor for breast cancer. Lancet 1996;348:1542–1546.
143 Lahmann PH, Gullberg B, Olsson H, et al: Birth weight is associated with postmenopausal breast cancer risk in Swedish women. Br J Cancer 2004;12:12.
144 Sanderson M, Shu XO, Jin F, et al: Weight at birth and adolescence and premenopausal breast cancer risk in a low-risk population. Br J Cancer 2002;86:84–88.
145 Sanderson M, Williams MA, Daling JR, et al: Maternal factors and breast cancer risk among young women. Paediatr Perinat Epidemiol 1998;12:397–407.
146 Sanderson M, Williams MA, Malone KE, et al: Perinatal factors and risk of breast cancer. Epidemiology 1996;7:34–37.
147 Mellemkjaer L, Olsen ML, Sorensen HT, et al: Birth weight and risk of early-onset breast cancer (Denmark). Cancer Causes Control 2003;14:61–64.
148 Vatten LJ, Maehle BO, Lund Nilsen TI, et al: Birth weight as a predictor of breast cancer: a case-control study in Norway. Br J Cancer 2002;86:89–91.

149 Hodgson ME, Newman B, Millikan RC: Birthweight, parental age, birth order and breast cancer risk in African-American and white women: a population-based case-control study. Breast Cancer Res 2004;6:R656–R667.

150 Innes K, Byers T, Schymura M: Birth characteristics and subsequent risk for breast cancer in very young women. Am J Epidemiol 2000;152:1121–1128.

151 Le Marchand L, Kolonel LN, Myers BC, Mi MP: Birth characteristics of premenopausal women with breast cancer. Br J Cancer 1988;57:437–439.

152 Singh GK; Yu SM: Birthweight differentials among Asian Americans. Am J Public Health 1994;84:1444–1449.

153 Service RF: New role for estrogen in cancer? Science 1998;279:1631–1633.

154 Vatten LJ, Romundstad PR, Trichopoulos D, Skjaerven R: Pregnancy related protection against breast cancer depends on length of gestation. Br J Cancer 2002;87:289–290.

155 Ekbom A, Erlandsson G, Hsieh C, et al: Risk of breast cancer in prematurely born women. J Natl Cancer Inst 2000;92:840–841.

156 Sanderson M, Williams MA, White E, et al: Validity and reliability of subject and mother reporting of perinatal factors. Am J Epidemiol 1998;147:136–140.

157 Panagiotopoulou K, Katsouyanni K, Petridou E, et al: Maternal age, parity, and pregnancy estrogens. Cancer Causes Control 1990;1:119–124.

158 Bernstein L, Depue RH, Ross RK, et al: Higher maternal levels of free estradiol in first compared to second pregnancy: early gestational differences. J Natl Cancer Inst 1986;76:1035–1039.

159 Janerich DT, Hayden CL, Thompson WD, et al: Epidemiologic evidence of perinatal influence in the etiology of adult cancers. J Clin Epidemiol 1989;42:151–157.

160 Forman MR, Meirik O, Berendes HW: Delayed childbearing in Sweden. JAMA 1984;252:3135–3139.

161 Rothman KJ, MacMahon B, Lin TM, et al: Maternal age and birth rank of women with breast cancer. J Natl Cancer Inst 1980;65:719–722.

162 Thompson WD, Janerich DT: Maternal age at birth and risk of breast cancer in daughters. Epidemiology 1990;1:101–106.

163 Janerich DT, Thompson WD, Mineau GP: Maternal pattern of reproduction and risk of breast cancer in daughters: results from the Utah Population Database. J Natl Cancer Inst 1994;86:1634–1639.

164 Newcomb PA, Trentham-Dietz A, Storer BE: Parental age in relation to risk of breast cancer. Cancer Epidemiol Biomarkers Prev 1997;6:151–154.

165 Weiss HA, Potischman NA, Brinton LA, et al: Prenatal and perinatal risk factors for breast cancer in young women. Epidemiology 1997;8:181–187.

166 Colditz GA, Willett WC, Stampfer MJ, et al: Parental age at birth and risk of breast cancer in daughters: a prospective study among US women. Cancer Causes Control 1991;2:31–36.

167 Zhang Y, Cupples LA, Rosenberg L, et al: Parental ages at birth in relation to a daughter's risk of breast cancer among female participants in the Framingham Study (United States). Cancer Causes Control 1995;6:23–29.

168 Odegard RA, Vatten LJ, Nilsen ST, et al: Risk factors and clinical manifestations of pre-eclampsia. Am J Gynecol 2000;107:1410–1416.

169 Broughton Pipkin F, Rubin PC: Pre-eclampsia – the 'disease of theories'. Br Med Bull 1994;50: 381–396.

170 Vatten LJ, Skjaerven R: Is preeclampsia more than one disease? Obstet Gynecol Surv 2004; 59:645–646.

171 Xiong X, Demianczuk NN, Buekens P, Saunders LD: Association of preeclampsia with high birth weight for age. Am J Obstet Gynecol 2000;183:148–155.

172 Odegard RA, Vatten LJ, Nilsen ST, et al: Preeclampsia and fetal growth. Obstet Gynecol 2000;96:950–955.

173 Goland RS, Tropper PJ, Warren WB, et al: Concentrations of corticotrophin-releasing hormone in the umbilical-cord blood of pregnancies complicated by pre-eclampsia. Reprod Fertil Dev 1995;7:1227–1230.

174 Parker CR Jr, Hankins GD, Carr BR, et al: The effect of hypertension in pregnant women on fetal adrenal function and fetal plasma lipoprotein-cholesterol metabolism. Am J Obstet Gynecol 1984;150:263–269.

175 Vatten LJ, Odegard RA, Nilsen ST, et al: Relationship of insulin-like growth factor-I and insulin-like growth factor binding proteins in umbilical cord plasma to preeclampsia and infant birth weight. Obstet Gynecol 2002;99:85–90.

176 Odegard RA, Vatten LJ, Nilsen ST, et al: Umbilical cord plasma leptin is increased in preeclampsia. Am J Obstet Gynecol 2002;186:427–432.

177 Troisi R, Potischman N, Johnson CN, et al: Estrogen and androgen concentrations are not lower in the umbilical cord serum of pre-eclamptic pregnancies. Cancer Epidemiol Biomarkers Prev 2003;12:1268–1270.

178 Halhali A, Tovar AR, Torres N, et al: Preeclampsia is associated with low circulating levels of insulin-like growth factor I and 1,25-dihydroxyvitamin D in maternal and umbilical cord compartments. J Clin Endocrinol Metab 2000;85:1828–1833.

179 Tamimi R, Lagiou P, Vatten LJ, et al: Pregnancy hormones, pre-eclampsia, and implications for breast cancer risk in the offspring. Cancer Epidemiol Biomarkers Prev 2003;12:647–650.

180 Laivuori H, Tikkanen MJ, Ylikorkala O: Hyperinsulinemia 17 years after preeclamptic first pregnancy. J Clin Endocrinol Metab 1996;81:2908–2911.

181 Polednak AP, Janerich DT: Characteristics of first pregnancy in relation to early breast cancer: a case-control study. J Reprod Med 1983;28:314–318.

182 Thompson WD, Jacobson HI, Negrini B, Janerich DT: Hypertension, pregnancy, and risk of breast cancer. J Natl Cancer Inst 1989;81:1571–1574.

183 Troisi R, Weiss HA, Hoover RN, et al: Pregnancy characteristics and maternal risk of breast cancer. Epidemiology 1998;9:641–647.

184 Vatten LJ, Romundstad PR, Trichopoulos D, Skjaerven R: Pre-eclampsia in pregnancy and subsequent risk for breast cancer. Br J Cancer 2002;87:971–973.

185 Innes KE, Byers TE: First pregnancy characteristics and subsequent breast cancer risk among young women. Int J Cancer 2004;112:306–311.

186 Paltiel O, Friedlander Y, Tiram E, et al: Cancer after pre-eclampsia: follow up of the Jerusalem perinatal study cohort. BMJ 2004;328:919.

187 Holdsworth RJ, Chamings RJ: Measurement of progestagen and oestrogen levels in human breast milk. Br Vet J 1983;139:59–60.

188 Bittner JJ: Some possible effects of nursing on the mammary gland tumor incidence in mice. Science 1936;84:162.

189 Spiegelman S, Burny A, Das MR, et al: Synthetic DNA-RNA hybrids and RNA-RNA duplexes as templates for the polymerases of the oncogenic RNA viruses. Nature 1970;228:430–432.

190 Hallam N, McAlpine L, Puszczynska E, Bayliss G: Absence of reverse transcriptase activity in monocyte cultures from patients with breast cancer. Lancet 1990;336:1079.

191 Levine PH, Mesa-Tejada R, Keydar I, et al: Increased incidence of mouse mammary tumor virus-related antigen in Tunisian patients with breast cancer. Int J Cancer 1984;33:305–308.

192 Sarkar NH, Moore DH: On the possibility of a human breast cancer virus. Nature 1972;236:103–106.

193 Hendershot GE: Trends in breast-feeding. Pediatrics 1984;74:591–602.

194 Ryan AS: The resurgence of breastfeeding in the United States. Pediatrics 1997;99:E12.

195 Ahluwalia IB, Morrow B, Hsia J, Grummer-Strawn L: M. Who is breast-feeding? Recent trends from the pregnancy risk assessment and monitoring system. J Pediatr 2003;142:486–491.

196 Forman MR, Fetterly K, Graubard BI, Wooton KG: Exclusive breast-feeding of newborns among married women in the United States: the National Natality Surveys of 1969 and 1980. Am J Clin Nutr 1985;42:864–869.

197 Forman S: Infant Nutrition. Philadelphia, Saunders, 1967.

198 Freudenheim JL, Marshall JR, Graham S, et al: Exposure to breastmilk in infancy and the risk of breast cancer. Epidemiology 1994;5:324–331.

199 Brinton LA, Hoover R, Fraumeni JF Jr: Reproductive factors in the aetiology of breast cancer. Br J Cancer 1983;47:757–762.

200 Ekbom A, Hsieh CC, Trichopoulos D, et al: Breast-feeding and breast cancer in the offspring. Br J Cancer 1993;67:842–845.

201 Winikoff B, Myers D, Laukaran VH, Stone R: Overcoming obstacles to breast-feeding in a large municipal hospital: applications of lessons learned. Pediatrics 1987;80:423–433.

202 Titus-Ernstoff L, Egan KM, Newcomb PA, et al: Exposure to breast milk in infancy and adult breast cancer risk. J Natl Cancer Inst 1998;90:921–924.

203 Michels KB, Trichopoulos D, Rosner BA, et al: Being breastfed in infancy and breast cancer incidence in adult life: results from the two nurses' health studies. Am J Epidemiol 2001; 153:275–283.

204 Butte NF: The role of breastfeeding in obesity. Pediatr Clin North Am 2001;48:189–198.

205 Gillman MW, Rifas-Shiman SL, Canargo CA, et al: Risk of overweight among adolescents who were breastfed as infants. JAMA 2001;285:2461–2467.

206 Dewey KG: Is breastfeeding protective against child obesity? J Hum Lact 2003;19:9–18.

207 Guo SS, Roche AF, Chumlea WC, et al: The predictive value of childhood body mass index values for overweight at age 35 y. Am J Clin Nutr 1994;59:810–819.

208 Whitaker RC, Wright JA, Pepes MS, et al: Predicting obesity in young adulthood and parental obesity. N Engl J Med 1997;337:869–873.

209 van den Brandt PA, Spiegelman D, Yaun SS, et al: Pooled analysis of prospective cohort studies on height, weight, and breast cancer risk. Am J Epidemiol 2000;152:514–527.

210 Birch LL, Fisher JO: Development of eating behaviors among children and adolescents. Pediatrics 1998;101:539–549.

211 Lucas A: Programming by early nutrition: An experimental approach. J Nutr 1998;128: 401S–406S.

212 Birch LL: Psychological influences on the childhood diet. J Nutr 1998;128(suppl): 407S–410S.

213 Birch LL, Fisher JO: Mothers' child-feeding practices influence daughters' eating and weight. Am J Clin Nutr 2000;71:1054–1061.

214 Hediger ML, Overpeck MD, Kuczmarski RJ, Ruan WJ: Association between infant breast-feeding and overweight in young children. JAMA 2001;285:2453–2460.

215 Ong KK, Ahmed ML, Emmett PM, et al: Association between postnatal catch-up growth and obesity in childhood: prospective cohort study. BMJ 2000;320:967–971.

216 Ong K, Kratzsch J, Kiess W, Dunger D: Circulating IGF-I levels in childhood are related to both current body composition and early postnatal growth rate. J Clin Endocrinol Metab 2002;87:1041–1044.

217 Fall CH, Pandit AN, Law CM, et al: Size at birth and plasma insulin-like growth factor-1 concentrations. Arch Dis Child 1995;73:287–293.

218 Fall CH, Clark PM, Hindmarsh PC, et al: Urinary GH and IGF-I excretion in nine year-old children: relation to sex, current size and size at birth. Clin Endocrinol (Oxf) 2000;53: 69–76.

219 Gunnell D, Okasha M, Smith GD, et al: Height and cancer risk: a systematic review. Epidemiol Rev 2001;23:313–342.

220 Adebamowo CA, Ogundiran TO, Adenipekun AA, et al: Obesity and height in urban Nigerian women with breast cancer. Ann Epidemiol 2003;13:455–461.

221 Li CI, Malone KE, White E, Daling JR: Age when maximum height is reached as a risk factor for breast cancer among young US women. Epidemiology 1997;8:559–565.

222 Li CI, Stanford JL, Daling JR: Anthropometric variables in relation to risk of breast cancer in middle-aged women. Int J Epidemiol 2000;29:208–213.

223 De Stavola BL, dos Santos Silva I, McCormack V, et al: Childhood growth and breast cancer. Am J Epidemiol 2004;159:671–682.

224 Alberman E, Filakti H, Williams S, et al: Early influences on the secular change in adult height between the parents and children of the 1958 birth cohort. Ann Hum Biol 1991;8: 127–136.

225 Zadik Z, Borondukov E, Zung A, Reifen R: Adult height and weight of breast-fed and bottle-fed Israeli infants. J Pediatr Gastroenterol Nutr 2002;37:462–467.

226 Position of The American Dietetic Association: promotion of breastfeeding (1997). J Am Diet Assoc 1997;97:662–666.

227 Weinderpass E, Girddley G, Persson I, et al: Risk of endometrial and breast cancer in patients with diabetes mellitus. Int J Cancer 1997;71:360–363.

228 Wolf I, Sadetzki S, Caton R, et al: Diabetes mellitus and breast cancer. Lancet Oncol 2005;6: 103–111.

229 Talamini R, Francheschi S, Favero A, et al: Selected medial conditions and risk of breast cancer. Br J Cancer 1997;75:1699–1703.

230 Michels KB, Solomon CG, Hu FB, et al: Type 2 diabetes and subsequent incidence of breast cancer in the nurses' health study. Diabetes Care 2003;26:1752–1758.

231 Nardon E, Buda I, Stanta G, et al: Insulin-like growth factor system gene expression in women with type 2 diabetes and breast cancer. J Clin Pathol 2003;56:599–604.
232 Schrezenmeir J, Jagla A: Milk and diabetes. J Am Coll Nutr 2000;19:176S–190S.
233 Perez-Bravo F, Oyarzun A, Carrasco E, et al: Duration of breast feeding and bovine serum albumin antibody levels in type 1 diabetes: a case-control study. Pediatr Diabetes 2003;4: 157–161.
234 Couper JJ, Steele C, Beresford S, et al: Lack of association between duration of breast-feeding or introduction of cow's milk and development of islet autoimmunity. Diabetes 1999;48: 2145–2149.
235 Ziegler AG, Schmid S, Huber D, et al: Early infant feeding and risk of developing type 1 diabetes-associated autoantibodies. JAMA 2003;290:1721–1728.
236 Virtanen SM, Rasanen L, Aro A, et al: Feeding in infancy and the risk of type 1 diabetes mellitus in Finnish children. The 'Childhood Diabetes in Finland' Study Group. Diabet Med 1992;9:815–819.
237 Kimpimaki T, Erkkola M, Korhonen S, et al: Short-term exclusive breastfeeding predisposes young children with increased genetic risk of type 1 diabetes to progressive beta-cell autoimmunity. Diabetologia 2001;44:63–69.
238 Pettitt DJ, Forman MR, Hanson RL, et al: Breastfeeding and incidence of non-insulin-dependent diabetes mellitus in pima Indians. Lancet 1997;350:166–168.
239 Yajnik CS: Early life origins of insulin resistance and type 2 diabetes in India and other Asian countries. J Nutr 2004;134:205–210.
240 Young TK, Martens PJ, Taback SP, et al: Type 2 diabetes mellitus in children. Arch Pediatr Adolesc Med 2002;156:651–655.
241 Ravelli AC, van der Meulen JH, Osmound C, et al: Infant feeding and adult glucose tolerance, lipid profile, blood pressure, and obesity. Arch Dis Child 2000;82:248–252.
242 Wasmuth HE, Hubert K: Cow's milk immune-mediated diabetes. Proc Nutr Soc 2000;59: 573–579.
243 Gerstein HC: Cow's milk exposure and type I diabetes mellitus. A critical overview of the clinical literature. Diabetes Care 1994;17:13–19.
244 Norris JM, Scott FW: A meta-analysis of infant diet and insulin-dependent diabetes mellitus: do biases play a role? Epidemiology 1996;7:87–92.
245 Norris JM, Barriga K, Klingensmith G, et al: Timing of initial cereal exposure in infancy and risk of islet autoimmunity. JAMA 2003;290:1713–1720.
246 Fronczak CM, Baron AE, Chase HP, et al: In utero dietary exposures and risk of islet autoimmunity in children. Diabetes Care 2003;26:3237–3242.
247 Dewey K: Is breastfeeding protective against child obesity? J Hum Lact 2003;19:9–17.
248 Lucas A, Blackburn AM, Aynsley-Green A, et al: Breast vs bottle: endocrine responses are different with formula feeding. Lancet 1980;1(8181):1267–1269.
249 Singhal A, Farooqi IS, O'Rahilly S, et al: Early nutrition and leptin concentrations in later life. Am J Clin Nutr 2002;75:993–999.
250 Bandini LG, Must A, Spadano JL, et al: Relation of body composition, parental overweight, pubertal stage, and race-ethnicity to energy expenditure among premenarcheal girls. Am J Clin Nutr 2002;76:1040–1047.
251 Kuczmarski RJ, Flegal KM, Campbell SM, et al: Increasing prevalence of overweight among US adults. The National Health and Nutrition Examination Survey, 1960–1991. JAMA 1994;272:205–211.
252 Sun SS, Schubert CM, Chumlea WC, et al: National estimates of the timing of sexual maturation and racial differences among US children. Pediatrics 2002;110:911–919.
253 Adair L, Gordon-Larsen P: Maturational timing and overweight prevalence in US adolescent girls. Am J Public Health 2001;91:642–644.
254 Herrinton LJ, Husson G: Relation of childhood height and later risk of breast cancer. Am J Epidemiol 2001; 154:618–623.

Lucas A, Sampson HA (eds): Primary Prevention by Nutrition Intervention in Infancy and Childhood.
Nestlé Nutr Workshop Ser Pediatr Program, vol 57, pp 203–221,
Nestec Ltd., Vevey/S. Karger AG, Basel, © 2006.

# Long-Chain Polyunsaturated Fatty Acids in Early Life: Effects on Multiple Health Outcomes

## A Critical Review of Current Status, Gaps and Knowledge

*Mary S. Fewtrell*

MRC Childhood Nutrition Research Centre, Institute of Child Health, London, UK

The efficacy and safety of long-chain polyunsaturated fatty acid (LC-PUFA) supplementation of infant formula has become one of the major and most controversial areas of infant nutrition research over the past 15 years. This paper reviews the current status of research into the effects of LC-PUFA supplementation during early life on functional outcome, and identifies the major areas that contribute to ongoing uncertainties in the field. A brief review of LC-PUFA biochemistry, function and status during fetal life and infancy is first provided as background.

## LC-PUFA Biochemistry and Functions

The long-chain fatty acids, docosahexaenoic acid (DHA; 22:6n-3) and arachidonic acid (AA; 20:4n-6) are synthesized from their parent 18-carbon precursors, α-linolenic acid (ALA; 18:3n-3) and linoleic acid (LA; 18:2n-6), respectively, by a process of desaturation and chain elongation (fig. 1). The two families of essential fatty acids, n-3 and n-6, are defined by the position of the double bond closest to the methyl terminal of the fatty acid. Mammalian cells are unable to insert double-bonds more proximal to the methyl terminal than the seventh carbon atom, hence ALA and LA are nutritionally essential. Once ingested, n-3 and n-6 fatty acids are not interconvertible, but the different families compete for the same enzymes in the metabolic cascade to their respective LC-PUFAs with n-3 having greater conversion efficiency, emphasizing the importance of the dietary ratio of 18:n-3 to 18:n-6.

The importance of LC-PUFAs as constituents of cell membranes has long been appreciated. LC-PUFAs of the n-3 family, especially DHA, are particularly

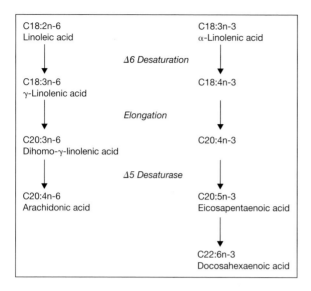

**Fig. 1.** Formation of LC-PUFA from essential fatty acid precursors.

important in the nervous system and retina where they are essential for normal functioning. In contrast, AA is more ubiquitous and found in cell membranes in a number of organs. It is increasingly recognized, however, that LC-PUFAs are not simply structural lipids, but highly bioactive substances with multiple actions [1]. For example, they affect membrane fluidity, influencing insulin sensitivity and, potentially, transmembrane signaling. Both families of LC-PUFAs are also precursors for the formation of prostaglandins and eicosanoids. In general, those derived from the n-6 family are both more potent and often antagonistic to those derived from the n-3 family. Thus n-6-derived eicosanoids are pro-inflammatory and adipogenic whereas n-3 eicosanoids are anti-inflammatory and may reduce fat deposition, again emphasizing the importance of balance between the two families. Polyunsaturated fatty acids also affect gene transcription, influencing the abundance or activity of transcription factors that play a major role in hepatic carbohydrate, fatty acid, triglyceride, cholesterol and bile acid metabolism. This is a rapidly evolving field in LC-PUFA research. Although currently the significance of these different actions of LC-PUFAs for functional outcomes may be unclear, the increasing appreciation of the bioactive nature of LC-PUFAs has served to highlight the multiple potential effects of supplementation. Thus, although historically studies of LC-PUFA supplementation in infants were directed at improving cognitive and visual outcomes, there is now increasing interest in plausible effects on other aspects of health.

## LC-PUFA Accretion in the Fetus and Infant

LC-PUFA accretion is maximal during late fetal life and infancy. The total amount of DHA in the brain increases approximately 30-fold during this period, coinciding with the most rapid period of brain growth. DHA accumulation also occurs in liver and adipose tissue during the last trimester and may be used to fuel rapid postnatal brain growth. It is thought that most LC-PUFA is obtained from the mother, possibly by selective placental transfer, rather than being synthesized by the fetus.

Breastfed infants receive a preformed supply of LC-PUFAs since both DHA and AA and their 18-carbon precursor fatty acids are present in human milk. Concentrations of AA are fairly constant across and within populations. In contrast, DHA concentrations show more marked variability depending on maternal diet, in particular the intake of fish and marine products. Thus, breast milk DHA concentrations in North America tend to fall between 0.2 and 0.4% whilst mean concentrations in Inuit and Japanese women may reach 1.4% [2]. The effect of ingested fish on breast milk DHA is acute and lasts 1–2 days.

Historically, infant formulas did not contain preformed LC-PUFAs, leaving the infant to synthesize them from ALA and LA. Both term and preterm infants possess the necessary enzymes to synthesize LC-PUFAs and initial concerns that these enzymes might be functionally immature in preterm infants appear to be unfounded. However, both ALA and LA are readily oxidized to provide energy, and if an infant is in negative energy balance it is unlikely that they will be used to synthesize LC-PUFAs.

The issue of whether preformed LC-PUFAs should be added to infant formulas has been extensively investigated over the past 15 years, whilst there has been more limited research into the effects of supplementing the mother during pregnancy or lactation. The following section summarizes the current status of this research.

## LC-PUFA Supplementation and Outcome

*LC-PUFA Supplementation during Pregnancy*

Randomized trials show that supplementing women with fish oil during pregnancy generally improves their LC-PUFA status and results in higher n-3 in cord blood. However, the evidence that improved biochemical status has functional benefits for the infant is less persuasive. Malcolm et al. [3] found no effect of maternal fish oil supplementation on infant visual outcomes up to 6 months post-term, although DHA status in cord blood itself predicted visual outcome. Helland et al. [4] randomized mothers to fish oil versus corn oil during pregnancy and lactation (up to 3 months postpartum) and showed no effect on infant growth or development. However, in a 4-year follow-up of a group of these children, those whose mothers had received fish oil during pregnancy had significantly higher scores on the Kaufmann ABC test of mental ability than those from the corn oil group. This finding emphasizes the importance of longer-term follow-up, both to detect 'emerging' effects and also to permit the use of more specific and discriminating tests of cognition.

There has been some interest in the possibility that maternal supplementation with n-3 might reduce the development of atopy in the infant, based on the hypothesis that a relative increase in proinflammatory n-6 fatty acids and a decrease in anti-inflammatory n-3 fatty acids might be involved in pathogenesis. In the large, prospective, population-based Avon Longitudinal Study of Pregnancy and Childhood cohort, maternal and cord blood fatty acid concentrations were not significantly related to the frequency of atopic symptoms in the offspring during early childhood [5]. However, in a randomized trial of fish oil supplementation during pregnancy in atopic mothers, fish oil resulted in increased n-3 status of the infant at birth and lower concentrations of some cytokines [6]. These infants were 3 times less likely to show a positive skin-prick reaction to egg at 12 months of age, and, although the frequency of atopic dermatitis was not significantly different between randomized groups, the fish oil group had less severe disease. These findings suggest a potential protective effect of n-3 supplementation on the development of atopy in high-risk infants.

### LC-PUFA Supplementation during Lactation

Breast milk n-3 concentrations are related to infant plasma and erythrocyte phospholipid DHA concentrations in a saturable curvilinear manner. Above a breast milk DHA content of approximately 0.8% fatty acids, no further increase in infant DHA status is seen [7]. Supplementation of lactating mothers with fish oil has also been shown to result in higher breast milk DHA content, but to date there is no evidence that this results in improved functional outcome in the infant. In Danish breastfeeding mothers, fish oil supplementation resulted in increased breast milk DHA content (a 3-fold increase at 4 months). However, although visual outcome was significantly related to breast milk DHA content, the fish oil group did not show improved visual outcome at 2 or 4 months [8].

### LC-PUFA and Infant Nutrition

Several observational studies in both term and preterm infants have shown that infants who are breastfed have higher LC-PUFA concentrations in blood [9, 10] and tissue [11, 12] than infants fed unsupplemented formulas. Furthermore, infants who receive LC-PUFA-supplemented formulas show improved blood and tissue LC-PUFA status [13]. However, it has been more difficult to establish that these undoubted biochemical effects are accompanied by beneficial effects on clinical and functional outcome in either group of infants.

Most research in this field has focused on adding preformed LC-PUFAs to infant formulas. The alternative strategy of increasing the concentration of the precursors, particularly ALA, has not been adequately investigated as no studies have compared formulas with enough difference in ALA content. Current recommendations for the levels and ratio of LA and ALA in infant formulas are based essentially on the ranges observed in samples of human milk, and were made in the absence of data on functional or clinical outcomes. In a randomized trial of healthy term infants assigned formulas with LA:ALA ratios of either 10:1 or 5:1, those fed the lower ratio formula had higher plasma and red blood cell DHA concentrations than those fed the higher ratio formula; however, concentrations did not reach those seen in a parallel group of breastfed infants [14]. No differences were seen in visual acuity or growth up to 34 weeks of age. These data, together with those from two other studies [15, 16] suggest that the LA:ALA ratio must be lowered to <6:1 to improve the DHA status of formula-fed infants.

## Randomized Trials of LC-PUFA Supplementation and Clinical Outcome

*Preterm Infants*

A systematic review for the Cochrane Library, last updated in November 2003, summarized the result of randomized trials of LC-PUFA supplementation and outcome in preterm infants [17]. Based on 11 identified trials, the authors concluded that no long-term effects of LC-PUFA supplementation were demonstrated on either developmental outcome or growth. However, they commented that infants enrolled in the trials were relatively mature and healthy preterm infants, and that marked differences in assessment schedules and methodology, dose and source of supplementation and fatty acid composition of the control formula between trials made direct comparisons difficult. Indeed, individual trials showed a range of beneficial, neutral or even apparently detrimental effects of supplementation on visual outcome, cognitive development and/or growth.

In a separate meta-analysis, SanGiovanni et al. [18] focused on short-term visual outcome and concluded that LC-PUFA supplementation was associated with short-term benefits for visual resolution acuity at 2 and 4 months, but whether supplementation confers lasting advantages remained to be determined.

The inconsistent results observed in LC-PUFA supplementation trials are well demonstrated by the results of three large studies that our own center has conducted or participated in. In the first study, supplementation was associated with improved cognitive development in the sub-group of infants with birth weights of <1,250 g, but had no effect on growth [19]. In a second trial, no effect of supplementation was seen on developmental outcome but supplemented infants were shorter than controls at 18 months post-term [20]. In the third study, published since the most recent update of the

Cochrane review, we showed that LC-PUFA supplementation was associated with greater weight and length gain up to 9 months [21]. Benefits were greater in boys, who showed greater length gain and higher Bayley Mental Development Index (MDI) at 18 months in boys. A further study published recently in abstract form [22] also reported significantly higher Bayley MDI and Psychomotor Developmental Index at 18 months post-term in preterm infants supplemented with LC-PUFAs during the first 12 months.

*Term Infants*

The Cochrane Systematic Review on LC-PUFA supplementation and outcome in term infants was last updated in June 2001 [23]. Based on 10 identified trials, it concluded that there was little evidence that supplementation produced benefits for visual or general developmental outcome, or influenced growth. However, as in preterm infants, the results of individual trials varied considerably. For example, a small randomized trial (approximately 20 infants per group) reported a 7-point higher Bayley MDI in supplemented infants [24] whereas our larger trial (approximately 150 infants per group) found no significant difference between groups using the same developmental test [25]. When the results of these two trials were combined, no overall effect on developmental outcome was observed. Another large trial (approximately 110 infants per group), reported in abstract form [26], also found no significant effect of LC-PUFA supplementation on developmental outcome at 12 months of age.

Since the last update of the Cochrane Systematic Review, data from an 18-month follow-up of infants randomized to unsupplemented versus LC-PUFA-supplemented formulas for the first 2 months of life have been published [27], showing no effect of supplementation on Bayley developmental scores, or on neurological status assessed using an examination specifically designed to detect minor abnormalities. A separate meta-analysis of trials evaluating effects on visual resolution acuity was also performed, and concluded there was some evidence of better visual outcome in LC-PUFA-supplemented infants at 2 months, but that longer-term effects remained to be determined [28].

Importantly, longer-term follow-up data are also now starting to appear. Auestad et al. [29] reported a 39-month follow-up of infants from one randomized trial in which no effect of either DHA or combined DHA/AA supplementation had been seen during the first year. At 14 months of age, infants supplemented with DHA alone had shown lower scores on tests of vocabulary production and comprehension than infants fed unsupplemented formula or those who were breastfed. At 39 months of age, about half of the infants were tested using a more comprehensive range of developmental tests (assessing overall IQ but also receptive and expressive vocabulary and visuomotor function). Scores were not significantly different between control and supplemented groups: in fact the 2 supplemented groups had both raw and adjusted IQ scores that were 3–4 points lower than those of the control and breastfed groups. The study had approximately 35 infants per randomized group, and was not powered to detect this effect size (approximately 0.3 SD).

Our own (unpublished) data from a 5- to 6-year follow-up of term infants randomized to LC-PUFA-supplemented versus unsupplemented formula during infancy shows a significant 5-point deficit in IQ for previously supplemented infants using the WISC-IQ (approximately 90 infants per group); no difference was seen between groups at the 18-month follow-up using the Bayley scales of infant development. It is not clear whether this finding reflects the emergence of an effect since the previous follow-up, or whether the global developmental test used during infancy was too insensitive to detect differences. It is possible that effects of LC-PUFA supplementation on cognitive outcome are subtle, perhaps affecting information processing. Willatts et al. [30] previously showed that term infants randomized to LC-PUFA-supplemented formula showed better performance on a specific test of problem-solving at age 10 months, and a more recent (unpublished) follow-up of this cohort shows that the supplemented group performs better on a test of information processing at age 5 years.

All of the studies discussed so far involved LC-PUFA supplementation of infant formula fed from birth. More recent studies have also addressed the effect of LC-PUFA supplementation later in infancy. In two separate trials, infants randomized to LC-PUFA-supplemented formulas when they stopped breastfeeding at either 6 weeks [31] of age or 4–6 months [32] of age had significantly better visual acuity up to 1 year of age than those weaned onto unsupplemented formula. These findings suggest that term infants may benefit from a supply of LC-PUFAs beyond the first few weeks or months of life, at least for visual outcome.

Two studies have examined the effects of providing additional DHA in weaning foods. Breast- and formula-fed infants who received DHA-enriched egg yolks four times per week from 6–12 months had higher red cell DHA levels at 12 months than those fed standard egg yolks or no egg [33]. Hoffman et al. [34] randomized breastfed infants to receive either 1 jar/day of weaning foods containing DHA-enriched egg yolk, or control baby food, between 6 and 12 months. Although many infants in both groups continued to breastfeed for a mean of 9 months, by 12 months those receiving the DHA-enriched weaning foods showed an increase in red cell DHA levels (compared to a fall in the control group). They also showed a greater increase in visual acuity resolution over the trial period.

## Current Status and Limitations of LC-PUFA Supplementation Trials

It is apparent from the preceding discussion that, despite good theoretical reasons to anticipate beneficial effects of LC-PUFA supplementation, and often despite clear evidence of biochemical effects, it has been difficult to establish clinical efficacy. A number of factors that may contribute to the inconsistent findings are discussed below.

(1)   The minimum requirement for LC-PUFA is unknown, making it difficult to determine an optimal level for supplementation. This difficulty is compounded by the variable concentrations of LC-PUFAs, particular DHA, in breast milk.

(2)   LC-PUFA supplementation trials are heterogeneous in terms of the intervention used. Although described generically as 'LC-PUFA-supplemented formulas', these products vary in so many respects that the value of directly comparing or pooling trials in a conventional meta-analyses is questionable. Thus 'LC-PUFA-supplemented formulas' differ in:

(a)   The content of precursor 18-carbon fatty acid and ratio of 18:n-3/18:n-6

(b)   The 'dose' of DHA and AA

The concentration of LC-PUFA in formulas used in intervention trials has varied considerably. The potential contribution of this factor to the inconsistent trial results has recently been considered by 2 groups, using a novel approach relating functional outcomes to the relative 'dose' of DHA [2, 35]. This necessitates making assumptions, for example, about the conversion efficiency of ALA to DHA, and the DHA content and intake of breast milk. Nevertheless, both analyses concluded that trials with the greatest difference in 'DHA equivalents' between control and intervention groups, or between breast- and formula-fed groups, showed the greatest difference in outcome. This provides some support for the concept of a 'dose response' between DHA intake (whether as ALA or DHA) and outcome.

(c)   The source of LC-PUFAs

It is plausible that factors associated with the LC-PUFA supplementation strategy used may influence outcome, independent of an actual effect of the LC-PUFAs themselves. Because it is not possible to simply add unesterified LC-PUFAs to infant formula, they are added as components of triglycerides and/or phospholipids in the form of oils which may derive from a number of sources. In each case, the introduction of the oil may add not only the desired LC-PUFA, but also other fatty acids and non-lipid components. For example, formulas may differ in the content of cholesterol, choline and other fatty acids and LC-PUFAs; it is not known whether these differences might themselves affect outcome.

A further issue relates to the positional distribution of LC-PUFAs. For example, in single-cell oils, triglycerides may be present with LC-PUFA esterified in the sn-1 position, or with two or three DHA or AA molecules. Such triglycerides are unphysiological and not seen in human milk. The extent to which the positional distribution of LC-PUFAs influences digestion, absorption or the subsequent actions of LC-PUFAs is unclear.

(3)   LC-PUFA supplementation trials are heterogeneous in terms of the outcome measures and testing methods used. Lauritzen et al. [2] found that those trials using an objective 'electrical' measure of visual function such as visual evoked response or electro-retinogram were more likely to report a positive effect of supplementation than trials that used behaviorally based tests such as Teller acuity cards. Similarly, the few studies using a more specific test of cognitive function, such as problem-solving ability, were more likely to see positive effects of LC-PUFA supplementation than those using a global test of infant development such as the Bayley.

(4)   Small sample size was undoubtedly an issue in the early supplementation trials which were generally powered to detect differences in biochemical outcomes, not clinical or functional endpoints. However, this criticism does not apply to many more recent studies which have shown similarly inconsistent results.

In addition to these problems, two further issues deserve mention. Firstly, there is currently a lack of long-term data on the efficacy and safety of LC-PUFA interventions. The limited longer-term cognitive data have in fact highlighted the potential for unexpected adverse effects that were either not present or undetectable during infancy. Such late emergence of programmed effects has previously been reported for other health outcomes in both animals and in humans.

Secondly, there are few data on the effects of LC-PUFAs on other aspects of health. Such effects are entirely plausible given the bioactive nature of LC-PUFAs. Areas that have received limited attention include the following.

*Cardiovascular Risk*

LC-PUFA supplementation was associated with lower low-density lipoprotein cholesterol concentrations at age 4 months in one study [36]. LC-PUFA intake may also influence the fatty acid composition of skeletal muscle membranes, which in turn affects insulin resistance. Baur et al. [37] found higher LC-PUFA concentrations in the skeletal muscle of breastfed infants, and this was associated with lower fasting blood glucose concentrations. Whether this has longer term consequences for glucose and insulin metabolism is unknown.

Forsyth et al. [38] reported lower blood pressure at age 6 years in children randomized to LC-PUFA-supplemented versus control formula during infancy. The magnitude of the effect (approximately 3-mm Hg) was similar to that reported in individuals who were breastfed rather than formula-fed. In contrast to these findings, in a randomized trial of maternal fish oil supplementation during lactation, offspring blood pressure at 2.5 years of age was not influenced by the assignment [39]. The studies differed not only in the age at follow-up, but also the study population; the Forsyth study enrolled formula-fed infants, and the control group received no LC-PUFAs, whereas in the second study, all infants were breastfed so the difference between groups in total LC-PUFA intake was less.

## Type-1 Diabetes

A case-control study in Norway [40] with 545 cases of childhood-onset type-1 diabetes and 1,668 controls reported a significantly lower risk of diabetes associated with taking cod liver oil supplements during the first year of life (OR 0.74; 95% CI 0.56, 0.99). This could represent an anti-inflammatory effect of n-3 LC-PUFAs present in cod liver oil.

## Atopy

The Childhood Asthma Prevention Study [41] involved 616 children at high risk of atopy who were enrolled antenatally in a two-by-two factorial randomized trial to examine the effect of both n-3 fatty acid supplementation and house dust mite allergen avoidance. There was a significant (10%) reduction in cough at 3 years of age in atopic children in the active diet group, but no difference in non-atopic children.

## Conclusions

There are good theoretical reasons why LC-PUFA supplementation should have beneficial effects on cognitive and visual outcome and, given the bioactive nature of LC-PUFAs, on other outcomes. Despite this, clinical efficacy and safety have not been established. Research into LC-PUFA supplementation has highlighted issues of more general relevance to the design and testing of infant formula. Firstly, there may be potential pitfalls in generically grouping 'supplemented' products, when the supplementation strategy and process may itself influence outcome. Secondly, the current situation in which LC-PUFAs are added to most infant formulas despite inconsistent effects on outcome in clinical trials raises the more difficult issue of what constitutes evidence of acceptable efficacy and safety for the addition of novel ingredients to formulas, as well as the potential role of post-marketing surveillance.

Differences in intervention, design and outcome measures between LC-PUFA supplementation trials make conventional meta-analyses difficult to interpret. Approaches relating the dose of LC-PUFAs to outcome across trials may be more useful, but currently it may be best to evaluate efficacy and safety for individual formulations. A final consideration is that, whilst formulas have been supplemented with LC-PUFAs with the objective of improving visual and cognitive outcome, the bioactive nature of LC-PUFAs and the effects on other health outcomes now being observed in longer-term follow-up studies raise the possibility that LC-PUFA supplementation may one day be recommended for other reasons entirely.

# References

1 Lapillone A, Clarke SD, Heird WC: Plausible mechanisms for effects of long chain polyunsaturated fatty acids on growth. J Pediatr 2003:143:S9–S16.
2 Lauritzen L, Hansen HS, Jorgensen MH, Michaelsen KF: The essentiality of long chain n-3 fatty acids in relation to development and function of the brain and retina. Prog Lipid Res 2001;40:1–94.
3 Malcolm CA, McCulloch DL, Montgomery C, et al: Maternal docosahexaenoic acid supplementation during pregnancy and visual evoked potential development in term infants: a double blind, prospective, randomized trial. Arch Dis Child Fetal Neonatal Ed 2003;88: 383–390.
4 Helland IB, Smith L, Saarem K, et al: Maternal supplementation with very-long-chain n-3 fatty acids during pregnancy and lactation augments children's IQ at 4 years of age. Pediatrics 2003;111:39–44.
5 Newson RB, Shaheen SO, Henderson AJ, et al: Umbilical cord and maternal blood red cell fatty acids and early childhood wheezing and eczema. J Allergy Clin Immunol 2004;114: 531–537.
6 Dunstan JA, Mori TA, Barden A, et al: Fish oil supplementation in pregnancy modifies neonatal allergen-specific immune responses and clinical outcomes in infants at high risk of atopy: A randomized, controlled trial. J Allergy Clin Immunol 2003;112:1178–1184.
7 Lauritzen L, Jorgensen MH, Hansen HS, Michaelsen KF: Fluctuations in human milk long-chain PUFA levels in relation to dietary fish intake. Lipids 2002;37:237–244.
8 Lauritzen L, Jorgensen MH, Mikkelsen TB, et al: Maternal fish oil supplementation in lactation: effect on visual acuity and n-3 fatty acid content of infant erythrocytes. Lipids 2004;39: 195–206.
9 Carlson SE, Rhodes PG, Rao VS, Goldgar DE: Effect of fish oil supplementation on the n-3 fatty acid content of red blood cell membranes in preterm infants. Pediatr Res 1987;21: 507–510.
10 Jorgensen MH, Hernell O, Lund P, et al: Visual acuity and erythrocyte docosahexanoic acid status in breast-fed and formula-fed term infants during the first four months of life. Lipids 1996;31:99–105.
11 Farquharson J, Cockburn F, Patrick WA, et al: Infant cerebral cortex phospholipid fatty acid composition and diet. Lancet 1992;340:810–813.
12 Makrides M, Neumann MA, Byard RW, et al: Fatty acid composition of the brain, retina and erythrocytes in breast- and formula-fed infants. Am J Clin Nutr 1994;60:180–194.
13 Auestad N, Montalto MB, Hall RT, et al: Visual acuity, erythrocyte fatty acid composition and growth in term infants fed formula with long chain polyunsaturated fatty acids for one year. Pediatr Res 1997;41:1–10.
14 Makrides M, Jeffrey B, Lien EL: A randomized trial of different ratios of linoleic to α-linolenic acid in the diet of term infants: effects on visual function and growth. Am J Clin Nutr 2000;71: 120–129.
15 Clark KJ, Makrides M, Neumann MA, Gibson RA: Determination of the optimal ratio of linoleic to α-linolenic acid in infant formulas. J Pediatr 1992;120:S151–S158.
16 Jensen CL, Prager TC, Fraley JK, et al: Effect of dietary linoleic:α-linolenic acid ratio on growth and visual function of term infants. J Pediatr 1997;131:200–209.
17 Simmer K, Patole S: Longchain polyunsaturated acid supplementation in preterm infants. Cochrane Review. The Cochrane Library. Chichester, Wiley, 2004, issue 3.
18 SanGiovanni JP, Parra-Cabrera S, Colditz GA, et al: Meta-analysis of dietary essential fatty acids and long-chain polyunsaturated fatty acids as they relate to visual resolution acuity in healthy preterm infants. Pediatrics 2000;105:1292–1298.
19 O'ConnorD, Hall R, Adamkin D, et al: Growth and development in preterm infants fed long-chain polyunsaturated fatty acids: a prospective, randomized controlled trial. Pediatrics 2001;108:359–371.
20 Fewtrell MS, Morley R, Abbott RA, et al: Double-blind randomised trial of long-chain polyunsaturated fatty acid supplementation in formula fed to preterm infants. Pediatrics 2002;110: 73–82.
21 Fewtrell MS, Abbott RA, Kennedy K, et al: Randomized double-blind trial of LCPUFA-supplementation using fish oil and borage oil in preterm infants. J Pediatr 2004;144:471–479.

22 Clandinin M, VanAerde J, Antonson D, et al: Formulas with docosahexaenoic acid (DHA) and arachidonic acid (AA) promote better growth and development scores in very-low-birth-weight infants. Pediatr Res 2002;51:187A–188A.
23 Simmer K: Longchain polyunsaturated fatty acid supplementation in infants born at term. Cochrane Review. The Cochrane Library, Chichester, Wiley, 2004, issue 3.
24 Birch EE, Garfield S, Hoffman DR, et al: A randomized controlled trial of early dietary supply of long-chain polyunsaturated fatty acids and mental development in term infants. Dev Med Child Neurol 2000;42:174–181.
25 Lucas A, Stafford M, Morley R, et al: Efficacy and safety of long-chain poly-unsaturated fatty acid supplementation of infant-formula milk: a randomised trial. Lancet 1999;354:1948–1954.
26 Carlson SE, Mehra S, Nagey WJ, et al: Growth and development of term infants fed formulas with docosahexaenoic acid (DHA) from algal oil or fish oil and arachidonic acid (ARA) from fungal oil. Pediatr Res 1999;45:278A.
27 Bouwstra H, Dijck-Brouwer DAJ, Boehm G, et al: Long-chain polyunsaturated fatty acids and neurological developmental outcome at 18 months in healthy term infants. Acta Paediatr Scand 2005;94:26–32.
28 SanGiovanni JP, Berkey CS, Dwyer JT, Colditz GA: Dietary essential fatty acids, long-chain polyunsaturated fatty acids, and visual resolution acuity in healthy fullterm infants: a systematic review. Early Hum Dev 2000;57:165–188.
29 Auestad N, Scott DT, Janowsky JS, et al: Visual, cognitive and language assessments at 39 months: a follow-up study of children fed formulas containing long-chain polyunsaturated fatty acids to 1 year of age. Pediatrics 2003;112:177–183.
30 Willatts P, Forsyth JS, DiModugno MK, et al: Effect of long-chain polyunsaturated fatty acids in infant formula on problem solving at 10 months of age. Lancet 1998;352:688–691.
31 Birch EE, Hoffman DR, Castenade YS, et al: A randomized controlled trial of long-chain polyunsaturated fatty acid supplementation of formula in term infants after weaning at 6 wk of age. Am J Clin Nutr 2002;75:570–580.
32 Hoffman DR, Birch EE, Castenade YS, et al: Visual function in breast-fed term infants weaned to formula with or without long-chain polyunsaturates at 4 to 6 months: A randomized clinical trial. J Pediatr 2003;142:669–677.
33 Makrides M, Hawkes JS, Neumann MA, Gibson RA: Nutritional effect of including egg yolk in the weaning diet of breast-fed and formula-fed infants: a randomized controlled trial. Am J Clin Nutr 2002;75:1084–1092.
34 Hoffman DR, Theuer RC, Castenada YS, et al: Maturation of visual acuity is accelerated in breast-fed term infants fed baby food containing DHA-enriched egg yolk. J Nutr 2004;134:2307–2313.
35 Uauy R, Hoffman DR, Mena P, et al: Term infant studies of DHA and ARA supplementation on neurodevelopment: results of randomised controlled trials. J Pediatr 2003;143:S17.
36 Agostoni C, Riva E, Scaglioni S, et al: Dietary fats and cholesterol in Italian infants and children. Am J Clin Nutr 2000;72(suppl):1384S–1391S.
37 Baur LA, O'Connor J, Pan DA, et al: The fatty acid composition of skeletal muscle membrane phospholipids: its relationship with the type of feeding and plasma glucose levels in young children. Metabolism 1998;47:106–112.
38 Forsyth JS, Willatts P, Agostoni C, et al: Long chain polyunsaturated fatty acid supplementation in infant formula and blood pressure in later childhood: follow up of a randomized controlled trial. BMJ 2003;326:953–958.
39 Ulbak J, Lauritzen L, Hansen HS, Michaelsen KF: Diet and blood pressure in 2.5-y-old Danish children. Am J Clin Nutr 2004;79:1095–1102.
40 Stene LC, Joner G, Norwegian Childhood Diabetes Study Group: Use of cod liver oil during the first year of life is associated with lower risk of childhood-onset type 1 diabetes: a large, population-based, case-control study. Am J Clin Nutr 2003;78:1128–1134.
41 Peat JK, Mihrdhahi S, Kemp AS, et al: Three-year outcomes of dietary fatty acid modification and house dust mite reduction in the Childhood Asthma Prevention Study. J Allergy Clin Immunol 2004;114:807–813.

## Discussion

*Dr. Björkstén:* Thank you for a very elegant presentation. I have some comments because we have been interested not in mental development but rather in immunology and allergy. As you may have noticed there is actually a difference in the composition of breast milk that affects the outcome of allergy in the babies, not only that the composition differs between allergic and non-allergic mothers but in fully breastfed babies we could identify certain associations with allergy development independent of maternal allergy. But it wasn't really the levels that we were interested in, it was the ratios between the longest n-3 and the 2–6 series rather than the absolute levels, and it seems quite clear that there is some sort of abnormality but again it is not the total levels. I was wondering to what extent some of these discrepancies that you are reporting are not necessarily the breast milk in different societies, and the other thing is it is the ratio rather than the levels?

*Dr. Fewtrell:* I talked about the approach of DHA equivalents to explain some of the inconsistent results, but another alternative would be to do the same thing with respect to the n-6/n-3 ratio. I suppose the problem is that if you wanted to compare formula-fed and breastfed infants you would not necessarily have the data on the n-6/n-3 ratios in the breastfed infants unless milk samples were collected prospectively.

*Dr. Björkstén:* Yes, but my suggestion is that perhaps in order to really sort things out one would have to go there and have to do that in a sort of multi-dose way.

*Dr. Fewtrell:* I agree and I think it could well be important. I deliberately didn't discuss any of the allergy data in my presentation so as not to overlap with Dr. Hanson's talk.

*Dr. Laron:* Head circumference is measured in babies as a measure of brain growth. Has any analysis been made to find out whether additions of LCPUFA influenced head circumference?

*Dr. Fewtrell:* In our own trials the head circumference hasn't been different between groups even when we have seen differences in weight and length. I am not aware of differences in head growth in other studies.

*Dr. Jensen:* I am not aware of a trial in which a difference in head circumference was observed between a LCPUFA-supplemented and a non-supplemented group.

*Dr. Bernardo:* Would you please comment on the addition of preformed LCPUFA among follow-on formula?

*Dr. Fewtrell:* I am not aware of any randomized trials looking at the effects of LCPUFA supplementation of follow-on formulas – that is, those designed for use beyond 6 months of age. The Birch group performed trials looking at supplementation when mothers stopped breastfeeding at either 6 weeks or 4–6 months and showed apparent benefits of LCPUFA supplementation for visual outcomes during infancy, but I think these trials used standard term formula. There have been two studies looking at LCPUFA supplementation of weaning foods with DHA-enriched eggs, again showing some benefits for DHA status and/or visual function.

*Dr. Saavedra:* Another trend has also arisen with regard to what to do with mothers either during pregnancy or during lactation. As we know there are very big differences between DHA contents in mothers which is particularly dependent on their diet and in many cases on their geographic location. From that point of view, and again with relatively few data, would you care to speculate on whether we should be looking at content in geographic areas and recommending, as we do for some salts and minerals, that mothers should either consume fish or DHA supplementation during pregnancy, lactation or both depending on the area they live in?

*Dr. Fewtrell:* I guess if you wanted to do that you would first need evidence, ideally from randomized trials, that supplementing mothers during pregnancy and lactation improves infant outcome and that the effect differed according to the mother's breast milk DHA content. Perhaps Dr. Jensen would like to comment on his soon-to-be-published trial that provides some evidence that supplementing mothers during lactation may improve their offspring's outcome?

*Dr. Jensen:* We actually used an analogy derived source of DHA. It was a very modest supplementation, 200 mg DHA, from shortly after delivery through 4 months postpartum. We administered some tests of neural development at 12 months of age and saw no differences between the two groups, but at 30 months of age those infants whose mothers had received the DHA supplement had about an 8.5 higher Bailey PDI than those infants whose mothers had received the placebo. What we did as supplementation was basically increase the amount of DHA in human milk from 0.2 to about 0.35% of total fatty acids. We also found that at 5–5.5 years of age those children whose mothers had received the DHA supplement performed better on a test of sustained attention than those children whose mothers received the placebo.

*Dr. Fewtrell:* With regard to pregnancy supplementation with fish or fish oil, ideally you would need to have trials in both low and high fish-consuming populations to see if habitual intake influenced the response to supplementation.

*Dr. Jensen:* I might ask, and this is an open-ended question, I am fishing for your comments, that in trials conducted in term infants the arachidonic acid to DHA ratio varied dramatically. In your large trial it was approximately 1, maybe a little under 1, in the Australian trial it was 1, in two large North American trials it was 3.2–3.5. Willets has pointed out that term trials in which the ratio was between 1.4 and 2 have shown some benefit on some measure of neurodevelopmental or neuropsychological status at least in trials in which the ratio falls outside that range either higher or lower. Any comments about that?

*Dr. Fewtrell:* Although I certainly would advocate looking at potential explanations for inconsistent results, it seems to me that we have to bear in mind the risk of identifying possible spurious explanations, especially when we are talking about one or two trials showing a particular effect, as is the case with the term studies showing positive neurodevelopmental or neuropsychological effects.

*Dr. Chad:* There seems to be an increased epidemic of attention deficit disorders in North America. A lot of children are on drugs to treat this and I was wondering if there are any trials under way to look at the association of DHA versus this as a possible outcome problem?

*Dr. Fewtrell:* Yes, there are certainly trials, and in the UK giving fish oil supplements to children with the aim of improving behavior and school performance is currently quite fashionable. This area wasn't one that I reviewed for the purpose of this presentation. I don't know if anyone else would like to expand on this.

*Dr. Jensen:* I will make a brief comment. We actually conducted a study of DHA supplementation in children with attention-deficit/hyperactivity disorder (ADHD) [1]. These were children between 6 and 11 years of age at strict DSM for our criteria for ADHD diagnosed by one of our developmental pediatricians. They were supplemented with 325 mg DHA/day for several months. The rating scale was given to both the parents and the teachers. They were administered the TOVA which is a computerized test of attention and impulse control, and we found no differences on any measure between the groups, granted this supplementation was started late in their lives, and it was several months of supplementation. There is study from the UK on a group of children with both ADHD and dyslexia as I recall and on a couple of measures, I believe reading ability, I don't recall the details. They did see some benefits perhaps not on attention per se, but I know no more about that.

*Dr. Lucas:* This is a very difficult area, the full-term infant. But it is interesting that advisory groups, for instance the group that advise the FDA, have not come to the conclusion that LCPUFA is established and certainly in term formulas. I think there is more a general agreement that it may be useful in the high-risk preterm infant, and I think that the evidence weighs slightly in favor of visual effects rather than not, but weighs slightly more in favor of adverse and neurodevelopmental effects than positive ones. Then there are two long-term trials showing adverse effects, 5- to 6-point deficit, and I think that the case is not proven. So the issue is whether we think there is enough evidence to make an ad hoc management decision that formula should contain LCPUFA in the present state of knowledge. I don't think that this group should be influenced by vested interests or anything else that should come to dispatch their view on that.

*Dr. Van Dael:* Based on the evidence that you have presented what would be your recommendation for regulations which, as you know, are currently quite a bit under revision. The European Union is revising its regulation for infant formula and follow-on formula and they may make recommendations for LCPUFA fortification. The same will happen at the CODEX level, which shows it to have a global implication. So based on the evidence you presented what would be your recommendation with respect to LCPUFA?

*Dr. Fewtrell:* As I understand it, the SCF, who advise on potential changes to the EU Directive are currently of the opinion that there isn't sufficient evidence to recommend the compulsory addition of LCPUFA to infant formulas, and they have recommended that addition should remain optional. My current reading of the literature is that the evidence for beneficial effects of LCPUFA supplementation in preterm infants may be growing but this is not the case for term infants. If I were evaluating the evidence from scratch, I don't think I would be recommending that LCPUFA be added to term formula, but possibly to preterm formula. I think there is a further generic issue here, and that is how we decide if and when something should be added to a formula. For example, we could specify in scientific terms that we require a certain number of trials in a minimum number of infants to show a desired effect, as was discussed in the context of hypoallergenic formulas yesterday. However, we are talking about evaluating specific products and performing long-term follow-ups. This may not be feasible in the real world. This seems to be a dilemma.

*Dr. Hamburger:* Are you answering that question in terms of required content or permissive content, the addition of LCPUFA?

*Dr. Fewtrell:* I certainly would not say they were required, and I'm not sure I would say they were permissive in term infants based on current evidence. That is my personal opinion.

*Dr. Haschke:* I would like to make a comment, which has probably nothing to do with science but which reflects the real world as it is. There is a parallel development which probably has not too much to do with science, it is marketing of infant formulas, and the train has left the station. Very clever, the producers of LCPUFA, the suppliers have informed the public directly about the benefits, and after a certain while this consistent message has reached the public. So when the consumers were asked, they said, 'yes, this is a perceived benefit, I am ready to pay extra for this perceived added value'. And from that moment onwards, when the first company started to add it, all the other companies, at least in the premium segment of infant formulas, followed. It is interesting, the differences between continents, how sensitive people are to this message. Here in the US it is definitely an issue, in the European Union it is mixed, in Asia it is definitely an issue, it is the main topic in infant formula. So in the near future we probably will not have the chance to make trials without LCPUFA supplementation because they will be everywhere.

*Dr. Fewtrell:* I totally agree that the train has left the station. When I gave a similar presentation recently, someone asked me why we couldn't just take LCPUFA out of infant formulas. In the real world, in the absence of a major demonstrable adverse effect, that is probably not going to happen and I was answering the earlier question as though LCPUFA had not yet been added to formulas. However, they have and I suspect they will stay there.

*Dr. Zeiger:* I am wondering why that train can't be derailed. Certainly faulty information have gone out with many other therapies such as hormonal replacement therapy for women has shown various detrimental effects, attitudes have changed, they are no longer being used to the degree they were used before. If some of the information that you presented today went into the public's hands I think they would be reeducated and I don't think the women would be using these supplemented formulas to feed their children due to great fears associated with it.

*Dr. Fewtrell:* I think it's a very difficult issue in practice because the data are not consistent. For example, some of the longer term effects may be beneficial whereas effects on other outcomes could be adverse. It is very difficult to distill the current data into a clear but simple message for parents.

*Dr. Haschke:* I think there is no reason to discuss this in an emotional way anyway; marketing and medical sciences do not always go hand in hand. I would agree with you, the train can be stopped if there are severe adverse effects of LCPUFA supplementation, then it will be stopped next day, but otherwise it will be very difficult even to deviate the train in a different area.

*Dr. Fewtrell:* It seems to me that in the meantime we should make sure we know what is happening in terms of longer term outcome in these trials. If we have raised some concerns about effects on certain outcomes we must investigate them further in the follow-up of other established studies, and we should also look at the potential benefits for other outcomes.

*Dr. Lucas:* Just to make a comment here, I think what happens here is that a number of things in the past were added to infant formulas such as taurine and nucleotides without any research because evidence-based practice was not the common thing at that time. LCPUFA occurred exactly on the cast of the development of evidence-based practices so most of the work that was done before it then became rather criticized. But nevertheless as has been said, the train left the station at that point and we ended up with that. In fact I think that if the LCPUFA field had just started 5 years later then it would have been caught up in a current of much greater scrutiny of evidence basis.

*Dr. Fewtrell:* I am not sure that even that would have prevented the current situation with LCPUFA supplementation because even if we had specified that we require a certain number of trials in a certain number of infants looking at a particular outcome, we would probably still be left with the same uncertainty. I'm not sure that specifying a certain number of trials is going to be a solution, particularly with something like LCPUFA where many of the issues have to do with the strategy of supplementation. Perhaps that brings us back to the issue of considering different formulations more and not grouping formulas generically.

*Dr. Lucas:* I think we would have been more critical. For instance we have one trial that has been particularly influential in the addition of infant formulas in the United States, it has got about 17–20 subjects in each follow-up and I think we would have been more critical about that now.

*Dr. Jensen:* Speaking of formulations the one large trial in which an adverse long-term effect was observed of course is your trial, and Dr. Lucas in his comments on Wednesday eluded to the fact that there may have been a source issue but no mechanism was tossed out. We do have another European trial and the results have yet to be published with respect to the neuropsychological outcome data but arguably there was what most of us would regard as a positive blood pressure effect at 6 years of age and if you look at the performance of the 6-year-olds on a test that theoretically assesses the speed of central nervous system information processing in a very targeted test, there was a benefit. So I am curious to know about the source, those of you who were involved in the trial feel it was a potential problem.

*Dr. Fewtrell:* Do you want to comment on that Dr. Lucas?

*Dr. Lucas:* We are talking about isolated trials so it is very difficult to have a statistical approach to what sources are good or bad. The problem is that everybody uses a slightly different strategy, this was an egg phospholipid source. We have another trial with a phospholipid source that showed reduced growth and a beneficial effect on neurodevelopment, and there was a trend in preterm infants. So you might say that on the basis of that phospholipids don't look like a very good way to go as far as LCPUFA supplementation is concerned. But really that is not a very well defendable view given that we don't have a very large experience of anything other than probably single-chain oils that are probably used now more than most.

*Dr. Moukarzel:* You answered almost all my questions. You know that the FDA has considered one source of LCPUFA as grass which is generally considered as safe, and this is a particular source. So of course when you talk to us about two studies showing some long-term potential side effects of adding LCPUFA we need really to think as you just said about the source of this LCPUFA. I wonder about this controversy, if we gather all the studies from the same source of LCPUFA, would this controversy still exist? I mean I have the feeling that if we collect all the studies using the same source of LCPUFA, one of these sources will be beneficial whereas the others won't be, and this is probably as you just said in your talk, one of the key questions that we need to look at, not only on how much we are adding but from which source we are adding it, what is the component we are adding, how much EPA we are adding? What would be your comment, and do you still consider the LCPUFA as safe?

*Dr. Fewtrell:* I agree that it is a sensible approach to look at the outcome of trials in relation to the LCPUFA source. In fact, the Gibson group has done a meta-analysis of the effects of LCPUFA supplementation on growth and they did consider the source. But unfortunately when you pool trials for such an analysis you end up looking at the short-term outcomes that are available for most trials, such as growth during the first year. Very few trials have followed the subjects beyond infancy so far, so I don't think it's possible to relate LCPUFA source to longer term outcomes which may potentially be of greater concern.

*Dr. Björkstén:* I have a comment about what Dr. Haschke said regarding this interaction between science and research. If it is indeed the case that the train has left the station and if indeed it is difficult to derail, which I am not sure I agree, then I think I would like to go back to our discussion of yesterday, and that is that probiotics are now on the way of being put into the products and getting on the train and the train is about to start. So I would actually urge people who are involved in these product developments to be quite sure of what they are doing because we don't know if they are entirely safe in early infancy for everyone under every circumstance, and certainly documentation is not there yet. So I would hate to hear in 2 or 3 years the same comment from Dr. Haschke that the train has left the station and we can't do anything about it, you can.

*Dr. Saavedra:* I agree totally with what Dr. Björkstén has just said. I think in part, we need to control the kind of work that we ultimately have to do because the interesting thing here is that if we had all the studies that we would have to do for LCPUFA in terms of doses, ratios, sources, we would end up with a table of permutations of clinical trials that would have essentially no ending. Half of it I do believe has to do with what you communicate and there is no question that when you go to buy food in a store there are foods with benefits and there are those with risks, and they both have benefits and risks, as a matter of fact probably all of them have some benefit and some risk. The way to solve the dilemma when something has already been out in the public versus how to solve dilemmas that may happen as we come to providing and making these foods and different new ingredients available to the public is to continue being as clear as possible as to what the degree of evidence there is, and ultimately that depends on the kind of claims and benefits that both clinicians as well as consumers are educated in. I don't think anybody buying chocolate needs to be educated on the benefits and the risks; would it be any different than what we do with any food and that certainly includes infant foods. The possibility of educating consumers and physicians to the point that both benefits and risks known to that point are there and the possibility of providing adequate choices for both, clinicians and consumers, so that they can decide if they want to take that benefit and know what the potential risks are is what we need to do. And having said that of course it is very complicated to educate everybody.

*Dr. Lucas:* If you were to take for instance the treatment of high blood pressure, it doesn't matter whether it is nice inhibitor or a β-blocker or whatever, we would all agree that dropping blood pressure in people with very raised blood pressure is going to reduce the incidence of strokes, and that is such an important outcome that we are prepared to take some risks and most drugs carry risks. But in infant nutrition risks are not terribly acceptable unless there really is a massive benefit and it is not obvious in the way that the reduction in blood pressure reduces strokes that the incorporation of LCPUFA in the formula produces cognitive benefits. There are data going in both directions, so is any risk acceptable in a situation where you don't have a very obvious benefit in a global public health situation like this, and I just pose that as a rhetorical question.

*Dr. Saavedra:* We should say no risk is acceptable if we know it. The problem is that we are living in a world where we don't know all the benefits and all the risks.

*Dr. Zeiger:* Dr. Saavedra, I would agree there are certainly risks and benefits associated with foods but the analogy with formula I don't think is as strong. With respect to formulas a real trust is expected by mothers that the formula is safe and not associated with risks. Before new nutrients/supplements are added to formulas, one would expect that strong evidence would exist for both safety and efficacy.

*Dr. Chad:* Is that the challenge, to identify if there are target groups that would benefit from this? In other words, as you presented the data globally in terms of meta-analyses there are pros and cons, whatever, but you can tease out certain groups that might benefit and I am not saying they do benefit but they might benefit, and is it the challenge now, if there is a role for this at all, to find which groups would benefit from this and use the educational initiatives to say that it would work for that and not for everybody else, and that is where you could possibly change the direction of the train.

*Dr. Fewtrell:* In an ideal world, yes. A lot of the studies have done sub-group analyses and some have shown for example that you get a greater effect of LCPUFA supplementation in lower birth weight infants, lower gestation infants, or in males. But the findings aren't consistent, so with the current state of knowledge I think it would be difficult to select particular groups of infants who should receive LCPUFA.

*Dr. Hursting:* I was wondering if a reverse translation approach might be useful here. We have had a couple of cases in the cancer field where a couple of trials had unusual findings. Going back to the animal models it has been very important and complex in the number of permutations you have got here, it depends on your animal models for the outcomes you are looking at. I don't know that, it is just a naïve question.

*Dr. Fewtrell:* I don't have particular knowledge of animal models in this field but in principle it sounds like a reasonable approach.

*Dr. Laron:* I would like to ask if reverse experiments have been done because there are no long-term studies on students who are excellent in their university studies and going back to see what their early nutrition was. In this country there are many Asian students with excellent records and I doubt that they had enriched formulas.

*Dr. Fewtrell:* I am not aware.

*Dr. Jensen:* Obviously you are talking about hundreds of potentially confounding factors in such a study.

*Dr. Saavedra:* Just one final comment. I think it is important to go back to the fact that we always want to know risk. We should be absolutely certain that what we try to do has no risk, and there is no question of that in the infant nutrition field, whether it is complementary foods, whether it is infant formula, that an even bigger precedent and almost anything else that we do particularly because of the reason for this meeting, that we are probably making differences that may have extremely long-lasting effects. Unfortunately, on the other hand, we have to accept that when we have taken that not so good path of not breastfeeding we have already accepted a risk, and from that point of view we need to do whatever is best to minimize that risk, and I think that is what we need to do.

*Dr. Fewtrell:* I think an important issue is whether there should be some requirement for long-term follow-up of intervention trials. As this currently isn't the case, it is entirely dependent on individuals to get funding and do the study.

## Reference

1   Voigt RG, Llorente AM, Jensen CL, et al: A randomized, double-blind, placebo-controlled trial of docosahexaenoic acid supplementation in children with attention-deficit/hyperactivity disorder. J Pediatr 2001;139:189–196.

Lucas A, Sampson HA (eds): Primary Prevention by Nutrition Intervention in Infancy and Childhood.
Nestlé Nutr Workshop Ser Pediatr Program, vol 57, pp 223–234,
Nestec Ltd., Vevey/S. Karger AG, Basel, © 2006.

# Perinatal PUFA Intake Affects Leptin and Oral Tolerance in Neonatal Rats and Possibly Immunoreactivity in Intrauterine Growth Retardation in Man

*Lars Å. Hanson*[a], *Marina Korotkova*[a,b], *Mirjana Hahn-Zoric*[a],
*Shakila Zaman*[c], *Aisha Malik*[d], *Rifat Ashraf*[e], *Sylvie Amu*[a],
*Leonid Padyukov*[a], *Esbjörn Telemo*[f], *Birgitta Strandvik*[a]

Departments of [a]Clinical Immunology and [b]Paediatrics, University of Göteborg,
Göteborg, Sweden; [c]Department of Social and Preventive Paediatrics, Fatima Jinnah
Medical College/Sir Ganga Ram Hospital, [d]Department of Obstetrics and Gynecology, King
Edward Medical College, and [e]Department of Social and Preventive Paediatrics,
King Edward Medical College, Lahore, Pakistan, and [f]Department of Rheumatology,
Göteborg University, Göteborg, Sweden

## Effects of Varied PUFA Intake by Pregnant and Lactating Rat Dams on the Neonatal Immune System

The importance of the essential fatty acids (EFAs) for early development has been illustrated in numerous studies. The essentiality of linoleic acid (C18:2n-6) and α-linolenic acid (C18:3n-3) depends on the fact that they cannot be produced by animal cells and that they play a major role in numerous critical tissues and functions. These two fatty acids are also precursors for such vital long-chain polyunsaturated fatty acids (PUFAs) of the n-6 and n-3 series as arachidonic acid and docosahexaenoic acid [1]. The EFAs also play an important role in the immune system for its protective as well as tissue-damaging capacities. EFAs are important components in all cell membranes and modify membrane fluidity, function and microenvironment [2]. Thus they are important for the number and function of cellular receptors, their binding to ligands and the signal transduction process. Several cellular receptors form the basis for the function of the innate as well as the adaptive immune system.

The EFAs are also required for production of several components with important functions, such as prostaglandins and leukotrienes. They are mediators of tissue reactivity forming part of the inflammatory processes, e.g. bronchial reactivity in asthma [3]. They also affect cells of the immune system, such as macrophages and lymphocytes, and may influence the production of cytokines and major effectors such as antibodies [4]. This forms the background to suggestions that dietary supplementation with α-linolenic acid may decrease the chemotactic response of neutrophils and monocytes and reduce their production of inflammatory mediators thereby dampening inflammation.

## Effects of EFAs on the Production of Leptin in Suckling Rat Offspring

The hormone leptin is mainly produced by white adipose tissue (WAT), and also by placenta [5], mammary glands [6], and neonatal adipose tissue [7]. In addition to the regulation of food intake and energy expenditure, leptin is involved in several physiologic processes, including immune responses. Being structurally similar to IL-6 cytokines, it binds to receptors which belong to the class-I cytokine receptors. Leptin stimulates proliferation and differentiation of hematopoietic cells [8] and upregulates monocyte/macrophage functions [9]. It modifies T-cell responses with increasing T-helper-1 (Th1: IL-2, IFN-γ) and suppressing T-helper-2 (Th2: IL-4, IL-10) cytokine production [10]. A recent study showed that increased serum leptin in mice was related to enhanced metacholine responsiveness and IgE responses on sensitization with ovalbumin (OA) [11]. This was proposed to link obesity and allergy in man.

Thus, leptin might play an important role in the induction and maintenance of immune and inflammatory responses, especially vital in the perinatal period. Dietary fat quantity affects perinatal serum leptin levels. Increased maternal fat intake raises plasma leptin concentrations in neonatal rats and affects hypothalamus-pituitary-adrenal responsiveness in neonates and prepubertal rats [12].

Recently, we have shown that dietary fat quality modulates serum leptin levels in rat offspring during the suckling period [13, 14]. During late gestation and throughout lactation, rats were fed a control, or an EFA-deficient (EFAD) diet. The weight of inguinal WAT depots and the serum leptin levels of the EFAD offspring were significantly lower than in the control pups during the whole suckling period. In addition, leptin mRNA levels in inguinal WAT were reduced in the EFAD pups compared with the control pups at 3 weeks of age. Milk leptin levels were higher in the EFAD dams than in the control dams at 3 weeks of lactation.

We have also demonstrated the effects of dietary n-6/n-3 PUFA ratios on serum leptin levels in the postnatal period [15]. During late gestation and throughout lactation the rats were fed a diet containing linseed oil (n-3 diet), sunflower oil (n-6 diet), or soybean oil (n-6/n-3 diet). As a result the ratio of n-6/n-3 PUFAs in breast milk and in the serum phospholipids of the offspring were significantly different in the n-3, the n-6/n-3 and the n-6 dietary groups (table 1). Decreased serum leptin levels were observed in the offspring receiving

**Table 1.** The major PUFA composition of breast milk lipids and serum phospholipids of the rat offsprings at 3 weeks of age from dams fed diets with different ratios of n-6 and n-3 fatty acids

| Fatty acids (mol%) | Dietary groups | | |
|---|---|---|---|
| | n-3 | n-6/n-3 | n-6 |
| Breast milk (n = 7–8) | | | |
| 18:2n-6 | $9.4 \pm 0.8^a$ | $31.1 \pm 2.7^b$ | $35.1 \pm 2.3^b$ |
| 18:3n-3 | $26.3 \pm 1.6^a$ | $3.1 \pm 0.4^b$ | $0.0 \pm 0.0^b$ |
| 20:4n-6 | $0.31 \pm 0.06^a$ | $1.6 \pm 0.4^b$ | $1.4 \pm 0.3^b$ |
| 22:6n-3 | $0.45 \pm 0.1^a$ | $0.62 \pm 0.1^b$ | $0.24 \pm 0.13^b$ |
| AA/DHA | $0.7 \pm 0.1^a$ | $2.5 \pm 0.6^a$ | $8.1 \pm 4.7^b$ |
| n-6/n-3 | $0.4 \pm 0.0^a$ | $8.9 \pm 0.7^a$ | $206.3 \pm 101.5^b$ |
| Serum at 3 weeks of age (n = 8–10) | | | |
| 18:2n-6 | $21.7 \pm 5.2^a$ | $28.0 \pm 1.5^b$ | $28.4 \pm 2.7^b$ |
| 18:3n-3 | $3.2 \pm 1.1^a$ | $0.42 \pm 0.1^b$ | $0.04 \pm 0.01^c$ |
| 20:4n-6 | $7.5 \pm 2.2^a$ | $13.2 \pm 1.0^b$ | $14.3 \pm 1.5^b$ |
| 20:5n-3 | $3.2 \pm 1.1^a$ | $0.09 \pm 0.01^b$ | $0.02 \pm 0.01^b$ |
| 22:6n-3 | $5.6 \pm 2.0^a$ | $4.6 \pm 0.4^a$ | $2.6 \pm 0.6^b$ |
| AA/DHA | $1.4 \pm 0.2^a$ | $2.9 \pm 0.2^b$ | $5.8 \pm 1.4^c$ |
| n-6/n-3 | $2.5 \pm 0.4^a$ | $8.3 \pm 0.7^b$ | $17.5 \pm 4.4^c$ |

Values given as mean ± SD. Different letters indicate significant differences between dietary groups ($p < 0.05$). Multiple comparisons made with Kruskal-Wallis and Dunn's tests.

Adapted from Korotkova et al. [15, 16].

the n-3 diet compared with the n-6/n-3 group (fig. 1). Body weight, body length, inguinal fat pad weight, and adipocyte size of the offspring receiving the n-3 diet were also significantly lower during the whole suckling period compared with n-6/n-3 fed offspring. The mean serum leptin levels of the n-6 offspring were between the other two groups, but not different from either group. No differences were observed in the milk leptin content between the groups.

These results suggest the importance of the EFA intake and the n-6/n-3 PUFA ratios in the maternal diet for adipose tissue growth and for maintaining adequate serum leptin levels in the offspring.

### Effect of EFAs on the Appearance of Oral Immunological Tolerance in Suckling Rat Offspring

During the neonatal period the gastrointestinal tract is exposed to a wide variety of microbial and food-related antigens. Usually, oral exposure to food antigens results in induction of oral tolerance, a state of specific immunological hyporesponsiveness upon further exposure to antigens [16]. Several

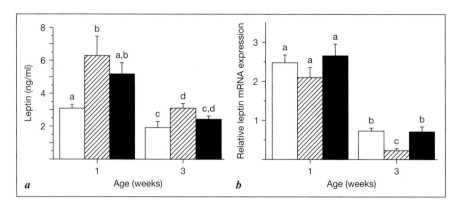

**Fig. 1.** The serum leptin levels (**a**) and the relative expression of leptin mRNA (**b**) in inguinal white adipose tissue (mean ± SE) of the offspring of dams on the n-3 diet (□), the n-6/n-3 diet (▨) or the n-6 diet (■). Values with unlike letters are significantly different: $p < 0.05$.

immunological mechanisms contribute to the induction and maintenance of oral tolerance such as anergy, clonal deletion and active suppression. In adult rats, active suppression is associated with the existence of regulatory suppressor cells (Treg/Th3) in the draining lymph nodes after immunization that are triggered by a specific antigen and responsible for the release of the antigen-non-specific suppressive cytokine TGF-β [17]. Consequently immune responses to other antigens in the close vicinity are diminished [18].

Failure to develop immunological tolerance may lead to an immune response resulting in allergic sensitization to food antigens [19]. Factors important for the induction or breakdown of oral tolerance in the neonatal period are poorly understood. In neonatal rodents oral exposure to antigen can induce tolerance or priming depending on antigen nature and dose, and on the maturity of the immune system [20].

Infant nutrition is one of the most powerful environmental factors that determine early growth and development. The breast milk contains numerous factors, including PUFAs, which may promote the development of the infant's immune system [21] and affect the immune responsiveness to antigens [4, 22]. The levels of n-6 and n-3 PUFAs in the breast milk are determined to a large extent by the maternal diet [23]. Thus, variation in the PUFA intake in the maternal diet might significantly modulate neonatal development of immunological tolerance and gastrointestinal sensitization to food antigens.

Dietary intake of PUFA has been shown to influence the tolerance induction in adult mice [24]. Furthermore, different effects of dietary n-6 and n-3 PUFA on Th1- and Th2-like responses and the mechanisms of oral tolerance to OA have been demonstrated [25].

Recently we found that the dietary intake of EFAs had no effect on the induction of oral tolerance in adult rats, but influenced the development of tolerance in neonatal rats to a food antigen fed to their dams during lactation [26]. During late gestation and throughout lactation rats were fed either a diet supplemented with EFAs, or an EFAD diet. The rat offsprings were subsequently exposed to OA either via the milk at 10–16 days (neonatal rats), or as adults via the drinking water at 7–9 weeks of age.

In rats, which were only exposed to these diets as adults, oral exposure to OA, lead to antigen-specific suppression of the delayed-type hypersensitivity (DTH) response and IgG antibody response to OA. Tolerance to OA was observed in both the EFA-supplemented and EFAD groups, and was accompanied by a reduction in DTH and IgG antibody responses to an unrelated antigen due to bystander suppression [18]. Thus, the oral tolerance was maintained and mediated at least partly by an active suppression mechanism in the adult animals of both the dietary groups.

In the offspring of the dams fed the EFAD diet, antigen exposure via the milk resulted in suppression of the serum antibody levels and DTH response against OA indicating induction of oral tolerance. Higher TGF-β mRNA levels in the draining lymph nodes suggested mediation via Treg cells. In contrast, OA exposure of the dams fed the EFA-supplemented diet did not result in suppressed OA responses of their offspring. Interestingly, a markedly higher ratio of n-6/n-3 PUFA in serum phospholipids was detected in the offspring of the dams fed the EFA-supplemented diet. Since they did not develop oral tolerance to the OA fed their dams, it seems that the dietary n-6/n-3 PUFA ratio is one factor important for the induction, or failure, of oral tolerance.

In further studies we demonstrated the effects of n-6/n-3 PUFA ratios in the maternal diet on the induction of neonatal oral tolerance in the rat offspring [27]. During late gestation and throughout lactation rats were fed the n-3, n-6 or n-6/n-3 diets. At 10–16 days of age the rat offsprings were subsequently exposed, or not, to OA via the milk. In the offspring on the n-3 diet the exposure to OA via the milk resulted in lower DTH and antibody responses against both OA and human serum albumin, compared to those offsprings not exposed to OA, indicating induction of oral tolerance (fig. 2). The lymph nodes draining the immunization site were also less enlarged in the offspring exposed to OA via their dams, suggesting that in the offsprings on the n-3 diet the tolerance was mediated, at least partly, by an active suppression mechanism. In contrast, the offsprings on the n-6/n-3 diet did not show tolerance. A further increase in the n-6 PUFAs in the maternal diet was associated with the induction of oral tolerance in the n-6 group of the offsprings. However, bystander suppression was not observed in the offsprings receiving the n-6 diet, suggesting that oral tolerance may be mediated by anergy. These results suggest that the ratio of the n-6/n-3 PUFAs in the maternal diet might affect the mechanisms of neonatal oral tolerance and are in line with the data of Harbige et al. [25] demonstrating that dietary levels of the n-6/n-3 PUFAs influence the mechanism of oral tolerance in adult mice.

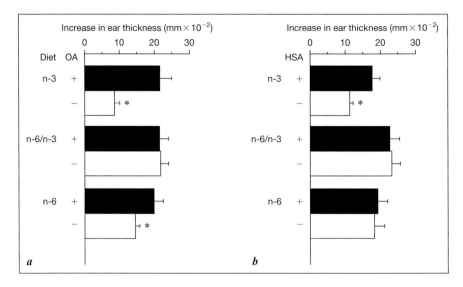

**Fig. 2.** DTH responses against OA (**a**) and human serum albumin (HSA; **b**) in the offspring of dams fed the diet with different ratios of n-6/n-3 fatty acids and either exposed to OA orally (+) before immunization or not (–) (mean ± SE). *Results are significantly different in the group exposed to OA orally ($p < 0.05$) from the group not exposed to OA within the dietary group. Multiple comparisons made with Kruskal-Wallis and Dunn's tests.

Thus the quality of fatty acid ingested by the mother may have effects on the development of immunological tolerance to dietary antigens in the offspring.

## Possible Role of PUFA and Cytokine Aberrations in Intrauterine Growth Retardation

Intrauterine growth retardation (IUGR) occurs in about 1–4% of Swedish deliveries, but is much more common in developing countries like Pakistan [28]. There are many known risk factors like maternal undernutrition, infections, etc., but the etiological mechanisms have not been definitely defined. Impaired outgrowth of trophoblasts into the decidua after implantation of the egg, remodeling the spiral arteries, has been considered crucial. At the same time it is clear that the maternal immune response against the fetus plays a central role in directing implantation, trophoblast growth, hormone production, etc. [28]. On the other hand the maternal response must be modified, or it can destroy the fetus. The likely role of regulatory CD4+CD25+ T cells is suggested by their abundance in human decidua and capacity to suppress

CD4+CD25– T cells by cell–cell contact [29]. The possible role during pregnancy of immunosuppressive cytokines from regulatory T cells such as IL-10 and/or TGF-β has not been defined.

## PUFAs in IUGR

The transformation of PUFAs from mother to fetus starts early in pregnancy and is of great importance for normal development. In IUGR, abnormalities of PUFAs have been described, both as EFAD in 20% of the infants [30] and as significantly changed ratios between fetal and maternal fatty acids compared to normal pregnancies [31]. The linoleic acid ratio was increased and the PUFA ratio was decreased, but a higher concentration of n-6 than n-3 fatty acids was reported in fetal serum phospholipids. Since PUFAs from phospholipids are substrates for prostaglandin synthesis, it might be of interest that significantly higher amounts of $PGE_2$ have been found in human amniotic fluid at the time when atopic sensitization might occur [32]. It is still highly controversial how atopy develops but additional data support an important role of fatty acids.

## Immunological Aberrations in IUGR

In the placentas of 34 normal Swedish mothers we found the expected predominance of Th2/Treg cytokines needed to balance the mother's immune response against the placenta/fetus. In 20 IUGR placentas the mRNA for IL-10 in the decidua was low ($p < 0.05$) and for IL-8 high ($p < 0.05$; table 2) [33]. It was debated whether the low maternal IL-10 might result in an increased immune attack against the fetus thus impairing the proper infiltration of the spiral arteries by trophoblasts inhibiting the formation of the placenta and hampering the nutrition of the fetus. IL-8, which is proinflammatory and a strong chemotaxin for neutrophils, may add to damaging inflammation. In the presence of preeclampsia together with IUGR, mRNA for IL-10 in the decidua was still low ($p = 0.05$) and the proinflammatory IL-6 elevated ($p < 0.05$). Without preeclampsia the IL-8 was increased ($p < 0.01$). Combining the data on mRNA for IL-8/IL-10 in the trophoblasts and decidua from the 20 IUGR and 7 cases of small-for-date deliveries gave an increased ratio ($p < 0.01$).

In another study of cytokines in the decidua from 45 IUGR and 55 non-IUGR pregnancies of Pakistani mothers with multiple risk factors for IUGR, we found decreases in mRNA for IL-10 ($p < 0.0001$) and IL-12 ($p < 0.008$) comparing IUGR to non-IUGR placentas (table 2). In contrast, TGF-β was increased ($p < 0.009$) [28] a similar decrease in mRNA for IL-10 ($p < 0.03$), but increase in TGF-β ($p < 0.009$), was found compared to non-IUGR placentas.

**Table 2.** Cytokine mRNA expression in IUGR placentas (with or without complications in pregnancy) and controls: summary of significant differences (p values)

| Groups | n | Decidua | | Trophoblast | | |
| --- | --- | --- | --- | --- | --- | --- |
| | | IL-10 | IL-8 | IL-8 | IL-6 | IL-10+TGF-β |
| *Swedish study* | | | | | | |
| IUGR vs. Controls | 20 34 | 0.05 (I<C) | 0.05 (I>C) | NS | NS | NS |
| IUGR+SGA vs. Controls | 27 34 | 0.05 (S<C) | 0.01 (S>C) | 0.05 (S>C) | NS | NS |
| IUGR+SGA+ PE vs. Controls | 12 34 | NS | NS | 0.01 (S+PE>C) | 0.05 (S+PE>C) | NS |
| IUGR+PE vs. Controls | 9 34 | 0.05 (I+PE<C) | NS | NS | 0.05 (I+PE>C) | NS |
| IUGR–PE vs. Controls | 11 34 | NS | 0.01 (I>C) | NS | NS | NS |
| IUGR+PE vs. IUGR–PE | 11 9 | NS | NS | NS | 0.02 (I+PE>I–PE) | 0.01 (I+PE>I–PE) |

| Groups | n | Decidua | | | Trophoblast | |
| --- | --- | --- | --- | --- | --- | --- |
| | | IL-10 | IL-12 | TGF-β | IL-10 | TGF-β |
| *Pakistani study* | | | | | | |
| IUGR vs. Controls Serum | 45 55 | 0.0001 (I<C) Mother | 0.008 (I<C) | 0.009 (I>C) | 0.03 (I<C) Infant | 0.009 (I>C) |
| IUGR vs. Controls | 45 55 | NS | NS | NS | NS | 0.05 (I<C) |

IUGR = Intrauterine growth retardation; SGA = small for gestational age; PE = preeclampsia; NS = not significant; I<C = IUGR<control; S<C = IUGR+SGA<control; S+PE>C = IUGR+SGA+PE>control, etc.

At this time it is not clear whether it is possible to relate any or some of these changes in IUGR placentas to the poor outcome of these pregnancies. Previous studies have illustrated that TNF-α and IFN-γ may inhibit growth, differentiation and survival of trophoblasts [34] and IFN-γ; TNF-α and IL-2 may cause fetal resorption, whereas IL-3 and GM-CSF can increase fetal survival and weight [35].

Obviously pregnancy outcome is determined by a complex set of cytokines balancing each other. Our findings of clearly aberrant production in IUGR placentas of certain cytokines presumably originating from the mothers' immune response against their fetuses/placentas may or may not be involved in the pathogenesis of IUGR. Maternal intake of PUFAs might be related to these aberrations, possibly impairing the normal development of sufficient maternal tolerance to her fetus.

## Conclusions

Our studies indicate the importance of PUFA intake both for the fetus/placenta in relation to the maternal immune system and for the neonate's immune capacity.

Giving lactating rats an EFAD diet decreased the weight of WAT and serum leptin in the pups during suckling compared to controls. At 3 weeks of age leptin-mRNA was still reduced in inguinal fat. Feeding an isocaloric diet with 7% linseed oil (n-3 diet) during late gestation and suckling, gave the offspring significantly lower serum leptin levels, body weight, inguinal fat pad weight and adipocyte size than those fed an isocaloric diet with soybean oil (n-6/n-3 diet). Leptin has cytokine structure and immunological effects.

An EFAD diet fed to rat dams during late gestation and lactation suppressed serum antibody and DTH in pups against OA given to the lactating rat dams. The increased TGF-β-mRNA in draining lymph nodes may explain the finding since bystander tolerance was also obtained in the pups against an unrelated antigen. No tolerance was noted in the control group. Using instead the n-3 diet mentioned above to the dams, oral tolerance both of DTH and serum antibody reactivity appeared against OA and an unrelated antigen. Feeding the n-6/n-3 diet to the dams, the pups did not become tolerant. Tolerance was also obtained on a diet with very high ratio of n-6/n-3, but seemingly via anergy. These data suggest that the ratio of n-6/n-3 in the maternal diet may be important for the appearance and form of oral tolerance in the neonate.

We measured mRNA for several cytokines in the decidua and trophoblasts from normal and IUGR placentas from Swedish mothers. The immunosuppressive cytokine IL-10 showed reduced expression in the decidua of the IUGR pregnancies ($p < 0.05$). Instead the proinflammatory cytokine IL-8 mRNA was increased ($p < 0.05$).

We performed a similar study in Pakistan where the prevalence of IUGR is 15–20%, with many maternal risk factors including undernutrition. A decrease was found in mRNA for IL-10 ($p < 0.0001$) and IL-12 ($p < 0.008$), but an increase in TGF-β ($p < 0.009$) compared to non-IUGR pregnancies. In the trophoblasts IL-10 mRNA was also lower ($p < 0.03$), but TGF-β mRNA was higher ($p < 0.009$). In the serum of IUGR newborns TGF-β levels were low ($p < 0.05$).

It may be considered that if maternal immunological tolerance against the fetus/placenta does not develop properly an increased risk of IUGR may follow. Our studies in rats suggest that the ratio of n-6/n-3 fatty acids may influence the capacity to develop immunological tolerance. A deficient capacity to develop tolerance may be followed by an increased risk of autoimmune and allergic diseases. Possibly IUGR should be included among these conditions since PUFAs seem to play an important role in the normal development and function of the placenta, and seemingly in the development of tolerance to the fetus [28].

**References**

1 Simopoulos AP: The importance of the ratio of omega-6/omega-3 essential fatty acids. Biomed Pharmacother 2002;56:365–379.
2 Uauy R, Mena P, Rojas C: Essential fatty acids in early life: structural and functional role. Proc Nutr Soc 2000;59:3–15.
3 Sellmayer A, Koletzko B: Long-chain polyunsaturated fatty acids and eicosanoids in infants – physiological and pathophysiological aspects and open questions. Lipids 1999;34:199–205.
4 Calder PC, Grimble RF: Polyunsaturated fatty acids, inflammation and immunity. Eur J Clin Nutr 2002;56(suppl 3):S14–S19.
5 Senaris R, Garcia-Caballero T, Casabiell X, et al: Synthesis of leptin in human placenta. Endocrinology 1997;138:4501–4504.
6 Aoki N, Kawamura M, Matsuda T: Lactation-dependent down regulation of leptin production in mouse mammary gland. Biochim Biophys Acta 1999;1427:298–306.
7 Hassink SG, de Lancey E, Sheslow DV, et al: Placental leptin: an important new growth factor in intrauterine and neonatal development? Pediatrics 1997;100:E1.
8 Mikhail AA, Beck EX, Shafer A, et al: Leptin stimulates fetal and adult erythroid and myeloid development. Blood 1997;89:1507–1512.
9 Santos-Alvarez J, Goberna R, Sanchez-Margalet V: Human leptin stimulates proliferation and activation of human circulating monocytes. Cell Immunol 1999;194:6–11.
10 Lord GM, Matarese G, Howard JK, et al: Leptin modulates the T-cell immune response and reverses starvation-induced immunosuppression. Nature 1998;394:897–901.
11 Shore SA, Schwartzman IN, Mellema MS, et al: Effect of leptin on allergic airway responses in mice. J Allergy Clin Immunol 2005;115:103–109.
12 Trottier G, Koski KG, Brun T, et al: Increased fat intake during lactation modifies hypothalamic-pituitary-adrenal responsiveness in developing rat pups: a possible role for leptin. Endocrinology 1998;139:3704–3711.
13 Korotkova M, Gabrielsson B, Hanson LÅ, Strandvik B: Maternal essential fatty acid deficiency depresses serum leptin levels in suckling rat pups. J Lipid Res 2001;42:359–365.
14 Korotkova M, Gabrielsson B, Hanson LÅ, Strandvik B: Maternal dietary intake of essential fatty acids affects adipose tissue growth and leptin mRNA expression in suckling rat pups. Pediatr Res 2002;52:78–84.
15 Korotkova M, Gabrielsson B, Lönn M, et al: Leptin levels in rat offspring are modified by the ratio of linoleic to alpha-linolenic acid in the maternal diet. J Lipid Res 2002;43:1743–1749.
16 Hanson DG, Vaz NM, Maia LC, et al: Inhibition of specific immune responses by feeding protein antigens. Int Arch Allergy Appl Immunol 1977;55:526–532.
17 Lundin BS, Karlsson MR, Svensson LA, et al: Active suppression in orally tolerized rats coincides with in situ transforming growth factor-beta (TGF-beta) expression in the draining lymph nodes. Clin Exp Immunol 1999;116:181–187.
18 Dahlman-Hoglund A, Dahlgren U, Ahlstedt S, et al: Bystander suppression of the immune response to human serum albumin in rats fed ovalbumin. Immunology 1995;86:128–133.
19 Mowat AM, Ferguson A: Hypersensitivity in the small intestinal mucosa. V. Induction of cell-mediated immunity to a dietary antigen. Clin Exp Immunol 1981;43:574–582.
20 Strobel S: Immunity induced after a feed of antigen during early life: oral tolerance v. sensitisation. Proc Nutr Soc 2001;60:437–442.
21 Hanson LÅ, Korotkova M, Telemo E: Breast-feeding, infant formulas, and the immune system. Ann Allergy Asthma Immunol 2003;90:59–63.
22 Harbige LS: Fatty acids, the immune response, and autoimmunity: a question of n-6 essentiality and the balance between n-6 and n-3. Lipids 2003;38:323–341.
23 Fidler N, Koletzko B: The fatty acid composition of human colostrum. Eur J Nutr 2000;39:31–37.
24 Cinader B, Clandinin MT, Hosokawa T, Robblee NM: Dietary fat alters the fatty acid composition of lymphocyte membranes and the rate at which suppressor capacity is lost. Immunol Lett 1983;6:331–337.

25 Harbige LS, Fisher BA: Dietary fatty acid modulation of mucosally-induced tolerogenic immune responses. Proc Nutr Soc 2001;60:449–456.
26 Korotkova M, Telemo E, Hanson LÅ, Strandvik B: Modulation of neonatal immunological tolerance to ovalbumin by maternal essential fatty acid intake. Pediatr Allergy Immunol 2004;15: 112–122.
27 Korotkova M, Telemo E, Yamashiro Y, et al: The ratio of n-6 to n-3 fatty acids in maternal diet influences the induction of neonatal immunological tolerance to ovalbumin. Clin Exp Immunol 2004;137:237–244.
28 Amu S, Hahn-Zoric MH, Malik A, et al: Cytokines in the placenta of Pakistani newborns with and without intrauterine growth retardation. Pediatr Res, 2005, in press.
29 Sasaki K, Sakai M, Miyazaki S, et al: Decidual and peripheral blood CD4+CD25+ regulatory T cells in early pregnancy subjects and spontaneous abortion cases. Mol Hum Reprod 2004;10: 347–353.
30 Vilbergsson G, Samsioe G, Wennergren O, Karlsson K: Essential fatty acids in pregnancies complicated by intrauterine growth retardation. Int J Gynaecol Obstet 1991;36:277–286.
31 Cetin I, Giovannini N, Alvino G, et al: Intrauterine growth restriction is associated with changes in polyunsaturated fatty acid fetal-maternal relationships. Pediatr Res 2002;52: 750–755.
32 Jones CA, Vance GH, Power LL, et al: Costimulatory molecules in the developing human gastrointestinal tract: a pathway for fetal allergen priming. J Allergy Clin Immunol 2001;108: 235–241.
33 Hahn-Zoric MH, Kjellmer H, Ellis I, et al: Aberrations in placental cytokine mRNA related to intrauterine growth retardation. Pediatr Res 2002;51:201–206.
34 Yui J, Garcia-Lloret M, Wegmann TG, Guilbert LJ: Cytotoxicity of tumour necrosis factor-alpha and gamma-interferon against primary human placental trophoblasts. Placenta 1994; 15:819–835.
35 Chaouat G, Menu E, Clark DA, et al: Control of fetal survival in CBA x DBA/2 mice by lymphokine therapy. J Reprod Fertil 1990;89:447–458.

## Discussion

*Dr. Sampson:* In that Pakistani group, do you have any idea about the LCPUFA intake?

*Dr. Hanson:* There are no formal studies, we are trying to look into it but I would say that in general the fat intake is very heavy, but at the same time undernutrition or malnutrition is common. But I would expect that the ratios are high.

*Dr. Björkstén:* I was interested in all that you said but to start with the first part, actually in the first set of experiments you had a control diet with or without oral ovalbumin and PUFA. From the slides I read that by giving oral ovalbumin you induced oral tolerance, but there was no difference in the control group given ovalbumin and the PUFA group given ovalbumin. Did I miss anything there?

*Dr. Hanson:* The difference you see is really between the groups with different ratios given ovalbumin.

*Dr. Björkstén:* But this was the first experiment there with 4 groups, and ovalbumin was really the factor?

*Dr. Hanson:* Are you asking for the study with the 3 ratios, the diet groups?

*Dr. Björkstén:* No. The difference here, as I saw it, was between those fed ovalbumin orally or not fed, rather than between the diet groups. Does this indicate an effect of the diet because if you compare columns 2 and 4, to me this indicates that feeding orally actually reduces the immune response but at first it doesn't look too convincing that it is actually the PUFA diet.

*Dr. Hanson:* If you compare, here you have the control diet and the response there and there, and there is no difference, and if you then look at the control diet with the ovalbumin you see no difference. If you look at the diet which is deficient then you see that both of these are reduced in responsiveness.

*Dr. Björkstén:* My point is, I am comparing panel 2 and panel 4, ovalbumin per-orally in the two groups, and to me it would indicate that the diet may not be as important.

*Dr. Hanson:* This is the only comparison which shows a difference.

*Dr. Björkstén:* I was also interested in the experiments where you had the 3 ratios, and you mentioned the possibility of regulatory T cells and TGF-β as explanatory. Did you measure them?

*Dr. Hanson:* You mean you would extract them and that would be very difficult, there would be very few. These are rat pups.

*Dr. Björkstén:* In principle pooling. I was just curious because if there is a pooled experiment for example of the group, then you could do it because it is a very interesting observation.

*Dr. Hanson:* 10 pups per group, you could mince the 10 pups. I agree with you.

*Dr. Haschke:* In your fist part of the experiments when you mentioned the ratio between n-6 and n-3 and the group which had the ratio of 0.4, this induced tolerance if I got it correctly. Could you speculate on whether their human milk doesn't have a ratio of 0.4? But one might look at this in terms of human milk with high ratios and human milk with low ratios where the outcome in terms of non-tolerance would be different.

*Dr. Hanson:* Yes, and this, I am sure, is behind some of the confusion that we have because the mother's diet will determine what is in her milk and that will have different effects on the baby. Perhaps we missed this, but we can now put it into the right perspective and then we can do more informatory experiments. This may include allergy studies with fish oil and others that may seem rather confusing presently. But if one determines the n-6/n-3 ratios used in these studies they may become easier to interpret. Those ratios may relate to the capacity to induce regulatory T cells.

*Dr. Haschke:* It would be logical to follow up with a trial perhaps where a low ratio of n-6/n-3 would be given to infants to induce oral tolerance.

*Dr. Hanson:* I would love to see that experiment, yes.

*Dr. Björkstén:* I would like to interact with what Dr. Hanson is saying. It is clear and we have shown that in breast milk from allergic and non-allergic mothers and also in the plasma of allergic children, so both in mothers, in their breast milk, in their serum, and in the babies, that the difference, related to allergy, is the ratios, not the absolute levels.

*Dr. Jensen:* By any chance have you looked at T-lymphocyte cell antigen markers in a preterm study in which at least longer chain PUFA intake seems to influence whether you have a more mature CD4+ lymphocyte population versus a more antigen naïve CD4+ lymphocyte population?

*Dr. Hanson:* It is a very relevant thing to do, but again the pups are very small and it would not be easy to get lymphocytes. But pooling as suggested might be a way to go. Certainly one needs to proceed from here on.

Lucas A, Sampson HA (eds): Primary Prevention by Nutrition Intervention in Infancy and Childhood.
Nestlé Nutr Workshop Ser Pediatr Program, vol 57, pp 235–245,
Nestec Ltd., Vevey/S. Karger AG, Basel, © 2006.

# The Crucial Role of Dietary n-6 Polyunsaturated Fatty Acids in Excessive Adipose Tissue Development: Relationship to Childhood Obesity

*Florence Massiera*[a], *Philippe Guesnet*[b], *Gérard Ailhaud*[a]

[a]ISDBC, Centre de Biochimie UMR 6543 CNRS, Faculté des Sciences, Nice, et, and
[b]Laboratoire de Nutrition et Sécurité Alimentaire, INRA, Jouy-en-Josas, France

## Introduction

Childhood obesity can be considered a non-infectious epidemic. According to the International Obesity Task Force's childhood obesity working group 'the epidemic of European Union childhood obesity appears to be accelerating out of control. Things are worse than our gloomiest predictions'. Consistent with this statement, cardiovascular risk factors are now becoming 'routinely reported' among children in many populations. Among the social trends favoring childhood obesity, increased energy intake and decreased energy expenditure have been substantiated. However the importance of qualitative changes (i.e. the fatty acid composition of fats) has been largely disregarded despite a dramatic alteration in the balance of essential polyunsaturated fatty acids (PUFAs). Since the 1960s, indiscriminate recommendations have been made to substitute vegetable oils, high in n-6 PUFAs and low in n-3 PUFAs, for saturated fats. Moreover significant changes in animal feed and in the food chain have been introduced. For example, the n-6/n-3 ratios in food commonly consumed in the American diet range from 17 to 41, largely above official recommendations. Among the consequences, these changes have led to a 4-fold increase in the supply of dietary arachidonic acid (ARA; 20:4n-6) in the last 50 years [1]. Importantly, these changes are translated into changes in the lipid composition of cell tissues and secretions in humans. Equally important, the requirement for linoleic acid (LA; 18:2n-6) for growth and development has been significantly overestimated [2] whereas the recommendation to reduce n-6 PUFAs even as the n-3 PUFAs are increased has not been followed [3]. Thus, in addition to a positive energy balance, qualitative changes in the fatty acid composition of fats may help to gain insight into the increasing prevalence of overweight and obesity in children and adults despite the slight decrease in energy and fat intake in the last decades [4], an observation which appears at odds with cross-sectional and longitudinal studies showing an association between a high fat intake and a subsequent fat mass enhancement [5]. The evidence from animal and human studies discussed herein favors the possibility that changes in the balance of essential PUFAs are altering the early stages of adipose tissue development, i.e. during fetal life and infancy which are life periods showing the highest adaptability and vulnerability to external factors.

## White Adipose Tissue in Early Life and Developmental Issues

How important is the development of white adipose tissue in early life? In humans, it is known that this tissue develops as early as the second trimester of pregnancy and more extensively during the last trimester and after birth. It is also well known that the cellularity of human subcutaneous adipose tissue from obese patients depends on the age at obesity onset, particularly the adipocyte number more than the adipocyte size [6]. It should be pointed out that cellularity measurements are taking place a posteriori, i.e. after excessive proliferation of precursor cells able to divide in vitro and in vivo, in contrast to non-dividing adipocytes. Clearly, proliferation of precursor cells remains an undetectable 'weightless' phenomenon as these cells exhibit a 30- to 50-fold smaller volume than adipocytes. Postnatally, white adipose tissue develops extensively in various depots. Available data show that clones of precursor cells may vary in their capacity to proliferate and differentiate into adipocytes in vitro but, although this ability differs between fat depots in rodents, it is highest in humans during the first year of life [6]. Thus, early age is a highly sensitive period during which the adipose tissue expands dramatically. Of note, the formation of mature adipocytes from precursor cells may take as long as a few weeks in rodents, i.e. up to a couple of years when extrapolated to humans. Of note also, the size and self-renewal of the adipose precursor pools in various depots as a function of age or in response to different diets is presently unknown. These issues are critical as subpopulations have recently been characterized in the stromal-vascular fraction of human adipose tissue where they likely represent the true potential of white adipose tissue development.

## Adipogenesis and Fatty Acids as Adipogenic Hormones

The differentiation of clonal and non-clonal precursor cells into adipocytes is a sequential process in which glucocorticoids, insulin and insulin-like

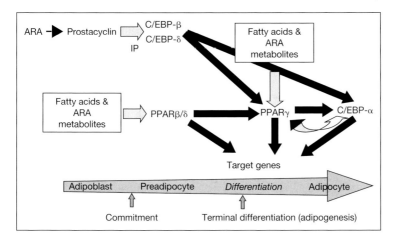

**Fig. 1.** Main transcription factors, nuclear receptors and activators/ligands of adipogenesis. Arachidonic acid gives rise in preadipocytes to prostacyclin which acts through its cognate cell surface receptor IP in upregulating C/EBP-β and δ, which in turn, upregulate PPARγ and promote adipogenesis. Arachidonic acid also gives rise to other metabolites which, as well as other dietary long-chain fatty acids, play the role of activators/ligands of PPARβ/δ and PPARγ, and also subsequently promote adipogenesis.

growth factor-1 have been identified as the major adipogenic hormones. However, both in rodents and humans, long-chain fatty acids act at the precursor stage and enhance the formation of adipocytes [7]. Fatty acids as well as eicosanoids arising from ARA metabolism through the action of cyclooxygenases and lipoxygenases, i.e. prostaglandins and leukotrienes, behave as activators/ligands of two members of the peroxisome proliferator-activator receptor (PPAR) family, i.e. PPARβ/δ and PPARγ which are sequentially expressed during adipocyte differentiation (fig. 1) [7]. In vitro, among dietary fatty acids promoting adipogenesis, ARA (arising in vivo from the metabolism of LA or directly from dietary sources) plays a unique role as a precursor of prostacyclin [8]. Once released from precursor cells, prostacyclin binds externally to its cognate receptor IP, activates the protein kinase A pathway via cAMP production and promotes adipogenesis of clonal precursor cells (fig. 1) [9, 10]. A tight correlation is observed between both short-term cAMP production and long-term adipogenesis induced by ARA ($r = 0.963$) [11]. Both the protein kinase A and extracellular signal-regulated kinase pathways are involved in these early events [12]. Importantly, only ARA triggers cAMP production, whereas eicosapentaenoic acid (EPA)>docosahexaenoic acid (DHA); arising in vivo from the metabolism of α-linolenic acid (ALA; 18:3n-3) or directly from dietary sources, inhibits the production of cAMP stimulated by ARA. Interestingly, in the presence of a specific PPARγ agonist, the ARA-mediated pathway is more potent than a specific PPARβ/δ agonist in promoting adipogenesis through the upregulation and activity of PPARγ2, the master gene of terminal differentiation [13]. Of note, dihomo-γ-linolenic acid (20:3n-6) also promotes adipogenesis (unpublished). In contrast to these n-6 PUFAs, saturated, monounsaturated and n-3 PUFAs (EPA and DHA) are no more adipogenic than a specific β/δ agonist, emphasizing the unique adipogenic role of prostacyclin which has been extended to adipose precursor cells isolated from human adipose tissue. Last but not least, the prostacyclin effect takes place only at the precursor stage as both the ligand production and the expression of functional IP cease in mature adipocytes [10].

## Fatty Acid Composition of Fats and Adipose Tissue during Development

Based upon in vitro data, in vivo experiments have been carried out to investigate whether a LA-enriched diet modulates fat mass. Under isoenergetic conditions, comparative experiments have been performed with wild-type (WT) mice and mice invalidated for the cell surface prostacyclin receptor (ip$^{-/-}$ mice). During pregnancy and the suckling period both WT and ip$^{-/-}$ mice were fed high-fat diets enriched with either 15% corn oil (LA predominant; LA diet) or 10% corn-oil and 5% perilla oil (LA and ALA predominant; LA/ALA diet). These studies have shown that (1) pups from WT mothers fed the LA diet are 40% heavier 1 week after weaning than those from mothers fed either the LA/ALA or standard diet. Thus inclusion of ALA in the LA-enriched diet counteracts the LA-induced enhancement of fat mass. (2) This enhancement is abolished in ip$^{-/-}$ mice, demonstrating the critical role of the prostacyclin receptor in this phenomenon, and (3) this enhancing effect of the LA diet on body weight and fat mass is confined to the gestation/lactation period; importantly, the weight difference between mice fed the LA or the LA/ALA diet is maintained in adult animals. In other words, PUFAs of the n-6 and n-3 series are *not* equipotent in promoting adipogenesis in vitro and adipose tissue development in vivo [13]. Feeding rats isocaloric diets with varying n-6/n-3 ratios for the last 10 days of gestation and throughout lactation has led to major changes in the milk fatty acid composition. A shift from 0.4 to 8.9 of this ratio increases by 52% the inguinal fat pad weight 1 week after birth [14]. Clearly, varying the proportions of these essential fatty acids in vivo may alter the proportion of ARA and its metabolites versus EPA and DHA (fig. 2). Evidence that ALA modulates ARA and prostacyclin production from LA has been obtained. In adult humans, a reduction in LA supply results in a decrease in prostaglandins measured in urine. Moreover, ALA intake severely decreases prostaglandin synthesis in human platelets but not the conversion of LA to ARA [15]. In normal term infants receiving 16%

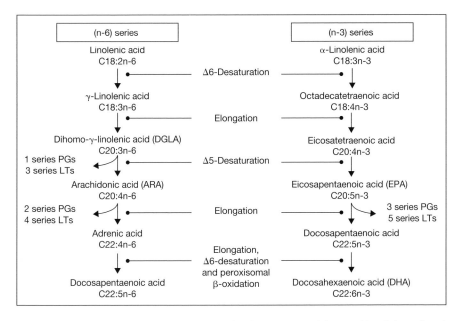

***Fig. 2.*** Metabolic pathways of the essential polyunsaturated fatty acids of the n-6 and n-3 series. Linoleic acid (LA) and α-linolenic acid (ALA) are both substrates of Δ6-desaturase. Thus absolute amounts of LA and ALA and the LA/ALA ratio modulate the fluxes of n-6 and n-3 PUFA metabolites.

LA and from 0.4 to 3.2% ALA (LA/ALA ratios from 44 to 5), lower ARA and higher DHA levels are observed in plasma phospholipids and, interestingly, are associated with lower body weight [11]. In mice increasing total fat (5–20% fat) and decreasing n-6/n-3 ratios (from >100 to 0.1) lead to a dramatic decrease in prostacyclin production in peritoneal macrophages which share many properties with preadipocytes [16].

A direct and important role played by ARA on prostaglandin production must be emphasized as ARA, present in tissue lipids and mainly derived from dietary sources [1], increases the amount of prostaglandins recovered in human urine [17] and in pig lung [18], whereas DHA [18] but not EPA [19] decreases it. As the fatty acid composition of adipose tissue lipids is a fair reflection of ingested fats [20] and as preadipocytes synthesize prostaglandins including prostacyclin [8], it is assumed that the modulation of prostaglandin synthesis by varying the amount and the balance between essential PUFAs may exhibit a pattern in adipose tissue similar to that observed in other tissues.

## Fatty Acid Composition of Fats in Early Life and Relationships to Childhood Obesity and Health

Considering the adipogenic role of the LA-enriched diet and the counteracting effect of ALA in rodents, the key question to be addressed in humans is whether the balance of PUFAs has changed over decades during the gestation/lactation period so that it could favor excessive adipose tissue development and subsequent metabolic disturbances. Comparative US data from the National Health and Nutrition Survey II (1976–1980) and the NAHNES III (1988–1994) indicate that the adiposity indices for 6- to 11-month-old infants of all races has increased 1.9- and 1.7-fold for boys and girls, respectively [21], i.e. at ages where a positive energy balance or the quality of carbohydrates [22] cannot be advocated. In contrast, these data suggest that qualitative nutrient changes have occurred during gestation and/or during breast milk/formula milk consumption. In humans, recent data show that low intrauterine availability of γ-linolenic acid (18:3n-6) is related to low birth weight and presumably to low fat mass, consistent with the important role played by LA metabolites in adipose tissue development. Interestingly, low birth weight is associated with increased body fatness and insulin resistance at 7 years of age [23]. The rate of weight regain to normalize the body weight of these newborns appears important and suggests that adipose tissue development then occurring rapidly is potentially harmful [24].

As shown earlier, the content of LA in the mature breast milk of US women has steadily increased from 6–7 to 15–16% of total fatty acids between the early 1950s and the mid-1990s, whereas the percentage of ALA has remained essentially unchanged (~1%) [25], consistent with the PUFA content of adipose tissue triglycerides in US women [20]. The tight correlation between the fatty acid composition of ingested fats and that of breast milk has indeed been demonstrated in female baboons [26]. A great variation in PUFA content has been reported in the breast milk of European women, but it should be noted that both the LA content and the LA/ALA ratio in the mature breast milk of US women are higher than those of European women. Furthermore, the ratio of ARA to DHA is 2-fold higher in the breast milk of US women because of its lower DHA content [25]. These differences are of interest if one considers the differences observed between school-age American and European children with regard to the prevalence of overweight (approximately 32 versus 19%) and obesity (approximately 7.5 versus 4%). Of note, comparisons of energy intake and prevalence of overweight and obesity in the late 1980s between US and French children of 1–2 years of age show that protein, carbohydrate and lipid intake are very similar but that the percentage of PUFAs are 1.5-fold higher in American than in French infants, consistent with a role of n-6 PUFAs in promoting excessive adipose tissue development (Rolland-Cachera MF, personal communication).

Although breastfeeding may help reduce the prevalence of overweight and obesity in childhood, it is not the most frequent way of feeding newborns in industrial countries, and the enhanced fatness has been attributed to the higher energy intake of formula-fed infants [25]. However, and unfortunately, the fatty acid composition of infant formula, enriched or not with n-3 PUFAs, indicates that the percentage of LA has remained very high ($\sim$16–18%), mimicking that of mature breast milk of US women. Last but not least, the food industry in the USA has recently advertised the use of preterm infant formulas supplemented with DHA and ARA for term infants, despite the fact that no clear-cut benefits for brain and eye development have been demonstrated with this fatty acid supplementation in normal term infants [27, 28], and despite the fact that ARA acts as a potent adipogenic nutrient in vitro [13]. Moreover, 5-day-old piglets supplemented for 2 weeks with ARA exhibit a 27% increase in body weight without a change in body length [5, 29].

## Conclusion

During the last decades, many changes have taken place with respect to the nutritional environment of human beings. The steady increase in the body mass index of children has been correlated with an early adiposity rebound which has been associated with high protein but not fat intake at age 2 years [30]. It has been suggested that eating more carbohydrates with a higher glycemic index has a major impact on the prevalence of childhood obesity in 2- to 8-year-old children [22]. We propose that unnoticed changes in the fatty acid composition of dietary fats during pregnancy, and that of mature breast and formula milk, are responsible at least in part of the dramatic increase in the prevalence of childhood overweight and obesity. In the worst-case scenario, since adipocytes once formed exhibit little or no turnover in the body [6], the continuous intake of n-6 PUFA-enriched food could only lead to further overweight and obesity in adolescents and adults.

## References

1 Taber L, Chiu CH, Whelan J: Assessment of the arachidonic acid content in foods commonly consumed in the American diet. Lipids 1998;33:1151–1157.
2 Cunnane SC: Problems with essential fatty acids: time for a new paradigm? Prog Lipid Res 2003;42:544–568.
3 Simopoulos AP, Leaf A, Salem N Jr: Workshop statement on the essentiality of and recommended dietary intakes for omega-6 and omega-3 fatty acids. Prostaglandins Leukot Essent Fatty Acids 2000;63:119–121.
4 Taubes G: Nutrition. The soft science of dietary fat. Science 2001;291:2536–2545.
5 Willett WC: Dietary fat plays a major role in obesity: no. Obes Rev 2002;3:59–68.
6 Ailhaud G, Hauner H: Development of white adipose tissue; in Bray GA, Bouchard C (eds): Handbook of Obesity: Etiology and Pathophysiology, ed 2. New York, Dekker, 2004, pp 481–514.

7 Amri EZ, Ailhaud G, Grimaldi PA: Fatty acids as signal transducing molecules: involvement in the differentiation of preadipose to adipose cells. J Lipid Res 1994;35:930–937.
8 Gaillard D, Negrel R, Lagarde M, Ailhaud G: Requirement and role of arachidonic acid in the differentiation of pre-adipose cells. Biochem J 1989;257:389–397.
9 Negrel R, Gaillard D, Ailhaud G: Prostacyclin as a potent effector of adipose-cell differentiation. Biochem J 1989;257:399–405.
10 Vassaux G, Gaillard D, Ailhaud G, Negrel R: Prostacyclin is a specific effector of adipose cell differentiation. Its dual role as a cAMP- and Ca(2+)-elevating agent. J Biol Chem 1992;267:11092–11097.
11 Jensen CL, Prager TC, Fraley JK, et al: Effect of dietary linoleic/alpha-linolenic acid ratio on growth and visual function of term infants. J Pediatr 1997;131:200–209.
12 Belmonte N, Phillips BW, Massiera F, et al: Activation of extracellular signal-regulated kinases and CREB/ATF-1 mediate the expression of CCAAT/enhancer binding proteins beta and -delta in preadipocytes. Mol Endocrinol 2001;15:2037–2049.
13 Massiera F, Saint-Marc P, Seydoux J, et al: Arachidonic acid and prostacyclin signaling promote adipose tissue development: a human health concern? J Lipid Res 2003;44:271–279.
14 Korotkova M, Gabrielsson B, Lonn M, et al: Leptin levels in rat offspring are modified by the ratio of linoleic to alpha-linolenic acid in the maternal diet. J Lipid Res 2002;43:1743–1749.
15 Adam O, Wolfram G, Zollner N: Effect of alpha-linolenic acid in the human diet on linoleic acid metabolism and prostaglandin biosynthesis. J Lipid Res 1986;27:421–426.
16 Broughton KS, Wade JW: Total fat and (n-3):(n-6) fat ratios influence eicosanoid production in mice. J Nutr 2002;132:88–94.
17 Adam O, Wolfram G, Zollner, N: Influence of dietary linoleic acid intake with different fat intakes on arachidonic acid concentrations in plasma and platelet lipids and eicosanoid biosynthesis in female volunteers. Ann Nutr Metab 2003;47:31–36.
18 Huang MC, Craig-Schmidt MC: Arachidonate and docosahexaenoate added to infant formula influence fatty acid composition and subsequent eicosanoid production in neonatal pigs. J Nutr 1996;126:2199–2208.
19 Li B, Birdwell C, Whelan J: Antithetic relationship of dietary arachidonic acid and eicosapentaenoic acid on eicosanoid production in vivo. J Lipid Res 1994;35:1869–1877.
20 Garland M, Sacks FM, Colditz GA, et al: The relation between dietary intake and adipose tissue composition of selected fatty acids in US women. Am J Clin Nutr 1998;67:25–30.
21 Ogden CL, Troiano RP, Briefel RR, et al: Prevalence of overweight among preschool children in the United States, 1971 through 1994. Pediatrics 1997;99:E1.
22 Slyper AH: The pediatric obesity epidemic: causes and controversies. J Clin Endocrinol Metab 2004;89:2540–2547.
23 Rump P, Popp-Snijders C, Heine RJ, Hornstra G: Components of the insulin resistance syndrome in seven-year-old children: relations with birth weight and the polyunsaturated fatty acid content of umbilical cord plasma phospholipids. Diabetologia 2002;45:349–355.
24 Rogers I: The influence of birthweight and intrauterine environment on adiposity and fat distribution in later life. Int J Obes Relat Metab Disord 2003;27:755–777.
25 Ailhaud G, Guesnet P: Fatty acid composition of fats is an early determinant of childhood obesity: a short review and an opinion. Obes Rev 2004;5:21–26.
26 Sarkadi-Nagy E, Wijendran V, Diau GY, et al: Formula feeding potentiates docosahexaenoic and arachidonic acid biosynthesis in term and preterm baboon neonates. J Lipid Res 2004;45:71–80.
27 Auestad N, Halter R, Hall RT, et al: Growth and development in term infants fed long-chain polyunsaturated fatty acids: a double-masked, randomized, parallel, prospective, multivariate study. Pediatrics 2001;108:372–381.
28 Makrides M, Neumann MA, Simmer K, Gibson RA: Dietary long-chain polyunsaturated fatty acids do not influence growth of term infants: a randomized clinical trial. Pediatrics 1999;104:468–475.
29 Weiler HA: Dietary supplementation of arachidonic acid is associated with higher whole body weight and bone mineral density in growing pigs. Pediatr Res 2000;47:692–697.
30 Rolland-Cachera MF, Deheeger M, Bellisle F: Early adiposity rebound is not associated with energy or fat intake in infancy. Pediatrics 2001;108:218–219.

## Discussion

*Dr. Hanson:* Thank you very much for that. It agrees in every detail with what I just talked about, not only as to the late outcome in the rats on high n-6/n-3 ratios having increased weight and insulin levels and blood pressure and all that, but also the failure to become tolerant. I think this is a very significant contribution you made and I believe we really have to listen to these findings and do something about them.

*Dr. Steenhout:* Thank you very much also for your nice talk. In your mouse models, you showed a reduction in weight with the addition of n-3 to the n-6 diet, but you didn't show us the results with only n-3. Did you do that or not?

*Dr. Massiera:* No, we didn't do only n-3. That is right.

*Dr. Jensen:* In our study, as you pointed out, infants received a very low α-linolenic acid formula in which the ratio of linoleic acid to α-linolenic acid was very very high, higher than anyone would do today. Those infants had higher rates of weight gain during the first 4 months than infants fed a formula containing 3.2% of total fatty acids as α-linolenic acid. When we did a follow-up study we obviously were not going to use a formula that contains as little as 0.4% of total fatty acid as α-linolenic acid. We used 3 formulas, two of which contained about 16% of total fatty acids as linoleic acid and either 1 or 2% of total fatty acids as α-linolenic acid and then another formula contained 8%, half of the amount of linoleic acid, and in that study we included the usual anthropometric measures outcomes, weight, length, head circumference, skin folds, etc., and measures of both total and resting energy expenditure, and found no differences between those groups. So it suggests that the range over which this operates may be a little more limited. But that does have relevance, because if you look at the diet that the low α-linolenic acid group infants were consuming in the first study, that is exactly what most toddlers, children, adolescents and adults Americans consume in the US, but it does appear that perhaps it is what would be considered, from an evolutionary stand point, the extremes of high relative linoleic acid intakes, i.e. exactly what we are consuming. I would be interested in your comments.

*Dr. Massiera:* I think the ratio is very important and the key because a previous study has been following total PUFAs in general, so we can't say that there are no effects. There is a lot of controversy regarding the human data, but we definitely must reconsider this n-6/n-3 ratio in a more balanced manner.

*Dr. Laron:* At the beginning when you listed the adipogenic hormones you listed insulin and IGF-1 in the same line. Do you think they have the same kind of mechanism?

*Dr. Massiera:* We don't know precisely whether they both act in the same way, but at high levels they interact with each other's receptors.

*Dr. Laron:* How do you think that IGF-1 acts as an adipogenic agent? The question is do growth hormone and IGF-1 act on adipose tissue by the same mechanism or do they act by differential mechanisms?

*Dr. Massiera:* I am not a specialist in the IGF-1-signaling pathway or even effect. I think it has been demonstrated that the effect is not the same but quite a redundant pathway.

*Dr. Laron:* I can tell you that IGF-1 has an adipogenic effect in men [1] but I don't understand the mechanism, and wonder whether it acts through insulin receptors.

*Dr. Massiera:* In cell culture, IGF-1 has an adipogenic effect but it is not very clear whether this effect is mediated through IGF or the insulin receptor.

*Dr. Lucas:* This is just a sort of spontaneous thought. DHA alone has been shown to suppress growth in at least 3 studies, and actually there is some evidence for growth suppression even with arachidonic acid (AA) plus DHA. But I am just speculating if

243

what we are seeing as a potential negative could be a plus as far as future metabolic syndrome risk is concerned.

*Dr. Massiera:* You mean supplementation by DHA?

*Dr. Lucas:* I mean in formulas that had DHA alone, in the early formulas that were just supplemented with fish oil, which had quite high EPA as well as DHA, there was great suppression. It was always argued to be due to unbalanced addition of DHA without AA, and in fact there have been a couple of studies with DHA and AA as a suppressor, but whenever this has occurred it has been seen as a negative. In view of the data it occurred to me that slow early growth is good probably at every stage in terms of metabolic syndrome risk and whether this could be a potential explanation.

*Dr. Massiera:* I think adipose tissue plays a central role in the metabolic syndrome in general, so if the decrease in adipose tissue development can be done in some way by DHA supplementation, it can be good for the metabolic syndrome as a consequence [2].

*Dr. Steenhout:* My first comment concerns the results of a paper by Clandinin et al. [3] studying formulas for premature babies with different mixtures of LCPUFAs. The group receiving algal-DHA 0.3% and Fungal-ARA 0.6% is reported to have a better growth and faster catch-up. But when you look at the results in detail you realize that this principally concerns the weight growth and not the height or head circumference. Even though it may not be the best indicator for obesity development, the BMI for this group is higher and this is probably not the best thing to do in terms of obesity prevention. My second comment concerns the feeding recommendations based on the wish to have infants following growth curve references that have been continuously adapted. I have the feeling that during that last 50 years we have indirectly induced a secular trend of increasing weight and consequently the risk of later obesity. Should we not come back to growth curves based on breastfeeding reference groups as recently suggested in a *British Medical Journal* editorial by Wright [4]? Would you like to comment?

*Dr. Massiera:* No.

*Dr. Hursting:* I have a comment and a question regarding the IGF question. We have seen in ASA BAF1 mice, the whole CBP family of transcription factors as well as in CEP-β knockout mice. We actually see very low fat white adipose tissue but high IGF-1 and high insulin levels, and in fact they are diabetic as adults. So there is something going on there but I don't fully understand it. My question relates to the PPARγ, a sort of central path, and I am wondering if you manipulate that pathway with agents or other dietary factors to interact with that, would that have the same effect as dropping the AA intake do you think?

*Dr. Massiera:* In fact it has been demonstrated that rosiglitazone treatment in mice in vivo increases adipose tissue development and that blocking PPARγ completely counteracts adipose differentiation. The best proof is the knockout mouse.

*Dr. Jensen:* I would just mention that at our institution t some animal studies were also done in which animals were given diets with rather extreme n-6 versus n-3 fatty acids in different directions and with gene arrays and so forth. Those genes that encode for enzymes would promote fatty acid synthesis and deposition seem to be upregulated, and in some cases enzymes responsible for fatty acid oxidation tend to be upregulated with high n-3 fatty acid intakes. However, these were rats, and when we actually did animal calorimetry, there were no differences in body composition or energy expenditure but there was almost a difference in the risk quotient. But these gene expression differences didn't seem to translate into physiologic effects so we felt disappointed.

*Dr. Massiera:* We have an explanation for that. I don't know if the nutritional manipulation should be during the lactation period or the pregnancy period, because if you compare those data to classical nutritional manipulation at weaning, giving high-fat diets to these rats, there is no significant effect even in our case with the mice.

*Dr. Jensen:* These were relatively young rats but the window of impact may be different from species to species.

*Dr. Massiera:* Yes, but we are giving the diets to the mothers during pregnancy and not only after birth. I think that is what makes the difference.

*Dr. Jensen:* We did not do prenatal intervention.

## References

1   Laron Z, Ginsberg S, Lilos P, et al: Body composition of IFG-I treated girls with Laron syndrome (abstract 183). Annual Meeting of the Pediatric Academic Society, Washington, 2005. PAS 2005;57:1029.
2   Carlson SE: Docosahexaenoic acid and arachidonic acid in infant development. Semin Neonatol 2001;6:437–439.
3   Clandinin MT, Van Aerde JE, Merkel KL, et al: Growth and development of preterm infants fed infant formulas containing docosahexaenoic acid and arachidonic acid. J Pediatr 2005; 146:461–468.
4   Wright CM: Growth charts for babies. BMJ 2005;330:1399–1400.

Lucas A, Sampson HA (eds): Primary Prevention by Nutrition Intervention in Infancy and Childhood.
Nestlé Nutr Workshop Ser Pediatr Program, vol 57, pp 247–255,
Nestec Ltd., Vevey/S. Karger AG, Basel, © 2006.

# -Omics for Prevention: Gene, Protein and Metabolite Profiling to Better Understand Individual Disposition to Disease

*M. Affolter*[a], *G.E. Bergonzelli*[a], *K. Blaser*[b], *S. Blum-Sperisen*[a],
*B. Corthésy*[c], *L.B. Fay*[a], *C. Garcia-Rodenas*[a], *L.V. Lopes*[a],
*L. Marvin-Guy*[a], *A. Mercenier*[a], *D.M. Mutch*[a], *A. Panchaud*[a],
*F. Raymond*[a], *C. Schmidt-Weber*[b], *A. Schumann*[a], *F. Spertini*[c],
*G. Williamson*[a], *M. Kussmann*[a]

[a]Nestlé Research Centre, Nestec Ltd., Lausanne; [b]Swiss Institute for Allergy and Asthma Research, Davos, and [c]Centre Hospitalier Universitaire Vaudois, Lausanne, Switzerland

Diet is evolving from nourishing populations via providing essential nutrients to improving health of individuals through nutrition. Modern nutritional research focuses on health promotion and disease prevention, on protection against toxicity and stress, and on performance improvement. The concept of developing nutritionally enhanced or functional food requires: (1) the understanding of the mechanisms of prevention and protection; (2) the identification of the biologically active molecules, and (3) the demonstrated efficacy of these molecules.

As a consequence of these ambitious objectives, the disciplines 'nutrigenetics' and 'nutrigenomics' have evolved. Nutrigenetics asks how individual genetic disposition, manifesting as single-nucleotide polymorphisms, copy-number polymorphisms and epigenetic phenomena, affects susceptibility to diet. Nutrigenomics addresses the inverse relationship, i.e. how diet influences gene transcription, protein expression and metabolism. The mid-term objective of nutrigenomics is integrating genomics (gene analysis), transcriptomics (gene expression analysis), proteomics (global protein analysis) and metabolomics (metabolite profiling) to define a 'healthy' phenotype. The long-term deliverability of nutrigenomics is personalized nutrition for maintenance of individual health and prevention of disease.

The major challenges for -omics in nutrition and health still lie ahead of us, some of which apply to -omic disciplines in general while others are specific

247

for -omic discovery in the food context: (1) the integration of gene and protein expression profiles with metabolic fingerprints is still in its infancy as we need to understand how to (a) select relevant sub-sets of information to be merged, and (b) resolve the issue of the different time scales, at which transcripts, proteins and metabolites appear and act; (2) the definition of health and comfort is less a clear-cut case than the one of disease; (3) -omics in nutrition must be particularly sensitive: it has to reveal many weak rather than a few abundant signals to detect early deviations from normality, and (4) in the food context, health cannot be uncoupled from pleasure, that is, food preference and nutritional status are interconnected.

Transcriptomics serves to put proteomic and metabolomic markers into a larger biological perspective and is suitable for a first 'round of discovery' in regulatory networks. Metabolomics, the comprehensive analysis of metabolites, is an excellent diagnostic tool for consumer classification. The great asset of this platform is the quantitative, noninvasive analysis of easily accessible human body fluids like urine, blood and saliva. This feature also holds true to some extent for proteomics, with the constraint that proteomics is more complex in terms of absolute number, chemical properties and dynamic range of compounds present. In theory, blood should bear a signature for most biological conditions and urine should reflect the majority of metabolic disorders. The challenge of targeting 'proteins in blood' and 'metabolites in urine' stems from the complexity regarding compound diversity and range of compound concentrations in which the diluted signals of interest may eventually 'disappear'.

Proteomics represents an established technology in the pharmaceutical industry mainly for biomarker and drug target discovery. The potential of proteomics for research in the food industry is increasingly being recognized and the employment of proteomic approaches to nutrition and health issues is now emerging. Proteomics in the context of nutrition and health has the potential to: (1) deliver biomarkers for health and comfort; (2) reveal early indicators for disease disposition; (3) assist in differentiating dietary responders from non-responders, and, last but not least, (4) discover bioactive, beneficial food components. Independent of the context of application, proteomics represents the only platform that delivers not only markers for disposition or condition but also targets of intervention: the only way to intervene in a biological condition and to modulate its outcome is interfering with the proteins involved.

It is evident that not only comprehensive analyses with one discovery platform (lateral integration of information) are required but also vertical integration between different -omic levels is indispensable for a deeper understanding of disposition, health, environment and diet [1]. A major 'vertical integration issue', to date unresolved, is given by different time scales of transcript production, protein expression and metabolite generation [2]. The transcript machinery usually responds fast to an external stimulus (seconds to minutes), the proteins may be expressed within minutes to hours (and have a half-life from minutes to even months) and metabolites vary significantly during the day and depend on latest dietary input. This means that data which seem to correlate qualitatively (e.g. reflecting the same pathway) may not necessarily be related time-wise. Rather, they may represent different responses at different time points and, possibly, to different stimuli.

Comprehensive -omic analysis is an essential building block of 'systems biology', which can be defined as follows [3]. Systems biology is the comprehensive analysis of the dynamic functioning of a biological system (cell, organ, organism or even ecosystem) at the gene, protein and metabolite (or higher organizational) level, achieved by comparison of two defined biological states of this system, typically before and after perturbation. While a comprehensive list of components (genes, proteins, metabolites) of a given biological system is a prerequisite for this kind of research, the main reasoning for the 'system view' is that only information on the interactions between the components gives clues to the function of the entire network. A systems biology approach has recently demonstrated the power of proteomics to dissect immunity and inflammation. Toll-like receptor recognition and signaling was elucidated and showed how bacterial 'barcodes' are read and interpreted in order to trigger an adapted immune response [4].

In order to address some of the challenging objectives of -omics-driven nutritional research, we have addressed: (1) the effect of early antibiotic administration on the maturation of intestinal tissues; (2) protein discovery in human milk; (3) the effects of polyunsaturated fatty acids on gene expression and lipid profile in the liver; (4) biomarkers for intestinal stress; (5) biomarkers for allergy disposition and tolerance induction, and (6) inflammation-related gene expression analysis.

(1) Antibiotics and gut maturation: the effects of early administration of antibiotics on intestinal maturation were assessed at the gene expression level in a rat model.

(2) Human milk: rapid enrichment and iterative, consolidated identification of immunologically relevant milk proteins was achieved through the employment of restricted-access media and a tailored proteomic strategy [5–7].

(3) Fatty acids and liver transcriptome/lipidome: epidemiological studies have correlated higher intakes of polyunsaturated fatty acids (PUFAs) with a lower incidence of chronic metabolic disease. The molecular mechanisms regulated by PUFA consumption were examined assaying the liver transcriptome and lipid metabolome of mice fed a control and a PUFA-enriched diet [8].

(4) Gut stress markers: we catalogued protein expression along the jejunum, ileum and colon of the rat intestine and found gut segment-specific proteins [9]. The innovative combination of a neonatal separation model with proteomic analysis allowed us to study whether early life psychological stress may impact the adult gut neuromuscular protein expression and the approach revealed specific protein biomarkers.

(5) Biomarkers for allergy and tolerance: a collaborative effort of combining clinical research and ex vivo/in vitro immunology with proteomic biomarker discovery is undertaken by the Nestlé Research Centre, the Centre Hospitalier Universitaire Vaudois and the Swiss Institute for Allergy and Research. The objective is to identify protein and peptide markers for allergy disposition (clinical samples) and tolerance induction (in vitro stimulation of ex vivo T cells) in defined immune cell populations. A first proteomic survey of human peripheral blood mononuclear cells is presented.

(6) Inflammation-related gene expression: inflammation is implied in a multitude of nutritionally relevant disease conditions. We aim to studying inflammation-related gene expression patterns through the implementation of a custom-array approach [10].

## References

1 Desiere F: Towards a systems biology understanding of human health: interplay between genotype, environment and nutrition. Biotechnol Annu Rev 2004;10:51–84.
2 Nicholson JK, Holmes E, Lindon JC, Wilson ID: The challenges of modeling mammalian biocomplexity. Nat Biotechnol 2004;22:1268–1274.
3 Clish C, Davidov E, Oresic M, et al: Integrative biological analysis of the APOE*3-leiden transgenic mouse. OMICS 2004;8:3–13.
4 Aderem A, Smith KD: A systems approach to dissecting immunity and inflammation. Semin Immunol 2004;16:55–67.
5 Labéta MO, Vidal K, Rey-Nores JE, et al: Innate recognition of bacteria in human milk is mediated by a milk-derived highly expressed pattern recognition receptor, soluble CD14. J Exp Med 2000;191:1807–1812.
6 LeBouder E, Rey-Nores JE, Rushmere NK, et al: Soluble forms of Toll-like receptor (TLR)2 capable of modulating TLR2 signaling are present in human plasma and breast milk. J Immunol 2003;171:6680–6689.
7 Panchaud A, Kussmann M, Affolter M: Rapid enrichment of bioactive milk proteins and iterative, consolidated protein identification by MudPIT technology. Proteomics 2005, in press.
8 Mutch D, Grigorov M, Berger A, et al: An integrative metabolism approach identified stearoyl-CoA desaturase as a target for an arachidonate-enriched diet. FASEB J 2005;19:599–601.
9 Marvin-Guy L, Lopes LV, Affolter M, et al: Proteomics of the rat gut: analysis of the myenteric plexus-longitudinal muscle preparation. Proteomics 2005;5:2561–2569.
10 Gunderson KL, Kruglyak S, Graige MS, et al: Decoding randomly ordered DNA arrays. Genome Res 2004;14:870–877.

## Discussion

*Dr. Saavedra:* Thank you very much, that was a great overview of what is being done, what might be done and hopefully what ideas we can take from all of you to begin and continue doing. I did have to ask that since English seems to be a risk factor, if having a French or a German accent confers some protection to any of the conditions that you talked about. This is open for discussion.

*Dr. Sorensen:* That was an excellent review. We talked a little bit about this but I am still puzzled by your approach to dealing with individuality, and you showed us experiments in mice that are all of the same genetic background. What is the difference in expression between individuals that are encountered in any human study and that due to disease or stimulation that is artificially introduced when cells are activated to get them to express certain proteins? How do you know what is due to that fact versus the genetic composition of each individual?

*Dr. Kussmann:* This is an extremely important point. It is not as though we overlooked this. Referring to this stress study, we believe that inter-individual variability is in that case less than if you look at humans. You can only master this problem by appropriate statistics. If you do mammalian gene expression studies you should at least have 5 or 10 biological replicates, for human gene expression studies you should probably have a lot more. You can only look at this from a statistical point of view because we do not genetically screen the animals beforehand. Statistical processing afterwards tells you something about the biological noise. There is another noise we have to deal with and this is experimental noise, and here we feel quite confident that with the platform we have in place the experimental variability is very much reduced. So wherever we can play on replicates we focus on different subjects and also on experimental repetition.

*Dr. Sorensen:* How specific are the metabolites? If you have 300,000 proteins you detect 3,000 metabolites, does it mean that the same metabolite may be part of 30 different proteins, and that you would not be able to determine what it really means if you find it in the urine because it could be derived from many different situations?

*Dr. Kussmann:* Yes, you are right also in this regard. Therefore I suggested in one of the slides that we have to think about what we want to integrate when we look at different -omic levels at the same time. It is simply not good enough to put everything into the same database because things may not be inter-related. The integration of changes in metabolite profiles and gene expression results is combining the most distant parts of the story. I would rather compare data from 'neighboring' platforms, that is to say proteins and metabolites and then proteins and genes and try to close this gap. Another approach to deal with this problem is to introduce causality. Imagine you do a transcript analysis and then you find regulators of transcription factors changed; that is a valuable piece of information because it is way up the cascade; then you would try to use this as a 'hub' and try to cascade down this finding to proteins and metabolites. But a lot of -omic information will not cross-correlate because the complexity levels are different and we may look at very distant effects at the same time. This situation is even a bit more complicated in the sense that metabolites respond in a much shorter time, so we have to think about how we deal with dynamics over time at these 3 -omic levels: your metabolite profile changes over the day significantly, the proteins react much more slowly and with the genes it is again different. You can do time monitoring of metabolites, this is the great advantage of metabolomics. In proteomics you can only take snapshots in which you freeze the biological condition and you get a picture at a given time. When you do cell culture experiments you can do time-course proteomics through metabolic labeling: you culture cells in isotopically enriched media and then you follow many proteins at the same time. I would say that it is fairly advanced, but it is possible.

*Dr. Hursting:* This is a clear presentation of the 3 -omics together that I never heard, so thanks for that. I am wondering what is your consideration in comparing experiment to experiment, or lab to lab, or platform to platform because sometimes when it comes up we have an opportunity to do things at different platforms beside Affymetrix. But what are the considerations from your experience in trying to compare across these platforms or even within a platform experiment to experiment?

*Dr. Kussmann:* Are you addressing the reproducibility and comparability of data derived from the same -omic level? It seems that we share the same -omic background. I think we were all blamed for the 'fact' that the biological answer you get depends on the platform you use. I think the true story behind this is the challenge of standardizing these studies and this is an issue in nutrition. The same holds for -omic technologies. We have to define the protocols not only on how to perform the laboratory experiment but also on how to treat the data. There was a recent comparative study published in *Nature Methods* where they looked into different gene expression platforms: for instance the Affymetrix which we have, Agilent and others, and then the so-called 'gold standard' reference methods like PCR [1]. They also looked into inter-laboratory comparability: if two laboratories applied the same platform, how do they compare? It is all about standardization, if the entire process from sample preparation down to data processing is defined, you get a nice overlap of regulated genes: typically two thirds correlate. You always find 'contradictory' results, but 'contradiction' can also mean complementation because any technology gives you only a part of the story. Data that do not overlap are not necessarily false-negatives or false-positives. On the proteomics side the situation depends on the mass spectrometry and the separation techniques we use. You can get two thirds of overlap between two different mass spectrometric platforms. The studies often differ in the sense that the upstream sample preparation is not always standardized: the biological origin of your sample and how you treat it. In proteomics the problem is rather that you rediscover the same proteome in different studies. Studies that had totally different objectives publish similar lists of proteins. So why is that? Because the dynamic range is so challenging. My recommendation is if you want to do something in the protein world you have to enrich for the things you want to look at. You may alter the picture a little bit but if you leave the sample as such, you just scratch the surface.

*Dr. Wang:* Just to follow your idea, to follow now our knowledge, can we go ahead and search for healthomics? In traditional Chinese medicine we pay a lot of attention to the whole body but not the genes, molecules. So we pay attention to health from another direction than in modern Western medicine where you go from molecules, from the organs and to the whole body.

*Dr. Kussmann:* I don't mind the invention of other -omics words, although healthomics is something I haven't thought about yet. It may be a far reach at the moment though. I think you are right in addressing the challenge of defining health at -omic levels which is of course much more difficult than defining disease, because the intrinsic variability is greater. We apply the -omic platforms in order to compare at the global molecular level defined biological conditions. That raises the issue of how defined this condition is. There is some other benefit of these -omic technologies: think about the studies that have been reported throughout the meeting, there are many conflicting results especially in the nutrition business. There is an issue of cohort definition. We may be able to help at an early stage to improve cohort definition; cohort definition at a molecular level and not so much at a phenomenological level; that can help to improve the study outcomes. While the 'hype' of -omic discovery is declining in the pharmaceutical world, in nutrition we can take advantage of these learnings and apply these technologies in order to better design studies. Any financial objections, because these technologies are costly, are not justified because there is nothing as expensive as a failed long-term clinical study.

*Dr. Hamburger:* Earlier in your talk you mentioned the desire for personalized nutrition and I wondered if in your studies you encountered an example of any genetic fixed issue that allows you to jump to a personalized nutrition. In other words is there an example that you are able to cite now that leads you to believe that this will ultimately result in a personalized nutrition.

*Dr. Kussmann:* I can only give you the examples of inborn metabolic defects for instance phenylketonuria. This is something which is well established and you can interpret this as an attempt to personalize nutrition because we have to avoid this amino acid. We would like to develop this further in the sense that we would like to have a better understanding of consumer groups; however I cannot give you mature examples at that level yet. There are a few examples where a single genetic defect leads to a metabolic problem and then you simply avoid an ingredient. You can extend this to the allergy field, the allergens are well characterized but the individual responses are less characterized. One aspect is to avoid allergens, another is how to induce tolerance. We are trying to come up with a more comprehensive set of explanatory markers that allow us to define these consumer groups, but it is not a matured concept you can find in supermarkets, except for these few clinical examples I have given.

*Dr. Laron:* I would like to contest the example you gave and the structure of your pyramid. I propose to turn it around: the upper wide platform is the genetic background, then you have the ethnic or familial customs and then the individual habits and environmental influences on nutrition. Would that be correct?

*Dr. Kussmann:* Yes, I think we are quite on the same line. However, I would like to add that genetic disposition is only one aspect. Many individual responses and dispositions can be traced down to SNPs and copy number polymorphisms.

*Dr. Laron:* But they don't apply to only one person.

*Dr. Kussmann:* Either using personalized or individualized nutrition you always run into conflicts about how this is interpreted. What we do not want and what we do not envisage is that you enter a restaurant with your gene chip and the menu is then printed out according to your chip. We have to think about how we can get access to sets of biomarkers that are accessible by noninvasive means. I am convinced that the biomarker sets are not comprehensive enough and they often derive only from one analytical level; individualized nutrition means divide the population into groups of people that share the same heritage, the same lifestyle and are exposed to a similar environment.

*Dr. Laron:* But why not go further, in modern medicine we think we should have a health card from conception on. This health card could also include advice for optimal nutrition for that individual.

*Dr. Kussmann:* I can see your point and scientifically this may make sense but don't forget that we are in nutrition and not in the pharmaceutical area, so for us all these nutritional recommendations cannot be uncoupled from pleasure, it should still be fun to eat. We don't want to create paranoia and consumers have to have their latest screen before they look at their plate. We can offer means of assessing personal needs, but it is only an offer for choice.

*Dr. Saavedra:* Then we hope that the array of snacks that await us during the break will actually cover all our potential needs. Thank you very much.

## Reference

1   Larkin JE, Frank BC, Gavras H, et al: Independence and reproducibility across microarray platforms. Nat Methods 2005;2:337–344.

## Discussion (Refers to the presentation "Mechanistic Research – Future Perspectives" by D.M. Bier)

*Dr. Bier:* Any specific questions about genomics, proteomics and metabolomics I am going to pass on.

*Dr. Kussmann:* Thank you for this nice wrap up of all these thoughts. I wanted to make a little comment about the amount of information that is already available. We may discuss whether it is necessary to generate all this -omics-derived information and that leads eventually to the term 'systems biology', to the understanding of a biological system in a holistic manner. There is already so much information available, it is just a major issue to interrogate this huge data set for particular purposes. There are many groups in the world that are practicing systems biology that there are now major research efforts undertaken to interrogate existing information and try to align it with ongoing studies. The problem we have is that we do global -omics-driven investigations, and then we look at this one study. We are still not capable of integrating it with the information that has already been created.

*Dr. Bier:* I don't disagree with that by the way. My comments on this are not meant to suggest that we should not go there because I think we should. My concern is what we will eventually be able to get out of it. What I see in the -omics field, in some way including what you said, is that there is promise that if we measure everything we are going to have an answer, and the answer is 42 for those of you who haven't read the book. It may be hard to get all the information but then when we get it, if we only look at a piece of it, there is going to be a lot of material. One of the issues about choosing what you look at is that you tend to throw away the really unexpected material that puts up those things that we have seen with the knockout mouse experiments. Things have happened that no one expected and that would very likely have been thrown away in a system where it was narrowed down to what you were thinking about. So I don't disagree with you, I think that there are some problems there.

*Dr. Lucas:* I think probably the greatest problem in pediatric research is not the interpretation of data or the amount of it, it is the ability to be able to do it and all the obstacles that have been put in our way. You discussed that a little. But what can we do as professionals or even as a workshop to make a statement about this? This is really a very serious problem.

*Dr. Bier:* It is a particularly difficult problem because all of us know that even among universities in the same country or even among EU boards in the same university there have to be answers over time. Somehow we have to try to get the pediatric research groups who have contributed to this issue, such as the academy groups that may exist in the EU, to come together to make some generic statements that are going to cross boarders in a very broad way, otherwise we might have difficulty here when we act individually. I think it is a very big problem and the remaining step is having the good scientist, the good question and the tools to carry it out, and in our case the tools are children, and without them we are never going to answer this question.

*Dr. Saavedra:* One of things that you alluded to it in a couple of the slides has to do with ethics. It is tied to what Dr. Lucas was just talking about. On the one hand we have those constraints that we can't do a lot of things in children because it is not ethical. On the other hand we have some science that is going, we have genetic experiments that are already occurring with no ethical constraints at all. I mean it is not just mature enough to be able to bring in this runaway science that is good, and we have considered it good in many instances, but on the other hand it is going to create problems that we may not be able to get back.

*Dr. Bier:* What kind of experiments do you mean?

*Dr. Saavedra:* Cloning, for example, is happening right now, and stem cell research. Much of it is happening with not only a lack of constraint with regard to the resources and where they are applied, but also with regard to the ethics and where they are applied. Because we perhaps have too many restrictions, we have done experiments or begun doing fewer experiments in children. We have no control on others or at least we don't feel there is sufficient control as to what, if any, ethics could or should be applied to this. Could you comment on that?

*Dr. Bier:* I think in the course of history there has probably never been a time when the human being was ahead of the ethics. The science of the human being was ahead of whatever the prior ethical rules existed for that society, and there is obviously a period of time when it is impossible to match the two. I think in the case of a very large fraction of pediatric research we have 30 or 40 or 50 years of what in fact has a long history of use, meaning safe use, for safe investigation. Those things obviously could be doable. Then there are others which are on the edge which become much more difficult and obviously cannot be dealt with now but maybe dealt with in 10 years. We got to the point where simple things that cause the problem become impediments to doing research or we have the important issues of privacy. By the way I don't think any of these things have simple answers, but we have privacy things now that are making it impossible to get your partner's medical records. It is extremely difficult.

*Dr. Saavedra:* Should resources be allocated and dedicated to the ethics of the research in parallel to the research?

*Dr. Bier:* Absolutely, in fact many of the ethics questions are being handled by internal review boards where people are spending immense periods of time, have no resources allocated to them, and make decisions without the resources. I think that is a problem.

*Dr. Sorensen:* I wonder if there is another skeleton in the closet. It may be the way we deliver health care, particularly in this country, even if it would be possible to really gather all the information and put it together. For instance in the case of the asthma guidelines, I think the NIH is the asthma guideline number 10, yet in any community when pediatricians are asked about asthma guidelines, surprisingly few know about them and even fewer ever follow them, and that for a simple thing like asthma. In our present health care system there are ever increasing differences in the kind of care that certain people get versus the care that the majority of our children get, and this is sorry situation for the US. Do you think that no matter how well we solve the issues that you have been discussing, the bigger issue is that we will be totally limited in the possible impact that we can have as health care professionals?

*Dr. Bier:* I obviously kept my remarks to the research side as that is what I do. I am not an expert in health care delivery, which involves a whole of a set of individuals including the people who pay for it, the American public in our case and congress. I think we have lots of examples where there is a change in health care delivery based on the way research is done. So I will use diabetes control in complication trials as an example: after 10 years and some hundreds of millions of dollars, it was convincingly demonstrated that maintaining normal glycemia decreased retinopathy and people with type-1 diabetes had a number of secondary outcomes. Even when that study was ongoing, we knew that it was impossible for the health care system to deliver that kind of care because these were almost individualized dieticians, social workers, phone access workers, but the demonstration of that effect has lead over the years to slow and steady changes in the health care delivery system: type-1 diabetic payments for more frequent visits, micrometers for measuring blood glucose, and on. So yes, it didn't cure the problem but it has made a tremendous dent in the average hemoglobin A1 one sees in children with diabetes. So I think there are going to be negative examples too, but there is one in which I think there was positive benefit.

Lucas A, Sampson HA (eds): Primary Prevention by Nutrition Intervention in Infancy and Childhood.
Nestlé Nutr Workshop Ser Pediatr Program, vol 57, pp 257–266,
Nestec Ltd., Vevey/S. Karger AG, Basel, © 2006.

# Concluding Remarks

It has been a very exciting meeting. Dr. Sampson is going to talk mainly about the second half of the presentations. So I would like to go through a number of the presentations and pick out a few points to remind you of some of the concepts that came across. Then I want to talk a little bit about some of the ideas and research issues that distill out of this.

At the beginning we discussed some thoughts and concepts on primary prevention in infancy and childhood nutrition. We agreed that primary prevention is both the prevention of disease before it occurs and the reduction of its incidence, but for this particular field we felt that this should be extended to prevent or reduce the risk of disease and prevent the impairment of *cognitive potential* because this a very important objective in pediatrics. Now primary prevention includes education, what we do as clinical scientists (clinical and public health practice or intervention) and what governments do (policy, legislation and regulation), though as professionals we need to have an influence on the latter. Now the key issue of this workshop was research and primary prevention and, as we heard in the last few lectures, this may have a fundamental basis, but Dr. Sampson is going to focus on that. My point is that ultimately primary prevention requires outcome research to prove that nutrition has an impact on health risk. This can be short-term, it can be long-term programming effects or effects of nutrition throughout childhood; and nutrition is also a vehicle for factors that influence health such as pathogens, toxins, nutraceuticals and so forth. I gave some examples of these, such as the use of human milk in neonatal intensive care in the short-term which has a major impact on the life-threatening condition necrotizing enterocolitis, and in the longer term the use of pharmaceutical trials to demonstrate that early nutrition has long-term programming effects on the brain, on bone health and cardiovascular disease risk with huge prevention potential.

Dr. Fewtrell talked about bones, and I am going to come back to that later; Dr. Singhal talked about cardiovascular risk, and I focused a bit more on the brain. It is remarkable that in some groups such brief periods of dietary manipulation can have such profound effects on important outcomes like motor and mental impairment, associated with major changes in the brain detected using sophisticated applications such as magnetic resonance imaging.

Dr. Singhal talked about the prevention of atherosclerosis and the metabolic syndrome. He pointed out that atherosclerosis begins in childhood, the risk factors are identifiable very early, and that the metabolic syndrome is really very common. He focused on the impact in human milk and pointed out that there is a wealth of observational studies showing that breastfeeding is associated with reduction of the key components of the metabolic syndrome, high blood pressure, raised LDL, obesity and insulin resistance. In preterm infants causation can be confirmed by dose-response relationships and more importantly randomized trials. He also pointed out the huge effect size here: the blood pressure effect size in some randomized trials is in the order of 3–4 mm whereas a 2-mm fold alone would produce 100,000 less cardiovascular events in the USA each year and 10% lowering of LDL cholesterol in adolescents previously fed breast milk, which would correspond in adults to a 25% reduction in cardiovascular disease risk. So there is a major potential here for prevention. He also talked about the importance of postnatal growth for cardiovascular programming, pointing out that in a wide variety of animal species fast early growth is at the cost of long-term health. He added humans to this list by giving us some very exciting data on the dangers of rapid growth in early life. So early growth and nutrition have become major factors for later health in all infants, not just small ones which have been the focus. These postnatal influences have a much larger effect than birth weight which has received so much attention recently. In fact birth weight may, to an extent, even be a proxy for postnatal growth and not prenatal growth. So favorable programming of cardiovascular disease is associated with breastfeeding and slow early growth. He pointed out that these were in fact unified in an early growth acceleration model, which has huge implications for prevention in terms of adjusting early growth rates to optimize long-term cardiovascular risk.

Dr. Maffeis talked about childhood obesity and considered the potential mechanisms for the prevention of an epidemic. Most of us were rather excited to discover that obesity is so strongly associated with inflammation because that gives us another route to prevention in this area. He also talked about the importance of signaling systems for appetite control and finished by considering the great importance of exercise and activity in the control of obesity.

Dr. Kroke rather disturbingly told us how much we didn't know about the relationship between prenatal and postnatal factors in the development of obesity. In the first phase she talked about the complex relationship between birth weight and adult BMI, showing how difficult this was to relate to obesity. She felt in the end that birth weight, although much focused on, is actually not a very good indicator here, and pointed out that despite sound theoretical considerations and experimental findings the human data are not convincing in this area. Her second area related to perinatal factors. She pointed out that there are many animal experiments and studies on maternal diet in relation to fetal growth, but in humans the evidence is really not there, except perhaps from the Dutch famine which gives us some important leads. The relationship between maternal diet and later weight in the offspring she felt was very difficult to interpret and the best route here is to exploit some of the trials that have been done in this area for long-term follow-up. She also pointed out this U-shaped curve where adequate nutrition, which might be defined as breastfeeding, was at the bottom of the curve as far as the risk for obesity is concerned, but undernutrition and overnutrition were risk factors, and potentially lead to prevention in that area. She summarized saying that the hypothesis on the early origins of obesity is well supported by physiological concepts and animal data but, due methodological constraints, the human data are really quite weak in this area. The one area that shone out was that breastfeeding appeared to be associated with an about 20% reduction in obesity risk. We argued whether this 20% was small or large as some of us felt that it was actually quite a large effect and could well amplify with time.

Dr. Laron talked about childhood diabetes with an emphasis on perinatal factors, and noted the really steep rise in both type-1 and type-2 diabetes and the importance of environmental factors, focusing on viral and nutritional factors for type-1 and changes in nutrition and lifestyle for type-2. He put forward the hypothesis that the onset of both types of childhood diabetes occurs in the perinatal period, the autoimmune process being triggered as early as in utero or postnatally by cow's milk proteins. This was an extremely important route into prevention after having made the point that secondary and tertiary prevention failed rather miserably and that primary prevention now must be a priority.

Dr. Fewtrell talked about osteoporosis and whether primary prevention possible. For instance she noted adequate vitamin D and calcium intake in mothers, and breastfeeding was beneficial in babies and preterm infants. She presented the results of randomized trials showing that nutrition actually increases bone formation and therefore might be an important risk factor for later bone disease. This needs to be followed up. She pointed out that calcium and vitamin D as intervention were somewhat disappointing, but physical activity and optimizing linear growth might be more promising solutions. Her ideas for future research were to follow up existing trials particularly to determine adult outcomes and the effects of interventions on bone structure and geometry, looking at sensitive periods, site specificity and optimal interventions, and gave us some very good clues as to where we might go with gene interactions and potential mechanisms. But the really important issue was whether there was going to be a useful quantitative effect here. She tried to estimate this pointing out that the effects observed on bone mass with calcium supplementation were in the region of 1–5% and with physical activity in the region of 3–5%; and that could delay the onset of osteoporosis by

6 years and reduce fracture risk by 10–20%. I think if those were feasible they would be very worthwhile aspects of prevention.

Dr. Hursting gave us a really inspiring talk on nutrition and cancer protection, and pointed out that in the transition from normal to neoplastic cells there are a number of factors: anti-initiation strategies which he listed and anti-promotion progression strategies which involve steps that were all theoretically influenced by early nutrition, thus leading to cancer. To be more specific about this he pointed out that nutrition has been identified as one of the key influences on cancer, that prior active food components can affect many aspects that are relevant to cancer, including DNA repair, hormonal regulation, inflammation, immunity, apoptosis, cell cycle carcinogen metabolism, and that we should eat more fruits. He pointed out the areas in which nutrition interfaced with cancer, IGF-1, leptin, obesity, inflammation, LCP-UFA and prostaglandins. The IGF-1 story is really interesting in the way that early growth and nutrition could actually, through IGF-1, form a link between both cancer risk and cardiovascular disease outcome risk.

The huge association between cancer and obesity is surprising to many of us here, at least raising the possibility that one of the ways of preventing cancer would be to attack obesity. With regard to real interventions that could be done, Dr. Hursting pointed out that human studies were really quite rudimentary but that there are a number of animal studies and animal models for effects on cancer that give us some important leads for future human research.

Against that background I want to remind you of some of the things that I discussed in my introduction which have become rather more relevant now that we have had 3 days of discussion. I want to consider some of the research issues in primary prevention for the future. I identified critical interactions which could be genetic, environmental, relating to subject characteristics, and the interaction between early diet and our subsequent Western environment, the importance of the timing of the window, the emergence of the effect which could be late, the quality of evidence required in this area, risk-benefits analysis and mechanisms. Just to focus on those points I have taken out of my lecture, some of the research messages that I put forward, and I thought it would be useful to review them again: Genetic characterization and family history may well be needed in some primary prevention studies to identify the best target groups for intervention. We identified a few areas overall where quite specific genetic groups would be affected by nutrition interventions. Then we pointed out that the effect of an intervention might be quite different in opposing subgroups, like males and females and small-for-gestational age babies and appropriate-for-gestational age babies. So looking at interactions overall, the impact of a health intervention can be highly influenced by genes, subject characteristics, and current and subsequent environment, and that clearly needs to be thought about when planning new studies. Another important message is that the efficacy of a prevention strategy may be highly influenced by its timing, and we talked about the timing of intervention to reduce the incidence of cardiovascular disease; in the examples we discussed it could be more effective and practical to intervene in the postnatal period rather than in the fetal period.

Another important issue was that long-term follow-up is essential in nutritional intervention trials. Quite a number of effects of our interventions do not emerge until late. Remembering the LCPUFA example we discussed earlier today, when they do emerge they may be the opposite to what was expected, raising a safety concern. Therefore long-term issues really need to be addressed in our studies. That came out in many of the speakers' work. In terms of the quality of evidence whenever they are possible, experimental studies are a more sound basis for practice than observational ones, and quite a number of the speakers, including myself, pointed out the difficulty of proving causation and the dangers of basing practice with observational data. Of course it is not always possible to have experimental studies but it should be a goal. I also pointed out that it may not be safe to devise primary prevention policies based only on the outcome of interest to the investigator. The same intervention can have beneficial effects on one system, such as cardiovascular health and detrimental effects on another, such as the brain, so that performing a balance of risks is a critical exercise in actually producing the best compromise for infants and children.

Dr. Bier and myself pointed out that multilevel mechanistic research may provide the best underpinning for prevention strategies, and we should not just think of mechanistic research at a genetic or molecular cell biological level but also at the physiological level. We talked about mechanism at a structural, behavioral, and social level; the latter being very important in the area of obesity. Finally we stepped outside the human species and considered evolutionary modeling to generate hypotheses for future human studies. In terms of assessing the prevention potential of a new area we considered the quality of evidence and noticed that in some areas this is very good and in other areas it is really poor, and set out a task list of areas that we need to be working on in the future. The size of the effect when we looked at it critically was trivial in some areas and probably not worth achieving, and extremely important in others. The feasibility of application varied hugely for different areas of prevention stragtegy and I think we would all agree if it depends on public education then this is often hard to achieve.

In an overview, primary prevention by infant and child nutrition was an area that we identified collectively as having immense potential and which could not have been contemplated 20 years ago. But the research in this area is highly complex with many pitfalls. Perhaps a really important overarching point, and this came out very much today in the discussions, is that primary prevention practice cannot be based safely on theory, politics, and uncontrolled observations. We as a profession have to resist political decisions that are not evidence-based. It is really a sound evidence basis that we need to optimize health and development.

*Alan Lucas*

I would like to thank the organizers at Nestlé again for inviting us and supporting this conference. What I would like to do then is to go ahead and review the allergy section that was done yesterday and then some of the later slides today. As you may have noticed I have been over here trying to make slides as people were giving their presentations. Dr. Lucas was much wiser; he picked the early speakers.

Yesterday we talked about the potential prevention of atopy and allergic diseases and 4 speakers addressed various topics in that area: Dr. Björkstén spoke about gut microbiota; Dr. Zeiger looked at studies that have been done related to breastfeeding; I took on the task of looking at what we know about the use of various modified formulas, and then Dr. von Berg talked about the introduction of solids. Just to review why we are so interested in this topic, this slide depicts the increasing prevalence of atopic disease, although I think one of the things I have learned in the course of this conference is that obesity or cardiovascular disease could be depicted in a similar way, so we are all attempting to prevent some fairly serious outcomes.

Dr. Björkstén started it off by giving us quite a bit of information about the gut microbiota; we all know now it is not flora, it is microbiota. We were thrilled to learn that we are all carrying around 1kg of bacteria in our gut, which consists of over 500 species. However, at this point in time, fewer than 50% of the strains in there are known. He emphasized the fact that this is really a very vibrant environment that, as he called it, is an ecosystem characterized by stable chaos, and I would add that it basically is living under controlled inflammation. So this is a very dynamic area that Dr. Bier also pointed out as a very exciting area of future research. There clearly have been demonstrations of interaction between the microbes in the host and between components of the microbiota and the host. This is a very dynamic and open ecosystem that maintains some functional stability, but it does have many factors which can affect it including nutrition, which we were talking about, drugs and infection, etc. Dr. Björkstén also introduced his new theory on the TH1/TH2 paradigm, which is probably much more on the mark than what we used to believe was the potential role of microbiota in the development of the immune response. So what are the potential health effects of early intervention, assuming that gut microbiota early in life are a major driving force for immunologic maturation and function? He gave us some examples including the changes over time, which may in fact underlie some of the increases that we are seeing in allergy, autoimmunity, inflammatory bowel disease and perhaps even obesity. The gut microbiota may offer a potential for disease prevention and treatment if we learn more about it, but what bugs we need, which show the most important effects, and can we really make alterations, I think remain up in the air. If we are going to take advantage of alterations in the gut microbiota to improve health, this probably will have to be done early in life.

The next series of discussions were about the results of breastfeeding, various formulas and solid foods, and one of the common themes in these three talks was the fact that there are divergent findings in many of the studies. This was due to several reasons including the differences in design, deficiency in many of the designs, confounding factors, some of which were not adequately controlled, sample size, factors that we just don't know about at this point, and the fact that most are observational studies, the influence of reverse causation, and then other factors that haven't really been looked into but have been alluded to throughout this conference. For example, the variations that do occur in breast milk from different mothers and the variation in the content of various hydrolysate formulas may lead to very different results.

Looking at some of Dr. Zeiger's conclusions in evaluating the effects of breastfeeding, there is evidence to suggest that it does promote less wheeze, less asthma and less eczema. The effect size is about 30%, which makes breastfeeding one of the most effective things that we can do for infants, similar to the effect of eliminating tobacco smoke from the environment of an infant. The data support exclusive breastfeeding through the first 3–4 months of life, and the beneficial effect occurs without altering the maternal lactation diet. In other words, we should not be imposing any kind of restriction on the maternal diet, and the effect is not lost if in fact the mother herself is atopic or asthmatic. At this point in time, as is apparent with many of the studies we have heard about at this conference, the effect of breastfeeding on atopy beyond 6 years of life is really not known, and like many of the areas, the studies are of too short a duration. Looking at infant formula feeding, it was my conclusion that there is certainly no evidence to support the use of any hydrolyzed formula in place of exclusive breastfeeding as long as exclusive breastfeeding can be done. In situations where that is not possible, where supplementation is needed, infants from high-risk families should be given hydrolyzed infant formulas for at least the first 6 months of life. There is some suggestion in the literature that this will prevent some cases of atopic dermatitis. Evidence from the GINI study would suggest that if there is no atopic dermatitis in the family, the partial whey hydrolysate formula appears to be as effective, but if there is atopic dermatitis in the family suggesting a more robust atopic predisposition, then the use of extensively hydrolyzed casein formula is probably necessary. At this point there is insufficient evidence to demonstrate any preventive effect for asthma or allergic rhinitis but this may be due in part to the fact that the studies have all been of short duration. Finally there is no evidence at this point for the benefit of hydrolyzed formula in low-risk infants and this is primarily because the long-term studies have not been done.

Looking at the timing of introduction of solid foods, Dr. von Berg concluded that the earlier studies showing an increased risk of atopic dermatitis with early introduction of solid foods have not been confirmed by more recent studies and that in fact some of the previous information may have been due to reverse causality. She also indicated that early nutritional antigen exposure does not necessarily parallel early sensitization. She looked at early hen's egg sensitization and gave us fairly striking evidence that this was a good marker for atopic disease, especially when combined with an atopic family history. She also presented some data from the GINI study related to the introduction of solid foods, which I think has really improved our understanding of this area. She concluded that the early introduction of solid foods seems to be less harmful than we previously thought and therefore many of the recommendations out there, especially those of the American Academy of Pediatrics should be far less rigid.

Today then we had some very interesting discussion on LCPUFAs, something I have to admit I know little about and hadn't really thought much about, but it is clearly a very interesting and exciting area for future research to investigate its multiple effects on health of young infants.

Dr. Fewtrell started off with a critical review and current knowledge in the area of the LCPUFAs, Dr. Hanson looked at the impact on the immune system and Dr. Massiera looked at the possible impact on body fat mass. So starting out, it appears that it is a fairly contentious area with lots of emotion behind it. However, I believe that the presentations gave us the impression that theoretically it seems to make sense that LCPUFA supplementation should be beneficial, but as pointed out, at this time the evidence is really all biochemical and the clinical efficacy may in fact be quite difficult to establish. One of the strong pleas was for good long-term follow-up studies to evaluate the effect of the n-6/n-3 ratio as opposed to just looking specifically at levels of these specific LCPUFAs. One of the other things that was pointed out was the fact that when we are doing these studies, just as we see in the hydrolysate studies for prevention of allergy, there are considerable variations in the different formula preparations. These differences may lead to potential pitfalls when we are just considering the generic effect of these particular formulas. It also was pointed out that minor differences can certainly affect these outcomes, again stressing the point that Dr. Lucas made in his opening remarks, i.e., there is a major need for long-term studies here because we may see differences as the studies are carried out longer term.

Then Dr. Hanson gave us some information about the potential effect of LCPUFAs on the immune system, showing that a deficiency of the n-6 and n-3 essential fatty acids in the maternal diet was able to decrease leptin in offspring and also the amount of inguinal white adipose tissue and its leptin messenger RNA. He also showed that essential fatty acid deficiency gave increased milk leptin, and then discussed the potential outcome in offspring from these animals. He also discussed the effects of tolerance induction, showing that a low ratio of n-6/n-3 in the maternal diet resulted in neonatal tolerance in the pups following ovalbumin exposure via the milk and speculated that this tolerance was possibly due to an effect on regulatory T cells and the production of TGF-β. He also showed that there was no tolerance in the group that had the high ratio of n-6/n-3 and in the very high ratio group there was evidence of tolerance but apparently due to a different mechanism, that of T cell anergy, thus suggesting a major interaction between diet and tolerance induction. Dr. Hanson then gave us some information on the potential effects of maternal diet on gestational immunity. He first showed data on IL-10 messenger RNA content in the decidua of Swedish mothers who had infants with intrauterine growth retardation, and then showed us data from his large cohort of Pakistani patients who had a significant decrease in IL-10 and increase in TGF-β in both decidua and trophoblast in those with intrauterine growth retardation. He suggested that this reduced IL-10 in the placenta may be involved in the pathogenesis of intrauterine growth retardation.

Then Dr. Massiéra went on to give us information about the potential effects of diet on body adipose tissue and showed us a comparison between animals that received a high n-6 diet compared to a standard diet and pointed out the fact that this group had much higher adipose levels. This was probably mediated through the IPR promoter since this phenomenon was not seen in IPR knockout mice. She then gave us some tentative conclusions on the effects of LCPUFAs on body fat indicating that dramatic changes in the fatty acid composition of the dietary fats probably have gone largely unnoticed over the years and that this may be leading to changes in white adipose tissue development of newborns and infants and potentially accounting for some of the increase in obesity that we are seeing. Whether or not the prevention of childhood obesity is the key issue, the fatty acid composition of dietary fat should be reconsidered and provided in a more balanced manner with the supplementation by n-3 polyunsaturated fatty acids being accompanied by a simultaneous reduction of the n-6 polyunsaturated fatty acids in formula, as well as other foods. She noted that this was a recommendation that was made previously by a NIH panel as well.

Then in the last series of discussions we heard presentations on the impact of nutrition from a more mechanistic aspect, Dr. Kussmann giving us a really excellent lecture on the different '-omics' and encouraging us to use '-omics' in everything, and then Dr. Bier followed it up with future prospects and even 'wholomics'; I think we are now getting a whole new vocabulary. I think Dr. Kussmann's presentation on the different aspects and the different ways to use genomics, proteomics and metabolomics was really one of the nicest presentations bringing all this together and giving us a unified concept. He stressed the complexity of this area, making us aware of the fact that where at one point we thought genomics was such a complex area, it really is pretty simple when we start looking into some of the other areas such as the proteomics and metabolomics. Looking at how these different approaches will be useful in the future will hopefully help us get to the bottom of many of the nutritional issues and other medical issues that are confounding us.

Then finally Dr. Bier gave us an outstanding final summary of some of the major issues that are coming up and need to be dealt with in the area of research, especially research in children. I think this whole area of ethical standards related to experimentation in children really has to be addressed face on, that as he pointed out, we are all experiencing more and more difficulty doing research on children. I definitely would agree with one of the statements in his slides, that it may be unethical for us not to be doing research in normal children. He also wants us to think about the field of epigenomics, and I was not aware of the two studies he presented demonstrating the major effect that environment can have on the expression of our genome. He then reviewed a number of the new technologies of the 21st century, again encouraging us to shift our way of thinking about these traditional approaches that we have taken in the past, something he has labeled the small science, and really start to think much more about the big picture. He indicated that the mathematics of this area may be somewhat of a limiting factor in the near future but hopefully this is something that we will be able to overcome. When it comes to the point where we will be able to apply some of these principles, human behavior may serve as a limiting factor.

So in wrapping up, I will take away from this meeting many common interests in all our areas of research. There is certainly a major need for well-designed, prospective multicenter trials in many areas of infant nutrition. Everyone has said there is this need for long-term studies and this is something that seems to be an area that is very difficult to get funded. It is not so difficult to get the first 5 years of a large study funded, it is trying to keep the cohort going beyond that. It looks to me, from what we have seen here, that this may be the most important information that we need to disseminate, and somehow we have to get the funding agencies to help with this.

Finally I would like to thank all the speakers who came and for their excellent presentations, and thank the audience for the great questions; I think many of them were quite stimulating and kept all the speakers thinking. I believe that this has been a good experience for all of us. Thank you.

*Hugh A. Sampson*

# Subject Index

# Subject Index

Subject Index

272